M. D. ANDERSON
CANCER CARE
SERIES

Series Editors

Aman U. Buzdar, MD   Ralph S. Freedman, MD, PhD

M. D. ANDERSON CANCER CARE SERIES

Series Editors: Aman U. Buzdar, MD, and
Ralph S. Freedman, MD, PhD

K.K. Hunt, G.L. Robb, E.A. Strom, and N.T. Ueno, Eds., *Breast Cancer*

F.V. Fossella, R. Komaki, and J.B. Putnam, Jr., Eds., *Lung Cancer*

J.A. Ajani, S.A. Curley, N.A. Janjan, and P.M. Lynch, Eds.,
Gastrointestinal Cancer

K.W. Chan and R.B. Raney, Jr., Eds., *Pediatric Oncology*

Ka Wah Chan, MB, BS
and R. Beverly Raney, Jr., MD
Editors

The University of Texas M. D. Anderson Cancer Center, Houston, Texas

Pediatric Oncology

Foreword by Eugenie S. Kleinerman, MD

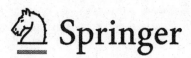 Springer

Ka Wah Chan, MB, BS
The University of Texas
M. D. Anderson Cancer Center
1515 Holcombe Blvd., Unit 87
Houston, TX 77030-4009, USA

R. Beverly Raney, Jr., MD
The University of Texas
M. D. Anderson Cancer Center
1515 Holcombe Blvd., Unit 87
Houston, TX 77030-4009, USA

Series Editors:
Aman U. Buzdar, MD
Department of Breast Medical
  Oncology
The University of Texas
M. D. Anderson Cancer Center
Houston, TX 77030-4009, USA

Ralph S. Freedman, MD, PhD
Immunology/Molecular Biology
  Laboratory
The University of Texas
M. D. Anderson Cancer Center
Houston, TX 77030-4009, USA

Cover illustration: © Gerald Bustamante/Images.com

Pediatric Oncology

Library of Congress Cataloging-in-Publication Data

A C.I.P. Catalogue record for this book is available
from the Library of Congress.

ISBN 0-387-24470-0   e-ISBN 0-387-24472-7   Printed on acid-free paper.
ISBN-13: 978-0387-24470-9

Printed in the United States of America.

9 8 7 6 5 4 3 2 1   SPIN 11327516

springeronline.com

FOREWORD

Childhood cancer was almost always fatal before 1970. Today, 80% of children diagnosed with cancer will survive at least 5 years; 70% will be cured. However, cancer continues to be the leading cause of nonaccident-related deaths in children. More children die each year from cancer than from cystic fibrosis, diabetes, asthma, AIDS, and congenital abnormalities *combined*. Nine children die from cancer every school day.

Despite the fact that pediatric cancers account for only a small percentage of the total cancer burden, more effective therapies are needed to improve mortality rates in children. Therefore, our research priority must be the development of new agents and new therapies for childhood cancer.

M. D. Anderson Cancer Center has been caring for children with cancer since its doors opened over 60 years ago. This institution has been home to several research and clinical pioneers whose innovative work has influenced and shaped the practice of pediatric oncology throughout the world. Notably, Drs. Wataru W. Sutow, Donald Pinkel, and Norman Jaffe have been credited with introducing curative therapies for children with leukemia and solid tumors.

Cancer treatment involves far more than administering chemotherapy and surgically excising tumors. It requires a multidisciplinary approach to patient management, particularly in the treatment of solid tumors, which pose the biggest challenge in cancer care today. Surgery and radiotherapy as well as radiographic and pathologic assessments of response are critical factors in the treatment of children with cancer.

This monograph describes the M. D. Anderson approach to treating children with a variety of malignancies. The book is organized by tumor type, and it is written by the clinicians who make up our multidisciplinary care teams. The book also includes sections on new therapeutic agents being used at our institution, supportive-care and behavioral medicine techniques, and our unique program for managing adolescent and young adult cancer patients.

Extensive experience and unique clinical perspectives are of limited value unless they are shared. We envision this book as an educational resource and a reference guide for clinicians challenged to choose optimal

care plans for their patients with childhood malignancies. This monograph
has been prepared with careful thought and great pride.

Eugenie S. Kleinerman, MD

PREFACE

Progress in pediatric oncology has antedated even some of the more recent accomplishments in adult oncology. Considerable advances have been made in the treatment of children and adolescents with leukemia, lymphoma, sarcoma, and other cancers, and this success has resulted in a significant improvement in the overall survival of these young patients.

Even when cured, however, young people who survive cancer often experience challenging physical and emotional consequences. The management of these consequences must be integrated with the treatment and follow-up strategies to ensure these patients the best possible quality-of-life.

The ongoing, unified research efforts of a single pediatric cooperative group can serve as a catalyst for further advances in this field. Many pediatric patients may benefit from evidence-based therapeutic and supportive-care approaches; however, they may not have access to research facilities or may not choose to be a part of ongoing research. This monograph provides an excellent overview of current treatment strategies in pediatric oncology. It delivers encouraging news to physicians, regardless of specialty, who see young patients in their medical practices. Pediatricians would especially benefit from reading this volume, but family physicians, oncologists, hematologists, neurologists, radiotherapists, behavioral scientists, and psychologists would also find it useful.

We would like to thank the following people for their very valuable contributions to this work: the volume editors; the chapter authors; Vickie J. Williams, managing editor; and Kim DuPree, Katie Matias, and Sandra Young of the Department of Scientific Publications.

Aman U. Buzdar, MD
Ralph S. Freedman, MD, PhD

CONTENTS

Contents

CONTRIBUTORS

Richard J. Andrassy, MD, Denton A. Cooley, MD, Chair in Surgery; Chairman and Professor, Department of Surgery, The University of Texas Houston Health Science Center

Martha A. Askins, PhD, Assistant Professor, Division of Pediatrics

Joann L. Ater, MD, Professor, Division of Pediatrics

Martin Blakely, MD, Assistant Professor, Department of Surgical Oncology

Ka Wah Chan, MB, BS, Professor, Division of Pediatrics

Eric L. Chang, MD, Assistant Professor, Department of Radiation Oncology

Mary S. Choroszy, RN, MSN, CPNP, Pediatric Nurse Practitioner, Division of Pediatrics

Donna R. Copeland, PhD, Professor, Division of Pediatrics

Hafeez Diwan, MD, PhD, Assistant Professor, Department of Pathology

Tina V. Fanning, MD, Professor, Department of Pathology

Misha Faustina, MD, Fellow, Section of Ophthalmology, Department of Plastic Surgery

Robert F. Gagel, MD, Head and Professor, Division of Internal Medicine

Dan S. Gombos, MD, FACS, Assistant Professor, Section of Ophthalmology, Department of Plastic Surgery

Cynthia E. Herzog, MD, Associate Professor, Division of Pediatrics

Norman Jaffe, MD, DSc, Professor, Division of Pediatrics

Sima S. Jeha, MD, Director, Leukemia/Lymphoma Developmental Therapeutics. Current affiliation: Associate Member, St. Jude Children's Research Hospital, Memphis, TN

Susannah E. Koontz-Webb, PharmD, Division of Pharmacy

Valerae O. Lewis, MD, Assistant Professor, Department of Orthopaedic Oncology

Renee M. Madden, MD, MSc, Assistant Professor, Division of Pediatrics. Current affiliation: Physician, Bone Marrow Transplantation, St. Jude Children's Research Hospital, Memphis, TN

Anita Mahajan, MD, Assistant Professor, Department of Radiation Oncology

Moshe H. Maor, MD, Professor, Department of Radiation Oncology

Bartlett D. Moore III, PhD, Associate Professor, Division of Pediatrics

Craig A. Mullen, MD, PhD, Chief and Professor, Division of Pediatric Hematology and Oncology, University of Rochester Medical Center, Rochester, NY

Margaret G. Pearson, MSN, Advanced Practice Nurse, Division of Pediatrics

Demetrios Petropoulos, MD, Assistant Professor, Division of Pediatrics

Victor G. Prieto, MD, PhD, Associate Professor, Department of Pathology and Department of Dermatology

R. Beverly Raney, MD, Professor, Division of Pediatrics

Nidra I. Rodriguez Cruz, MD, Fellow in Pediatric Oncology, Division of Pediatrics

Merrick I. Ross, MD, Professor of Surgery and Chief, Melanoma Section, Department of Surgical Oncology

Michael E. Rytting, MD, Assistant Professor, Division of Pediatrics

John Stewart, MD, PhD, Assistant Professor, Department of Pathology

Rena Vassilopoulou-Sellin, MD, Professor, Department of Endocrine Neoplasia and Hormonal Disorders

Jeffrey S. Weinberg, MD, Assistant Professor, Department of Neurosurgery

Laura L. Worth, MD, PhD, Assistant Professor, Division of Pediatrics

Donna S. Zhukovsky, MD, Associate Professor, Department of Palliative Care and Rehabilitation Medicine

1   ACUTE LEUKEMIA

Michael E. Rytting, Mary S. Choroszy,
Demetrios Petropoulos, and Ka Wah Chan

CHAPTER OVERVIEW

Leukemia is the most common malignancy in childhood. There have been major advances in our understanding of the biology of leukemia. Better supportive care and increased treatment intensity have led to significant improvements in the outcome of children with acute lymphoblastic and myelogeneous leukemias. Hematopoietic stem cell transplantation is used as treatment for patients in whom conventional-dose chemotherapy fails to induce a response. It is also used for patients in whom high-risk features are noted during first complete remission.

INTRODUCTION

This chapter describes the diagnostic, therapeutic, and supportive care measures used at M. D. Anderson Cancer in the treatment of pediatric patients with acute leukemia. The primary types and subtypes of acute leukemia are covered, and the clinical features and prognostic factors associated with these leukemias are discussed. Novel treatments and special considerations with respect to certain patient groups are also explained.

ACUTE LYMPHOBLASTIC LEUKEMIA

Acute lymphoblastic leukemia (ALL) is the most common of all childhood malignancies, and it accounts for about three fourths of all diagnoses of leukemia (regardless of tumor type) in children each year. About 3,000 new cases of ALL are diagnosed each year in the United States, with a peak age at diagnosis of 4 years old. Over the past 3 years, the prognosis for pediatric patients with ALL has improved substantially (Gaynon et al, 2000). The current treatment approach is risk-adapted therapy, which means that treatment is determined on the basis of the biologic characteristics and risk status of each patient. Through the use of molecular diagnostic techniques, disease categories have become better defined, and the intensity of therapy can be appropriately adjusted. The goal of therapy is to improve the cure rate of high-risk disease while reducing treatment toxicity for patients whose risk of relapse is low. Currently, ALL relapse occurs in 20% to 25% of children, and their prognoses are poor (Chessels et al, 2003).

Etiology and Predisposing Factors

In the majority of cases of pediatric ALL, there is no clear etiology; rather, the condition appears to arise spontaneously. However, ALL is associated with some known risk factors. For example, the incidence of ALL increased in children exposed to atomic radiation in Japan in the 1940s; infection with the Epstein-Barr virus is associated with endemic Burkitt's lymphoma and B-cell leukemia; patients with congenital immunodeficiency have an increased incidence of leukemia; and children with defective DNA repair mechanisms, such as those that occur with Fanconi anemia, develop leukemia at an abnormally high rate. Children with trisomy 21 are at an increased risk for both ALL and acute myeloid leukemia (AML). However, the exact mechanism of leukemogenesis in these patients is not yet known.

Molecular Genetic Abnormalities

The genetic aberrations of ALL are complex (Pui et al, 2004). The most common chromosomal abnormality is the t(12;21) or TEL-AML1 translocation, which is present in about 25% of cases and is associated with a good prognosis. About 30% of patients are as hyperdiploid. The modal number peaks at 55 chromosomes (DNA index greater than 1.16). The chromosomal abnormality is often numeric but has no specific structural abnormality. In infants, the t(4;11) translocation is very common and is associated with a poor outcome. Other common chromosomal abnormalities include rearrangements of the *myc* proto-oncogene and the T-cell receptor gene and translocations of E2A/PBX. Almost 30% of children with ALL appear to have a diploid karyotype or random genetic abnormalities. Chromosomal abnormalities are important for predicting prognosis and are now used to determine the best therapy; therefore, careful cytogenetic evaluation is essential for all pediatric patients with leukemia.

Chromosomal analysis using G-banding may detect abnormalities that are present in as few as 1% of cells. However, G-banding frequently does not detect the t(12;21) abnormality; thus, special techniques such as fluorescence in situ hybridization (FISH) or polymerase chain reaction (PCR) assays are required to detect this abnormality. FISH uses DNA probes tagged with a fluorescence marker to look for abnormal cells with specific genetic abnormalities. FISH is also helpful in diagnosing Philadelphia chromosome-positive (Ph+) ALL and some subtypes of AML. FISH results are available in 24 to 48 hours and can detect 1 leukemic cell per 1,000 cells evaluated. Serial FISH analysis is useful for following treatment response.

Other molecular genetic abnormalities such as immunoglobulin (Ig)-gene rearrangements can be followed using PCR technology. Through the use of sequence-specific probes, PCR can detect 1 leukemia cell in 10^5 to 10^6 normal cells. PCR is a useful method of detecting minimal residual disease in the peripheral blood or bone marrow. Use of such information to modify therapy has yet to be widely incorporated into pediatric therapeutic strategies, but it will likely be used eventually in ALL.

Diagnosis

Symptoms frequently encountered with childhood ALL include bone pain, fatigue, pallor, and tendency to bruise easily. Mild to moderate lymphadenopathy is common. Patients with T-cell ALL may present with respiratory problems resulting from massive thymic enlargement. Liver and spleen enlargement are often detected on physical examination and may result in nonspecific abdominal symptoms. Occasionally, visual disturbances resulting from ocular or cranial nerve involvement and headaches resulting from meningeal infiltration are the initial symptoms. Fever is not uncommon and may be caused by the leukemic process or an underlying infection. A complete blood count may initially be normal or near normal. Disturbances in the coagulation cascade along with thrombocytopenia can result in bleeding manifestations. These symptoms are less common in patients with ALL than in patients with AML.

The initial diagnosis of acute leukemia is made by light microscopy and supported by cytochemical stains. Morphologic findings should be compared to the patient's medical history and physical examination results. Exact classification of a leukemia depends on specialized testing, including immunophenotyping, cytogenetic studies, and molecular analyses.

Classification Using Flow Cytometry

Flow cytometry is an essential tool for reliable identification of the subtypes of acute leukemia. Extensive panels of antibodies are used to detect lineage-related antigens on the surface of blast cells. Immunophenotyping of leukemias can usually be completed on the day of bone marrow aspiration. The panel of antibodies used should be broad so that a diagnosis can be resolved even in morphologically ambiguous cases. On occasion, leukemia cells express antigens from multiple cell lineages; these cases require more detailed investigation to determine the treatment strategy.

Multiparameter flow cytometry can detect 1 leukemia cell in 10,000 cells analyzed. Because of its level of sensitivity, this technique can also detect minimal amounts of residual leukemia cells. The use of multiparameter flow cytometry to detect residual leukemia is being studied at M. D. Anderson and may be useful for systematically guiding patient care in the future.

Treatment and Prognosis

On the basis of National Cancer Institute criteria (initial white blood cell count and patient age), pediatric patients with ALL are classified as standard risk or high risk at the time of diagnosis. Children 1 to 9 years of age with a white blood cell count less than 50,000/μL and no adverse cytogenetic features are treated on standard-risk protocols. The inclusion of a delayed intensification phase for these patients improves their prognosis. The cure rate for these children approaches 80%. Children who have white blood cell counts greater than 50,000/μL and those who are older than 10 years of age are classified as high risk. Treatment for patients at high risk is determined on the basis of the speed of response on a bone marrow examination on days 7 and 14 (Nachman et al, 1998). Additional treatment intensification appears to improve the outcome of patients in whom response is slow.

The event-free survival rate for older children and adolescents ranges from 55% to 75%. In an effort to improve cure rates, we offer these patients an augmented protocol of cyclophosphamide, vincristine, doxorubicin, and dexamethasone (hyperCVAD) alternated with intermediate-dose methotrexate and high-dose cytarabine. This protocol was pioneered by the Department of Leukemia at M. D. Anderson. HyperCVAD therapy is intensified for patients who experience relapse by adding pegylated L-asparaginase and weekly vincristine during cycles. In addition, rituximab (a monoclonal antibody against the CD20 antigen) is added if more than 20% of blasts express CD20. Imatinib mesylate, a tyrosine kinase inhibitor, is extremely effective in patients with Ph+ ALL and chronic myelogenous leukemia (CML) and is now included in the chemotherapy regimen if Ph chromosome t(9;22) is identified. The addition of these agents to the hyperCVAD regimen has been well tolerated, and preliminary results suggest improved event-free survival rates for adult patients (Thomas et al, 2004).

Many of the prognostic factors for childhood ALL have disappeared with contemporary intensive chemotherapy protocols. Patients with T-lineage ALL and mature B-cell leukemia now have almost the same long-term survival rate as patients with precursor B-cell ALL. Treatment response has become the paramount factor for determining eventual outcome. Patients who have more than 25% blasts at the end of induction therapy or more than 5% blasts at the end of consolidation therapy are considered to be at very high risk of relapse. Biologic features that continue to confer high-risk status are the Ph+ translocation, very high white blood cell count, low hypodiploidy (≤44 or fewer chromosomes), and mixed lineage leukemia (MLL) gene rearrangement. Infants with MLL gene rearrangements are also at high risk.

Hematopoietic Stem Cell Transplantation

Allogeneic hematopoietic stem cell transplantation (HSCT) is used to treat children who are at very high risk of treatment failure. Therefore, it is recommended that HSCT be used during the first complete remission for the following pediatric ALL patient groups.

- Patients with Ph+, irrespective of initial white blood cell count
- Infants with ALL who have the 11q23 or t(4;11) abnormality (even as evidenced by molecular probes)
- Patients with hypodiploidy cytogenetics
- Patients whose disease responds slowly to induction therapy, with more than 25% blasts at the end of induction therapy or more than 5% blasts at the end of consolidation therapy (Uderzo, 2000)

Allogeneic HSCT is also the treatment of choice for patients in second complete remission who have any of the following conditions (Uderzo et al, 2000).

- Any T-cell phenotype, irrespective of the time to relapse
- Precursor B-cell ALL if the patient has had a relapse within 6 months after completing initial therapy
- Isolated extramedullary relapse followed by a marrow relapse
- Slow disease response to reinduction therapy

The decision to perform an allogeneic HSCT for a late relapse, defined as occurring more than 6 months after the completion of initial therapy, is more controversial. HSCT may be considered if a matched sibling donor is available, especially if the patient has been exposed to intensive chemotherapy during first remission. A transplant using an alternative donor is normally not recommended.

The outcome for children who have 3 or more relapses is poor; however, the likelihood of disease-free survival is greater for patients who undergo allogeneic HSCT than for those who continue with further conventional chemotherapy.

Finally, for patients in whom initial induction fails but who do not have rapidly progressive leukemia, HSCT should be performed if an appropriate related or unrelated donor is available.

Certain conditions are contraindications for allogeneic HSCT, including persistent relapse; specific viral infections, such as human immunodeficiency virus; an active infection; poor performance status; and impaired organ functions.

At M. D. Anderson, we use either a chemotherapy-based or a total-body irradiation-based preparative regimen. The chemotherapy-based regimen consists of triethylenethiophosphoramide, busulfan, and cyclophosphamide for children 3 years old or younger and for patients who have undergone prior craniospinal or total-body irradiation. The total-body irradiation-based regimen consists of 9- to 12-Gy radiation administered in 3 to 6 fractions and combined with cyclophosphamide, melphalan, or etoposide. This regimen is given to patients with T-cell leukemia, children older than 3 years of age, or patients with concurrent extramedullary relapse. We have pioneered individualized busulfan dosing on the basis of first-dose pharmacokinetic measurement. Children are treated with this drug before receiving an allogeneic HSCT. Recently, an intravenous formulation of busulfan became available, making the administration of this agent more convenient and tolerable.

A fludarabine-based reduced-intensity conditioning regimen combined with once-daily intravenous busulfan or melphalan resulted in donor-cell engraftment in adult patients with poor performance status or borderline organ functions (Giralt et al, 2001). The goal of this treatment is to harness the graft-versus-leukemia effect without imposing intolerable toxicity. This approach allows the transplant procedure to be extended to pediatric patients who may not otherwise qualify for this treatment modality.

The stem cell sources used are bone marrow, peripheral blood cells, and umbilical cord blood cells from either a related or unrelated donor. Because only 25% to 30% of patients have a matched family-member donor, most cases require a search for an unrelated stem cell donor. In this regard, umbilical cord blood units mismatched up to 2 human leukocyte antigens can be used. This is a major advantage to patients of some ethnic groups for whom it is often hard to find a fully histocompatible volunteer marrow donor. Additionally, umbilical cord blood units can become available within a few weeks after initiating a search. Because disease progression may occur in up to 40% of patients within 6 months of the first relapse, faster accrual of unrelated umbilical cord blood units makes managing these patients easier. The infusion of multiple or ex vivo expanded umbilical cord blood units for adolescents and young adults is being actively investigated at M. D. Anderson.

Supportive Care

At M. D. Anderson, as soon as a diagnosis of acute leukemia is made, the patient and the family receive counseling, and patient/family education and supportive care begin. Treatment-plan discussions are held with the oncologist, and educational materials are provided. Social workers assist by assessing the family's resources and support systems. Nurses begin teaching patients and family members about the treatment process. Patients and their parents are encouraged to participate in research protocols, if available.

A large amount of information must be communicated, and frequent follow-up meetings with the family are required. Teenage patients are encouraged to participate in all discussions and are offered copies of educational materials. Adolescents are encouraged to communicate openly and are assured that all conversations will remain confidential. Because leukemia chemotherapy regimens can result in impaired spermatogenesis, sperm banking is explained and offered to all pubertal boys as a possible solution to infertility. Emotional stress and depression are common, and the psychiatrist, clinical psychologist, teacher, and child-life worker can help the patient and the family handle this difficult time.

Insertion of a central venous device, such as a mediport, greatly facilitates the many phlebotomies and intravenous medications required for ALL therapy. If at all possible, we recommend the placement of a mediport after the patient has completed induction therapy to avoid wound dehiscence during administration of high-dose corticosteroids. Drawing blood through the mediport is discouraged because it could increase the risk for infection.

Current ALL treatment includes repeated bone marrow examinations to assess response to treatment and lumbar punctures to deliver chemotherapeutic drugs into the spinal fluid. These procedures are performed under short anesthesia (propofol) in a controlled environment. These arrangements are especially important when a traumatic lumbar puncture is performed at diagnosis because this procedure could be a diagnostic dilemma and could adversely affect treatment outcome (Howard et al, 2002).

Throughout treatment for leukemia, patients are at increased risk for infections and are placed on prophylaxis for *Pneumocystis carinii* pneumonia during therapy and for 4 to 6 months after completion of therapy. During the induction or delayed intensification phases of treatment, antiviral and antifungal prophylaxes are commonly used. Patients who are neutropenic and febrile require immediate evaluation and admission for intravenous antibiotics. These patients are subsequently discharged with oral antibiotics if the total phagocytic count exceeds $300/\mu L$. Patients with recurrent or persistent fevers frequently undergo extensive evaluation to detect fungal or viral infection. High-resolution computed tomography scans of the chest are often ordered to detect occult pneumonia. Aspergillus antigen (galactomannan) testing is now available to guide antifungal treatment. The management of fevers during other phases of therapy depends on the patient's medical history and physical examination as well as the absolute neutrophil count. Outpatient oral antibiotic therapy may be adequate for treating carefully monitored patients.

Special Considerations for Infants

ALL in infants represents a small but clinically unique subset of the disease. Despite intensive chemotherapy, the prognosis for infants is considerably worse than that for older children. However, recent reports have shown that intensive chemotherapy may improve the outcome of infants with ALL (Gaynon et al, 2000). The specific chromosomal translocation t(4;11), which is present in up to 60% of infants with ALL, confers a particularly poor prognosis. An evaluation for a possible bone marrow transplantation should be initiated at the time of diagnosis for all infants with this cytogenetic abnormality. Infants do not typically receive a mediport because their subclavian vein is often not large enough to allow mediport placement. In such patients, a semipermanent catheter is used.

MATURE B-CELL LEUKEMIA

Mature B-cell leukemia is a subtype of ALL. This subtype accounts for about 2% of all pediatric ALL cases. This subtype is part of the spectrum of noncleaved small-cell lymphomas in children. The pathology of these lymphomas has been categorized as "Burkitt's" or "Burkitt-like" in the revised European-American Lymphoma classification system. About 20 years ago, a diagnosis of mature B-cell leukemia was particularly gloomy. Since then, tremendous strides have been made in the therapy for this leukemia, and its cure rate now approaches that of the other variants of childhood ALL (Patte, 2003).

Clinical Features

Mature B-cell leukemia is the biologic equivalent of the leukemia phase of sporadic Burkitt lymphoma. It is defined as the presence of more than 25% of blasts in the bone marrow. Mature B-cell leukemia is associated with rapid cell division, and the risk of tumor lysis is particularly high. Some children may even have frank renal failure at the time of diagnosis. Masses in the nasopharynx, cranial nerve palsies, and other central nervous system manifestations may be present. A rapidly expanding abdominal mass in a patient with abnormal blood studies should raise the suspicion of mature B-cell leukemia. As with other forms of acute leukemia, bone pain and unexplained fevers may also be prominent.

Diagnosis

Mature B-cell leukemia is frequently suspected when blasts (referred to as L3 lymphoblasts) appear on light microscopy as strikingly vacuolated dark-blue cytoplasm with prominent nucleoli. Confirmation of the diagnosis depends on the detection of cell-surface IgM with light-chain restriction. The B-lineage markers CD20, CD19, and CD22 can be demonstrated on flow cytometry. Cytogenetic analysis of the tumor cells usually shows nonrandom translocations involving the *myc* proto-oncogene on chromosome 8 and heavy- or light-chain Ig genes, i.e., t(8;14), t(2;8), or t(8;22). Mature B-cell leukemia is one of the fastest growing tumors. Diagnostic evaluation should be completed as quickly as possible.

Treatment for Primary Disease

Because of the threat of tumor lysis, vigorous fluid hydration and urine alkalinization should begin immediately. Allopurinol (oral or intravenous) should be started, even if the initial uric acid level is normal, to help prevent the formation of uric acid crystals with subsequent renal impairment. Allopurinol can usually be discontinued after 3 to 5 days. Recently, recombinant urate oxidase, rasburicase, has been shown to be effective in lowering uric acid levels and in minimizing the need for dialysis (Wossman et al, 2003). Nonetheless, a nephrology consultation should be obtained early in the event that dialysis becomes necessary. Electrolyte, uric acid, serum calcium, and phosphorus levels should be checked frequently. Potassium should not be added to the intravenous fluid, but calcium replacement is often required.

Patients with mature B-cell leukemia often benefit from the placement of a central venous catheter or a long line to provide venous access and to protect soft tissues from injury associated with calcium extravasation. As with patients newly diagnosed with other acute leukemias, broad-spectrum antibiotics should be started in the event of a significant fever. If the white blood cell count is extremely high, leukapheresis may be considered. Cranial nerve palsies frequently resolve with intrathecal chemotherapy, and emergency radiotherapy is rarely required for these patients.

Intensive chemotherapy of short duration is the current treatment strategy. Patients undergo initial tumor reduction therapy to help avoid tumor lysis and are treated with intensive chemotherapy using combinations of vincristine, prednisone, cyclophosphamide, doxorubicin, etoposide, high-dose methotrexate, and cytarabine. Frequent lumbar punctures with instillation of intrathecal chemotherapy are used as central nervous system prophylaxis, and cranial radiotherapy is not necessary. Using this approach, most cooperative groups have reported a long-term, event-free survival rate exceeding 80% in patients with mature B-cell leukemia (Reiter et al, 1999). Teenagers may be treated on an M. D. Anderson protocol that uses cyclophosphamide, vincristine, L-asparaginase, doxorubicin, methotrexate, cytarabine, and intrathecal chemotherapy (an augmented hyperCVAD regimen). In addition, all patients whose leukemic blasts are positive for the CD20 antigen also receive rituximab. Preliminary results of studies evaluating rituximab regimens in adults with CD20+ leukemia suggest that the drug might improve survival.

Treatment for Relapsed Disease

Relapse of mature B-cell leukemia tends to occur early, usually within 12 months of completion of therapy. For these patients, an attempt to induce remission using intensive chemotherapy followed by bone marrow transplantation is the usual approach. Even with such aggressive therapy, the cure rate remains very low. Current investigational treatments for pediatric and teenage patients with relapsed B-cell ALL include liposomal formulations, vincristine, and other investigational agents.

MYELOID LEUKEMIA

The bulk of myeloid leukemias in pediatric patients are AMLs. CML is rare, although its frequency increases with age. Approximately 400 children in the United States are diagnosed each year with AML. Because there are currently more intensive chemotherapy regimens and better supportive care, the outcomes of these children have improved progressively over the past 30 years (Arceci, 2002). Still, fewer than half of all children diagnosed with AML are cured. Escalating the intensity of the chemotherapy is unlikely to increase current cure rates considerably, and such aggressive treatment may not be tolerated well. Instead, inclusion of novel chemotherapeutic, immunotherapeutic, and differentiation agents may be more attractive options. For patients in whom the disease relapses, cure rates are very poor. The expansion of treatment options for such patients, especially those who are not eligible for HSCT, is an active research initiative at M. D. Anderson.

Diagnosis

Therapeutic approaches for patients with AML differ according to subtype, so an accurate and timely diagnosis is essential. Light microscopy and standard cytohistochemistry can establish a diagnosis of AML morphologically. Immunophenotyping by flow cytometry may be needed to differentiate ALL from undifferentiated myeloid leukemia (M0) or megakaryocytic leukemia. Cytogenetic analysis by standard karyotyping and molecular techniques can detect nonrandom chromosomal aberrations that are present in many patients with AML and that have important implications for treatment outcome (Grimwade et al, 1998). Specific molecular abnormalities, such as the FLT-3 internal duplication, are routinely searched for at diagnosis because they have considerable prognostic implications (Kottaridis et al, 2001). Electron microscopy is used to help make a diagnosis of acute megakaryoblastic leukemia. Minimal residual disease can be monitored using PCR and FISH. In patients with acute promyelocytic leukemia (APL) and CML, therapeutic decisions are guided by testing minimal residual disease.

Some rare forms of myeloid leukemia occur only in children and require special attention. Newborns with the trisomy 21 abnormality may have a transient proliferation of immature myeloid cells that are indistinguishable from myeloblasts. For the majority of these infants, this condition resolves spontaneously, but about 20% will develop acute megakaryocytic leukemia (M7) within 2 to 3 years and will require chemotherapy. Juvenile myelomonocytic leukemia (JMML) is an unusual disease that is characterized by thrombocytopenia, lymphadenopathy, splenomegaly, and rash. This form of leukemia is particularly likely to develop in patients with neurofibromatosis type I. The current preferred therapy for JMML is bone marrow transplantation. CML may occur in children, although it is very rarely encountered. On the basis of results from extensive studies done at M. D. Anderson in adult patients, imatinib mesylate therapy has been used and found to be effective in pediatric patients with CML.

Supportive Care

Patients with AML frequently become extremely ill, either because of the disease itself or the required intensive therapy. A pediatric intensivist and an infectious disease expert must collaborate in managing complications. Patients with AML who have a white blood cell count greater than $200,000/\mu L$ are particularly prone to leukostasis. The manifestations of tissue hypoxia may include a change in mental status or dyspnea. These patients are managed with fluid hydration and urgent cytoreduction by leukapheresis. Other options include the administration of hydroxyurea or exchange transfusion. In the latter procedure, the intravascular volume should be replaced with a mixture of colloid and packed red blood cells to avoid further increase in blood viscosity. Definitive chemotherapy is also started as soon as possible in these patients. As described in the section on mature B-cell leukemia, tumor lysis syndrome is managed with intravenous fluid hydration, urine alkalinization, and reduction of uric acid load. Patients with AML are also prone to hemostatic abnormalities. Disseminated intravascular coagulation is a frequent complication, especially in patients with high white blood cell counts and those with a diagnosis of APL. Fresh-frozen plasma and cryoprecipitate are required to replenish the coagulation factors. For patients at risk of hemorrhage, maintaining a platelet count of 50,000 to $100,000/\mu L$ and a fibrinogen level greater than 100 mg/mL is recommended.

Infection is a major concern in patients with AML, especially at diagnosis and initiation of therapy. Because of encouraging results from preventive strategies in adult patients, all pediatric patients are placed on prophylactic antifungal therapy with either fluconazole or itraconazole. Prophylaxis against herpes simplex is also started at the time of diagnosis. Either trimethoprim-sulfamethoxazole or a late-generation quinolone is added. In patients suspected of being at increased risk for fungal infection, treatment with lipid formulations of amphotericin, voriconazole, or capsofungin is started. Combination antifungal therapy is sometimes used, but the efficacy of this practice has yet to be confirmed. Galactomannan testing is performed on most patients with AML and is used as a guide to antifungal therapy. Adult patients housed in a protected environment during induction chemotherapy have fewer serious infectious complications than patients treated in the regular hospital ward; however, this practice is not widely used in pediatric patients. Because of the supportive-care services available at our institution, the number of deaths attributed to induction therapy has been reduced.

In addition to the support services described here, patients and family members should be provided the same ancillary services described for patients with ALL.

Treatment for Primary Disease

Prior studies of AML in adults have established daunorubicin and cytarabine as 2 of the most effective agents in treating this tumor. The standard induction regimen consists of 3 days of daunorubicin and 7 days of cytarabine. The inclusion of high-dose cytarabine in postinduction therapy has been shown to improve the long-term survival rate. The Children's Cancer Group reported that intensive-timed induction therapy for treatment of children with newly diagnosed AML increases the rate of remission and long-term outcome (Woods et al, 1996). In the United Kingdom, trials conducted by the Medical Research Council have produced excellent results using cytarabine- and daunorubicin-based induction treatments and by consolidation with alternating cycles of amsacrine, cytarabine, and etoposide as well as mitoxantrone plus cytarabine (Hann et al, 1997). Overall induction success and disease-free survival rates were very similar in these studies.

At M. D. Anderson, induction chemotherapy is stratified according to the molecular and cytogenetic aberrations associated with each type of leukemia. Patients for whom neither an inversion 16 nor a t(8;21) abnormality is evident on molecular genetic testing are eligible for the intensive-timed therapy used by the Children's Cancer Group. Patients with an inversion 16 or a t(8;21) abnormality are offered a combination of fludarabine and cytarabine, which takes advantage of the increased sensitivity of these subtypes of AML to cytarabine. Exposure to cytarabine metabolites is enhanced by the inclusion of fludarabine or similar nucleoside analogs in the regimen.

The World Health Organization's new classification system divides AML into distinct subgroups based on the morphologic, immunophenotypic, genetic, and clinical features present. Pediatric oncology cooperative groups have used this classification system to design a protocol for treatment of APL.

APL with t(15;17) is the first leukemia to be treated with differentiation therapy. All-trans retinoic acid (ATRA) specifically targets leukemia cells and causes them to differentiate. ATRA is extremely effective in treating APL, and remission rates are as high as 90% with ATRA when it is used alone. The coagulopathy associated with APL is rarely encountered. Instead, about 25% of patients develop hyperleukocytosis, fever, respiratory distress, and fluid retention (ATRA syndrome), which is treated with steroids. Additionally, arsenic trioxide has been shown to induce second remissions in a high percentage of patients with APL who experience relapse after initial therapy (Laxo et al, 2003). At diagnosis, patients with APL are eligible for therapy using differentiating agents alone; conventional chemotherapy is not used. Preliminary results in adult patients have shown an induction-chemotherapy remission rate that appeared to be at least equivalent to that of historic controls. It is hoped that pediatric and adolescent patients who are treated similarly can avoid the potential long-term cardiac problems associated with traditional cytotoxic therapy.

Gemtuzumab ozogamicin is a toxin linked to an antibody against CD33, a common antigen present on more than 80% of AML cells. CD33 is particularly prominent in APL. Gemtuzumab ozogamicin is therefore included in regimens for patients with relapsed APL. For newly diagnosed patients, gemtuzumab ozogamicin is added if the response to initial differentiation therapy is not optimal.

Treatment for Relapsed Disease

As previously noted, defining better treatment options for patients with relapsed AML is a major goal of research in the Division of Pediatrics at M. D. Anderson. We have shown that clofarabine, a new chemotherapeutic agent developed at M. D. Anderson, can notably increase the concentration of cytarabine metabolites in leukemic cells. Data from a phase I study indicate that clofarabine is well tolerated and useful for reinduction chemotherapy (Jeha et al, 2004). A phase II trial is ongoing.

Many children 15 years old and older are eligible for treatment with new agents being investigated by the adult leukemia department of this institution. For relapsed APL, patients may be treated with a combination of ATRA, arsenic trioxide, and gemtuzumab ozogamicin. Those who have not responded to arsenic trioxide may be treated with homoharringtonine.

Novel Therapies

As the pathogenesis of AML becomes better understood, therapy that targets specific genetic mutations is being developed. The prototype for this approach is imatinib mesylate, which targets the specific tyrosine kinase activated by the mutation in CML. Other tyrosine kinase-activating mutations are known to occur in AML. One such mutation, FLT-3, occurs in up to 30% of patients. The FLT-3 internal tandem duplication is particularly common in patients with resistant and relapsed disease. Currently, small molecule inhibitors of FLT-3 are being tested at our institution. The farnesyl transferase inhibitors are another group of targeted-therapy drugs that act specifically upon a number of pathways, including the *ras* pathway, which has been particularly implicated in the evolution of AML and myelodysplastic syndromes.

Some cases of AML are characterized by silenced tumor suppressor genes. The silencing of tumor suppressor genes occurs as a result of increased DNA methylation of the promoter regions, leading to leukemia progression. Another mechanism of gene silencing occurs via aberrant deacetylase activity. With the reversal of histone acetylation suppression, open chromatin formation is induced, and normal gene function is restored. Drugs that inhibit methylation (such as decitabine) or that prevent deacetylation (such as valproic acid) allow expression of silenced genes, which in turn leads to differentiation of leukemia cells (Issa et al, 2004).

HSCT

Allogeneic HSCT from a human leukocyte antigen-matched donor or an antigen-mismatched family donor reduces the risk of relapse and usually improves overall survival for patients in first complete remission of AML (Woods et al, 2001). A recent report from the Children's Cancer Group (Neudorf et al, 2004) showed that up to 75% of children with AML in first complete remission are long-term survivors following receipt of a related-donor HSCT. A graft-versus-leukemia effect was also demonstrated in this population. The survival curve for patients who received an HSCT was stable at the 4-year follow-up evaluation, whereas that of patients receiving chemotherapy alone was not stable at this follow-up period. In addition, there was no advantage to administering any postremission therapy to patients who were to undergo allogeneic HSCT. However, certain subgroups of patients fare well with conventional chemotherapy and are not candidates for initial transplantation, for example, patients with APL and children with Down syndrome. Autologous HSCT is not recommended in pediatric AML (Woods et al, 2001) except possibly for patients with APL who are in second molecular remission.

HSCT is recommended for all patients in second complete remission following bone marrow or extramedullary relapse. If a matched related donor is immediately available, then patients in whom induction chemotherapy has failed or who have an early untreated relapse can receive HSCT in lieu of reinduction chemotherapy. This is also applicable to patients with refractory relapse if the leukemic process is smoldering and not rapidly progressive, i.e., there are fewer than 25% blasts in the bone marrow and no circulating blasts in the peripheral blood.

In the absence of a matched related donor, an unrelated-donor transplantation can be performed for de novo patients with AML who have: a) high-risk features, such as monosomy 5 or 7 syndrome; b) a del (5q) or del (3q) abnormalities; and c) slow response to induction therapy. In children with myelodysplastic syndrome, JMML, monosomy 7 syndrome, and therapy-related myelodysplasia, the outcome of conventional chemotherapy is typically very poor. Early allogeneic HSCT, including the use of alternative donors, is indicated. In these cases, we use either a chemotherapy-based regimen (except in patients with extramedullary relapse) or a total-body irradiation-based regimen for concurrent extramedullary relapse or for a second transplant.

Because Ph+ CML is rare in children, current practice guidelines are derived from clinical experience with adults. We recommend an allogeneic HSCT for patients in first chronic-phase CML if a matched sibling donor is available. If the patient or the family is not prepared to proceed with immediate transplantation, a trial of imatinib mesylate is initiated. HSCT should also be performed if a complete cytogenetic response is not achieved after an adequate trial period (usually about 6 months). On the other hand, patients who do not have a matched sibling donor but achieve a molecular remission with imatinib mesylate may have autologous marrow cryopreserved so that it may be used later if there is evidence of disease progression.

A transplantation from an allogeneic (related or unrelated) donor is indicated for all patients in second chronic-phase or accelerated-phase CML. Patients in blast crisis whose disease responds to chemotherapy or imatinib mesylate may also proceed to transplantation. The regimens used for CML are based exclusively on chemotherapy. Reduced-intensity conditioning and post-transplant use of imatinib mesylate are being explored.

LONG-TERM FOLLOW-UP

Survival rates continue to improve steadily for pediatric patients with leukemia. As these patients enter adulthood, follow-up with physicians who are familiar with the long-term side effects of cancer chemotherapy and who understand the special needs of cancer survivors is essential. M. D. Anderson has a long-term follow-up clinic where cancer survivors are assessed. Comprehensive specialty care is provided with particular emphasis on the orthopedic, endocrine, pulmonary, and cardiology problems that may occur in these patients. Patients' psychosocial, developmental, educational, and career issues are also addressed. The care of a childhood cancer survivor should be coordinated through the patient's primary pediatric oncologist who will be familiar with the medical history and any related problems.

KEY PRACTICE POINTS

- Cytogenetic and molecular studies are essential for the diagnosis and management of childhood leukemia.
- Supportive care and intensification of therapy are the major reasons the prognosis for children with leukemia has improved in the past few decades.

SUGGESTED READINGS

Arceci RJ. Progress and controversies in the treatment of pediatric acute myelogenous leukemia. *Curr Opin Hematol* 2002;9:353–360.

Chessels JM, Veys P, Kempski H, et al. Long-term follow-up of relapsed childhood acute lymphoblastic leukemia. *Br J Haematol* 2003;123:396–405.

Gaynon PS, Trigg ME, Heerema NA, et al. Children's Cancer Group trials in childhood acute lymphoblastic leukemia: 1993–1995. *Leukemia* 2000;14:2223–2233.

Giralt S, Thall PF, Khouri I, et al. Melphalan and purine analog-containing preparative regimens: reduced-intensity conditioning for patients with hematologic malignancies undergoing allogeneic progenitor cell transplantation. *Blood* 2001;97:631–637.

Grimwade D, Walker H, Oliver F, et al. On behalf of The Medical Research Council Adult and Children's Leukemia Working Parties The importance of diagnostic cytogenetics on outcome in AML: analysis of 1,612 patients entered into the MRC AML 10 trial. *Blood* 1998;92:2322–2333.

Hann I, Stevens R, Goldstone A, et al. Randomized comparison of DAT versus ADE as induction chemotherapy in children and younger adults with acute myeloid leukemia. Results of the Medical Research Council's 10th AML trial (MRC AML 10). *Blood* 1997;89:2311–2318.

Howard SC, Gajjar AJ, Chang C, et al. Risk factors for traumatic and bloody lumbar puncture in children with acute lymphoblastic leukemia. *JAMA* 2002;288:2001–2007.

Issa JP, Garcia-Manero G, Giles FJ, et al. Phase I study of low-dose prolonged exposure schedules of the hypomethylating agent 5-aza-2'deoxycytidine (decitabine) in hematopoietic malignancies. *Blood* 2004;103:1635–1640.

Jeha S, Gandhi V, Chan KW, et al. Clofarabine, a novel nucleoside analog, is active in pediatric patients with advanced leukemia. *Blood* 2004;103:784–789.

Kottaridis PD, Gale RE, Frew MR, et al. The presence of a FLT-3 internal tandem duplication in patients with acute myeloid leukemia (AML) adds important prognostic information to cytogenetic risk group and response to the first cycle of chemotherapy: analysis of 854 patients from United Kingdom Medical Research Council AML 10 and 12 trials. *Blood* 2001;98:1752–1759.

Lazo G, Kantarjian H, Estey E, et al. Use of arsenic trioxide (AO₃) in the treatment of patients with acute promyelocytic leukemia. *Cancer* 2003;97:2218–2224.

Nachman JB, Sather HN, Sensel MG, et al. Augmented post-induction therapy for children with high risk acute lymphoblastic leukemia and a slow response to initial therapy. *N Engl J Med* 1998;338:1663–1671.

Neudorf S, Sanders J, Kobrinsky N, et al. Allogeneic bone marrow transplantation for children with acute myelocytic leukemia in first remission demonstrated a role for graft-versus-leukemia in the maintenance of disease-free survival. *Blood* 2004;103:3655–3661.

Patte C. Treatment of mature B-ALL and high grade B-NHL in children. *Best Pract Res Clin Haematol* 2003;15:695–711.

Pui CH, Relling RV, Downing JR. Acute lymphoblastic leukemia. *N Engl J Med* 2004;350:1535–1548.

Reiter A, Schrappe M, Tiemann M, et al. Improved treatment results in childhood B-cell neoplasms with tailored intensification of therapy: a report of the Berlin-Frankfurt-Munich trial NHL-BFM 90. *Blood* 1999;94:3294–3306.

Thomas DA, Faderl S, Cortes J, et al. Treatment of Philadelphia chromosome-positive acute lymphoblastic leukemia with hyper-CVAD and imatinib mesylate. *Blood* 2004;103:4396–4407.

Uderzo C. Indications and role of allogeneic bone marrow transplantation in childhood very high risk acute lymphoblastic leukemia in first complete remission. *Haematologica* 2000;85:9–11.

Uderzo C, Dini G, Locatelli F, et al. Treatment of childhood acute lymphoblastic leukemia after first relapse: curative strategies. *Haematologica* 2000;85:47–53.

Woods WG, Kobrinsky N, Buckley JD, et al. Timed-sequential induction therapy improves postremission outcome in acute myeloid leukemia: a report from the Children's Cancer Group. *Blood* 1996;87:4979–4989.

Woods WG, Neudorf S, Gold S, et al. A comparison of allogeneic bone marrow transplantation, autologous bone marrow transplantation, and aggressive chemotherapy in children with acute myeloid leukemia in remission. *Blood* 2001; 97:56–62.

Wossman W, Schrappe M, Meyer U, et al. Incidence of tumor lysis syndrome in children with advanced stage Burkitts lymphoma/leukemia before and after introduction of prophylactic use of urate oxidase. *Ann Hematol* 2003;82:160–165.

2 HODGKIN LYMPHOMA AND NON-HODGKIN LYMPHOMA

Ka Wah Chan, Demetrios Petropoulos, Eric L. Chang, and Michael E. Rytting

CHAPTER OVERVIEW

Lymphomas account for 10% to 15% of malignancies in pediatric patients. The most common subtypes are Hodgkin lymphoma and non-Hodgkin lymphoma. The prognosis of both forms of lymphoma has improved significantly in the past 30 years. They are now the most "curable" forms of pediatric cancer. This chapter describes the diagnostic and treatment protocols used at M. D. Anderson Cancer Center in the management of lymphomas in children.

INTRODUCTION

Lymphoma is the third most frequently occurring cancer in children. The percentage of childhood cancers that are lymphomas varies by age, from 3% for children younger than 5 years old to 24% for 15- to 19-year-olds. In general, approximately 10% to 15% of malignancies in pediatric patients are lymphomas. Hodgkin lymphoma and non-Hodgkin lymphoma are the 2 predominant subtypes. Non-Hodgkin lymphoma occurs more frequently in younger children than Hodgkin lymphoma, whereas the reverse is true for adolescents.

HODGKIN LYMPHOMA

In the United States, about 800 to 900 cases of Hodgkin lymphoma are diagnosed each year in patients younger than 20 years old. Hodgkin lymphoma is rare in children under 5 years of age. In children under age 10, it is more common in boys than girls, although among adolescents and young adults, boys and girls are equally affected.

Clinical Presentation

The vast majority of patients diagnosed with Hodgkin lymphoma present with indolent, painless lymphadenopathy in the lower cervical and supraclavicular regions. The size of these nodes may appear to fluctuate over time. About 60% of patients also have mediastinal involvement; however, inguinal lymph nodes are affected in less than 5% of cases. Up to 25% of the children also present with constitutional ("B") symptoms, which are associated with more aggressive disease. In contrast to non-Hodgkin lymphoma, bone marrow involvement at diagnosis is rare with Hodgkin lymphoma, affecting no more than 2% of patients, and it is confined exclusively to those with advanced disease.

Pathology and Prognostic Factors

The new World Health Organization (WHO) classification system separates Hodgkin lymphoma into 2 distinct entities: classical Hodgkin lymphoma and the nodular lymphocyte-predominant variant. The former includes the nodular sclerosis, mixed cellularity, lymphocyte-rich, and lymphocyte-depleted subtypes. According to the National Cancer Institute's Surveillance, Epidemiology, and End Results database, the frequency of nodular sclerosis in children is 70%; mixed cellularity, 16%; lymphocyte-rich, 7%; and cases not otherwise specified, 6%. The lymphocyte-depleted subtype is very rare, constituting less than 2% of all cases. It should be noted that the mixed cellularity subtype has been reported in up to 30% of pediatric patients in series outside the United States. The nodular lymphocyte-predominant variant is very rare. It tends to be localized, and it exhibits a slowly progressive course.

The diagnosis of classical Hodgkin lymphoma requires evidence of Reed-Sternberg cells, which are derived from B lymphocytes and are positive for CD15 and CD30. There is also evidence of immunoglobulin gene rearrangement. Lymphocytic and histiocytic cells are found in the nodular lymphocyte-predominant variant of Hodgkin lymphoma. These cells express CD20 and other B-cell antigens but are negative for CD15 and CD30. Late relapses are more common in this variant than in the classical subtypes, and some cases of the nodular lymphocyte-predominant variant may progress to large B-cell non-Hodgkin lymphoma.

Several prognostic factors have been identified in pediatric Hodgkin lymphoma. Most studies have shown that clinical features such as advanced stage (IIIB and IV); bulky mediastinal adenopathy; nodular sclerosis; B symptomatology, such as fever and weight loss; and laboratory abnormalities, including anemia, leukocytosis, and hypoalbuminemia, adversely affect treatment outcome. Prognostic indexes using a combination of these factors have been proposed, but they have not been validated in prospective clinical trials. It should also be remembered that the predictive value of the prognostic factors is decreased by effective therapy.

Diagnosis and Staging

A detailed history should be taken to quantify signs and symptoms related to lymphadenopathy. Despite the size of mediastinal involvement, respiratory compromise is rare. It is also important to elicit evidence of B symptomatology. Studies should then be performed to establish a diagnosis, to investigate the extent of disease, to assess the prognosis, and to establish baseline organ functions. The required laboratory and radiographic tests are excisional biopsy of primary site, complete blood cell count, sedimentation rate, serum ferritin level, albumin level, liver and renal profiles, bilateral marrow biopsies (may be reserved for advanced stages with constitutional symptoms), computed tomography (CT) scans, bone scans, gallium scan by single photon-emission computed tomography, echocardiogram, and pulmonary function studies. Recent reports show that metabolic function studies using whole-body positron-emission tomography (PET) may detect more disease sites than CT or gallium scans. Lymphangiography, although sensitive, has been abandoned in favor of the more sophisticated modalities. It is useful to obtain baseline hormone profiles. Sperm banking should be discussed with adolescent boys before the start of chemotherapy.

Clinical staging, according to the Ann Arbor classification system, is still used in pediatric Hodgkin lymphoma. This system is being combined with other clinical and laboratory parameters to develop various prognostic

Table 2–1. Risk Categories of Hodgkin Lymphoma in Pediatric Patients

Categories	Clinical Features	5-year EFS	5-year OS
Favorable	Stage I and II non-bulky disease, no "B" symptoms	≥95%	≥99%
Intermediate	Stage I–II A or B bulky or extranodal disease, stage IIIA disease	80%–94%	90%–98%
High	Stage IIIB and IV disease	68%–91%	88%–94%

Abbreviations: EFS, event-free survival; OS, overall survival.

groups for clinical trials. Table 2–1 shows one of the schemas used by the Children's Oncology Group for risk stratification.

Treatment

The management of Hodgkin lymphoma in pediatric patients has evolved over the past 4 decades. Accumulated experience from clinical trials has provided the following information.

- When radiotherapy is used alone, relatively high doses and large fields are required. The local control rate of early-stage Hodgkin lymphoma is lower with radiotherapy alone than with radiotherapy plus chemotherapy, but the overall survival rate resulting from these 2 treatment approaches is about the same.
- Multiagent chemotherapy allows lower doses and smaller fields of irradiation to be used, limiting the treated volume to areas of known involvement rather than extending fields to cover nearby lymph node groups.
- Involved field (IF) radiotherapy (less than 25 Gy) combined with chemotherapy improves the event-free survival rate compared with chemotherapy alone in advanced Hodgkin lymphoma (Children's Cancer Group study 5942 and Pediatric Oncology Group study 8725). However, the overall survival rates of these 2 treatment options are similar.
- It is not necessary to prolong therapy after complete remission is achieved.
- The gonadotoxic and leukemogenic potentials of alkylating agents led to attempts to modify chemotherapy. Mechlorethamine and procarbazine have now been replaced by less toxic drugs.
- Because of the possibility of late relapses and the confounding effects of late complications, reports with a median follow-up of less than 5 years from diagnosis should be interpreted with caution.
- Although conventional chemotherapy with or without radiotherapy produces excellent results for the majority of patients with Hodgkin lymphoma, hematopoietic stem cell transplantation (HSCT) can play

an important role in the management of patients for whom frontline therapy fails to produce a response.

Therapy for Primary Disease

The current treatment approach for children with Hodgkin lymphoma involves risk-adapted, combined-modality therapy. A dose-intense strategy is also being investigated and is aimed at reducing the duration of therapy and lowering the cumulative doses of individual chemotherapeutic agents.

In ongoing clinical trials, therapy is determined on the basis of tumor response at the end of the second or third cycle of chemotherapy. With this response-based strategy, the dose of subsequent radiotherapy, subsequent chemotherapy, or the combination of these is determined by the result of a disease evaluation at that point in time. Patients with 70% or greater reduction in tumor burden are considered rapid early responders (RERs), and patients with less reduction in tumor burden are considered slow early responders (SERs).

An increase in the intensity of induction chemotherapy appears to improve treatment outcome in adults with advanced-stage Hodgkin lymphoma. In the current North American pediatric trial (not yet published), patients receive 2 cycles of dose- and time-intensive chemotherapy. After disease evaluation, RERs receive further therapy; the strategy for the supplemental therapy is sex specific. Girls receive 4 additional cycles of maintenance chemotherapy, but radiotherapy is omitted. This approach is designed to avoid the high incidence of breast cancer among girls given mediastinal irradiation. Boys receive a nonalkylator chemotherapy regimen that includes doxorubicin, bleomycin, vincristine, and dacarbazine (ABVD) plus IF irradiation. The goal of this treatment is to preserve fertility. SERs continue receiving 4 additional cycles of induction chemotherapy along with IF irradiation. For intermediate-risk Hodgkin lymphoma, RERs are randomly assigned to receive or not receive IF irradiation. All SERs receive radiotherapy, and half of them are treated with augmented chemotherapy.

The nodular lymphocyte-predominant variant of Hodgkin lymphoma is usually localized and runs an indolent course. Treatment with rituximab alone produces a high response rate, but the durability of the remission is not known.

Therapy for Recurrent Disease

Patients with primary treatment failure (defined as either disease progression or incomplete response to initial therapy, unequivocal radiographic disease progression after achievement of a partial response, or presence of biopsy-documented residual Hodgkin lymphoma after primary treatment) and those with a brief initial remission (less than 12 months) have a particularly poor prognosis. Single-center studies have shown that high-dose chemotherapy followed by autologous stem cell rescue can improve these patients' long-term disease-free survival rate. Overall, 31% to 67% of patients remain disease-free after HSCT; therefore, it is considered the treatment of choice for these patients.

Children with recurrent or relapsed Hodgkin lymphoma should first receive re-induction chemotherapy. The regimens usually consist of non-cross-resistant agents such as cisplatin, cytosine arabinoside, and ifosfamide. Newer agents, including gemcitabine and vinorelbine, when given individually or in combination often produce a good response. We have also included rituximab, an anti-CD20 antibody, in our regimen. Rituximab has been shown to produce some response, although most cases of Hodgkin lymphoma are CD20 negative. The positive effect of rituximab is thought to relate to its effect on the cellular milieu surrounding the lymphoma cells. At M. D. Anderson, we are also testing the activity of the anti-CD30 monoclonal antibody in refractory Hodgkin lymphoma. PET can be used to decide metabolic activity in any residual lesions detected on CT or magnetic resonance imaging scan. PET is often used to decide the optimal time to begin the transplant phase of treatment.

The conditioning regimen most commonly used in the Division of Pediatrics at M. D. Anderson consists of carmustine (or BCNU), etoposide, cytosine arabinoside, and melphalan (BEAM). Following hematologic recovery, we administer interferon alfa as maintenance therapy. The starting dose is 0.5 million units/m^2 given subcutaneously 3 times a week, which is increased gradually to 1 to 1.5 million units/m^2 5 times a week. This treatment is continued for 1 year after the transplant. Early results suggest that this approach results in an increased disease-free survival rate. Additionally, local radiotherapy to sites of previous disease involvement is recommended.

Patients whose recurrent Hodgkin lymphomas do not respond completely (incomplete response) after reinduction chemotherapy and patients with marrow involvement have a very grave prognosis, even after autologous HSCT. Allogeneic HSCT with conventional myeloablative conditioning is associated with a very high transplant-related mortality rate. Any potential benefit from a graft-versus-lymphoma effect may be negated. More recently, a reduced-intensity preparative regimen based on fludarabine in combination with melphalan or cyclophosphamide has been used. Preliminary results have shown regular donor-cell engraftment and encouraging short-term outcome.

Long-Term Side Effects

Because most children with Hodgkin lymphoma have an excellent outcome, the mortality rate associated with complications of therapy is about the same as the mortality rate associated with the primary tumor. The major late effects of radiotherapy include atherosclerotic heart disease, thyroid dysfunction, soft-tissue hypoplasia, and retardation of bone growth. The most devastating complication is the incidence of second malignant neoplasms, which continues to increase with extended follow-up. The risk for breast cancer in girls who receive thoracic irradiation is high, and we recommend that annual mammography begin 10 years after treatment. Breast self-examination should be practiced once the girl reaches puberty. The incidence of late effects, especially second malignant neoplasms, following treatment with low-dose IF irradiation is yet unknown, but it is expected to be lower than that associated with higher doses of irradiation.

Serious late effects can also be caused by certain chemotherapy drugs (for example, sterility can result from alkylating agents, secondary leukemia from alkylating agents and etoposide, pulmonary fibrosis from bleomycin, and cardiomyopathy from anthracyclines). It should be emphasized, however, that the treatment of relapse can itself increase the risk for a second malignancy; therefore, the danger of inadequate frontline therapy cannot be ignored.

NON-HODGKIN LYMPHOMA

Sixty percent of all lymphomas in pediatric patients are non-Hodgkin lymphomas. This disease represents 3% of all malignancies in children less than 5 years of age and 8% to 9% of malignancies in patients between 5 and 19 years of age. Boys with non-Hodgkin lymphoma outnumber girls with this disease by a ratio of 3 to 1. An increased risk for non-Hodgkin lymphoma, especially B-cell lymphoma, is seen in children with primary or acquired immunodeficiency states.

Clinical Presentation

In children, non-Hodgkin lymphoma manifests as a heterogeneous group of tumors, with Burkitt's lymphoma predominating in patients 5 to 14 years old and diffuse large-cell lymphomas predominating in patients 15 to 19 years old. Unlike Hodgkin lymphoma, the majority of patients with non-Hodgkin lymphoma present with extranodal manifestations. The clinical presentation correlates strongly with the tumor's immunophenotype and histologic features. For example, most patients with Burkitt's lymphoma have abdominal involvement, although these tumors are also common in the head and neck region. At diagnosis, lymphomatous infiltration is present in the bone marrow and central nervous system (CNS) in 23% and 12% of the children, respectively. Precursor T-lymphoblastic lymphoma most commonly affects the anterior mediastinum. Lymph nodes in the upper body may also be involved. On the other hand, early precursor-B lymphoblastic lymphoma tends to present with peripheral lymphadenopathy and cutaneous infiltrates. At diagnosis, large-cell lymphoma may be localized or disseminated. Bone marrow and CNS involvement are very rare, affecting only 5% and 2% of patients, respectively. Lymphomas affecting the CNS are usually of B-cell origin. They are associated with Epstein-Barr virus reactivation and are encountered in acquired immunodeficiency syndrome and in children on prolonged immunosuppressive therapy (such as organ-transplant recipients). Systemic symptoms, such as fever and weight loss, are less common in pediatric non-Hodgkin lymphoma, but may occur in patients with large-cell lymphoma, especially anaplastic large-cell lymphoma (ALCL).

Pathology and Prognostic Factors

Nearly all pediatric non-Hodgkin lymphomas are diffuse, aggressive, and high-grade malignancies. Pathologically, they can be grouped into 3 categories. Approximately 35% to 50% are small non-cleaved cell lymphomas (Burkitt's or Burkitt-like). Another 30% to 40% are lymphoblastic lymphomas of either precursor T- or precursor B-cell origin. Large-cell lymphomas comprise the remaining 15% to 20%; two-thirds of these are ALCL, and the rest are large B-cell lymphomas and peripheral T-cell lymphomas. Current classifications of non-Hodgkin lymphoma also rely on immunodiagnostic and cytogenetic tests, but treatment continues to be based on histologic features.

Nonrandom chromosomal translocations are found in various subtypes of non-Hodgkin lymphoma. These may have etiologic implications. In Burkitt's lymphoma, the *c-myc* oncogene on chromosome 8q24 is juxtaposed with a gene of an immunoglobulin chain on chromosome 2, 14, or 22. Translocations of T-cell receptor genes on chromosomes 7 and 14 are found in precursor-T lymphoblastic lymphoma. ALCL demonstrates CD30 (Ki-1) positivity and is associated with translocation of the *ALK* gene on 2p35 with a number of partner genes.

Diagnosis and Staging

When a child is suspected of having non-Hodgkin lymphoma, the evaluation needs to proceed speedily and systematically. A histologic diagnosis should be established by obtaining tissue from the most accessible site of involvement such as pleural or ascitic fluid or the bone marrow. Care must be exercised, particularly in patients with a compromised airway, because further tissue trauma by a biopsy may lead to complete obstruction. Posteroanterior and lateral chest radiographs and CT scans are vital for identifying airway obstruction. Symptoms may include inability to breathe well when lying supine, cough, or swelling in the face (due to superior vena cava obstruction). Immunophenotypic and cytogenetic studies will help identify the lineage and progeny of the tumor. This is particularly useful for the large-cell subgroup of non-Hodgkin lymphoma. Molecular diagnostic techniques are increasingly being used to aid in diagnosis and may also have prognostic implications, especially for patients with ALCL.

Imaging studies are essential to document the extent of disease involvement; however, they should not delay the onset of chemotherapy, as childhood non-Hodgkin lymphoma is one of the most rapidly proliferating

Table 2–2.   The St. Jude Children's Research Hospital's Staging System for Pediatric Non-Hodgkin Lymphoma

Stage	Extent of Disease
I: Localized	A single tumor site (nodal or extranodal), excluding the mediastinum
II: Localized	One of the following: • Two or more nodal areas on the same side of the diaphragm • A single tumor (extranodal) with regional node involvement • A primary gastrointestinal tumor with or without regional node involvement, grossly resected
III: Disseminated	One of the following: • Two or more nodal areas on opposite sides of the diaphragm • Two single tumors (extranodal) on opposite sides of the diaphragm • Primary intra-thoracic tumors • All extensive primary intra-abdominal disease • Any paraspinal or epidural tumors
IV: Disseminated	Any of the above with more than 25% involvement of the central nervous system, bone marrow, or both

tumor types in humans. In addition to standard radiologic studies, PET scans have been useful in detecting metabolic activity in otherwise occult sites of tumor involvement.

Bone marrow examination is routinely performed, and lymphomatous involvement is defined as greater than 5% but less than 25% of tumor cells in the marrow aspirate (the higher percentage is used if multiple specimens are taken) or as focal infiltration detected in a marrow biopsy. Diagnosis of nervous system involvement may be difficult. It may include cerebrospinal fluid pleocytosis (5 or more white blood cells/µL) and the presence of lymphoma cells, cranial nerve palsy, spinal cord compression, and isolated brain metastasis. In a number of series, the lactate dehydrogenase level at presentation had prognostic significance. Patients with an initial lactate dehydrogenase level at or above 500 IU/L had a worse outcome.

The most widely used staging system is the system reported by St. Jude Children's Research Hospital (Table 2–2). The system has therapeutic and prognostic implications and is more applicable to pediatric non-Hodgkin lymphoma than the Ann Arbor staging system.

Treatment

Contemporary multiagent chemotherapy is curative for the majority of children with newly diagnosed non-Hodgkin lymphoma. However, therapeutic success depends as much on initial supportive care and tumor reduction efforts as on aggressive chemotherapy.

Treatment for Primary Disease

Treatment for pediatric non-Hodgkin lymphoma is determined on the basis of the histologic subtype of the tumor and the extent of disease (localized versus disseminated). With the intensity and the length of therapy adjusted according to disease stage and tumor burden, many previously identified prognostic factors have lost their significance.

The management of Burkitt's lymphoma should be regarded as an oncologic emergency. Tumor lysis is common, and effective supportive care is paramount. Rasburicase, a recombinant urate oxidase, can dramatically lower the uric acid level and is the uricolytic agent of choice. Aggressive management of electrolyte imbalance (including dialysis and percutaneous nephrostomy) pave the way for prompt antineoplastic therapy. An initial low-dose cytoreduction phase is followed shortly by high doses of cytarabine, methotrexate, and cyclophosphamide combined with other conventional agents. CNS prophylaxis is accomplished by intrathecal chemotherapy. The treatment duration is now less than 6 months, with some protocols being completed within 7 to 8 weeks from initiation. For a description of the leukemia phase of treatment for Burkitt's lymphoma (mature B-cell leukemia), see chapter 1, "Acute Leukemia."

Precursor T-cell lymphoblastic lymphoma is treated similarly to T-cell acute lymphoblastic leukemia. The duration of therapy is significantly longer than for patients with other types of pediatric non-Hodgkin lymphoma. Intrathecal chemotherapy appears adequate for CNS prophylaxis, and cranial irradiation is not necessary. A short course of steroids may be needed in patients with airway obstruction caused by a large mediastinal mass and superior vena cava compression. The rare cases of precursor B-cell lymphoblastic lymphoma are treated on the same protocol as Burkitt's lymphoma. The same intensive therapy of short duration is also effective for B-cell large-cell lymphoma. On the other hand, cases of ALCL are frequently of T- or null-cell origin. These subtypes respond well to an intensive combination of doxorubicin, prednisone, and vincristine. Vinblastine has shown activity against disease relapse.

Therapy for Recurrent Disease

In general, the few patients in whom frontline therapy fails usually have aggressive disease, and therapeutic rescue is rarely feasible, even with HSCT. This is especially true in cases of Burkitt's lymphoma and lymphoblastic lymphoma. Allogeneic transplantation (related and unrelated) has not produced any survival advantage to suggest that a graft-versus-lymphoma effect can be induced. If there is active progressive disease or uncontrolled CNS involvement, even high-dose therapy and HSCT do not improve the patient's prognosis and should not be performed under these circumstances.

On the other hand, patients with intermediate-grade lymphoma who have an incomplete response to initial treatment or who are in second remission (complete or partial) may benefit from high-dose chemotherapy followed by autologous stem cell rescue. This approach has been used successfully as treatment for anaplastic large-cell lymphoma, primary B-cell mediastinal lymphoma with sclerosis, and peripheral T-cell lymphoma. The inclusion of rituximab, an anti-CD20 antibody, in a high-dose chemotherapy regimen (e.g., BEAM) provides additional antitumor activity in patients with B-cell malignancies. Rituximab is now considered a standard part of our transplant regimen. For these diagnoses, a second transplant using an allogeneic donor (related or unrelated) has also been performed successfully in patients in whom previous autologous HSCT failed.

KEY PRACTICE POINTS

- The new WHO classification describes a nodular lymphocyte-predominant Hodgkin lymphoma variant. It has a distinct biologic behavior and can be distinguished by unique surface markers.
- The current treatment strategy for Hodgkin lymphoma is risk-based. The rapidity of response to the first few cycles of chemotherapy is used to determine the subsequent treatment modality and intensity.
- Autologous stem cell transplantation followed by adjuvant interferon therapy produces excellent outcome in relapsed Hodgkin lymphoma.
- Allogeneic stem cell transplantation using a reduced-intensity preparative regimen is increasingly used for patients with relapsed Hodgkin lymphoma and non-Hodgkin lymphoma.
- Treatment of non-Hodgkin lymphoma in pediatric patients is determined by the histologic subtype and the extent of disease. Intensive chemotherapy of several months' duration results in a cure rate of more than 85% in all patients.
- Careful management of the metabolic complications and prompt initiation of cytoreduction chemotherapy are critical to the success of treatment.

Suggested Readings

Cairo MS, Sposto R, Hoover-Regan M, et al. Childhood and adolescent large-cell lymphoma (LCL): a review of the Children's Cancer Group experience. *Am J Hematol* 2003;71:53–63.

Cairo MS, Sposto R, Perkins SL, et al. Burkitt's and Burkitt-like lymphoma in children and adolescents: a review of the Children's Cancer Group experience. *Br J Haematol* 2003;120:660–670.

Donaldson SS. A discourse: the 2002 Wataru W. Sutow Lecture. Hodgkin disease in children—perspectives and progress. *Med Pediatr Oncol* 2003;40:73–81.

Jaffe ES, Harris NL, Stein H, et al. Pathology and genetics of tumors of haematopoietic and lymphoid tissues. In: Kleihues P, Sobin LH, eds. *World Health Organization Classification of Tumors*. Lyons: IARC Press; 2001.

Nachman JB, Sposto R, Herzog P, et al. Randomized comparison of low-dose involved-field radiotherapy and no radiotherapy for children with Hodgkin's disease who achieve a complete response to chemotherapy. *J Clin Oncol* 2002;20:3765–3771.

Patte C. Treatment of mature B-ALL and high grade B-NHL in children. *Bailliere Best Practice Clin Haematol* 2003;15:695–711.

Schwartz CL. The management of Hodgkin disease in the young child. *Curr Opin Pediatr* 2003;15:10–16.

Smith RS, Chen Q, Hudson MM, et al. Prognostic factors for children with Hodgkin's disease treated with combined-modality therapy. *J Clin Oncol* 2003;21:2026–2033.

Weitzman S, Suryanarayan K, Weinstein HJ. Pediatric non-Hodgkin's lymphoma: clinical and biologic prognostic factors and risk allocation. *Curr Oncol Rep* 2002;4:107–113.

Williams DM, Hobson R, Imeson J, et al. Anaplastic large cell lymphoma in childhood: analysis of 72 patients treated on the United Kingdom Children's Cancer Study Group chemotherapy regimens. *Br J Haematol* 2002;117:812–820.

3   Brain Tumors: Diagnosis, Surgery and Radiotherapy, and Supportive Care

Joann L. Ater, Jeffrey S. Weinberg, Moshe H. Maor,
Bartlett D. Moore, III, and Donna R. Copeland

Chapter Overview

This chapter covers the approach taken by the M. D. Anderson Cancer Center Division of Pediatrics in the diagnosis, treatment, and supportive care of children with central nervous system (CNS) tumors. The unique aspects of state-of-the-art radiotherapy and neurosurgery techniques available to children are discussed as well as our comprehensive supportive-care program. The specialized care of children with neurofibromatosis and CNS tumors are described. Chemotherapy programs and clinical trials for children with CNS tumors are discussed in Chapter 4, "Brain Tumors: Chemotherapy and Investigational Therapy."

INTRODUCTION

Primary central nervous system (CNS) tumors are the most common solid tumors in childhood, and brain tumors are the second most common malignancy in that age group (exceeded only by leukemia). The incidence of brain tumors is 28 per 1,000,000 children younger than 15 years old (Gurney et al, 1999). In the United States alone, approximately 2,200 brain tumors are diagnosed annually in children and adolescents, and the peak in incidence occurs in children 4 to 5 years old (Kuttesch and Ater, 2004).

The treatment of pediatric patients with brain tumors differs from treatment for adult patients because of the unique supportive-care needs of children and the unique tumor-related and treatment-related differences in childhood brain tumors compared with brain tumors in adults. Brain tumors in children, as opposed to those in adults, are characterized by lower incidence, more diverse tumor types, and a prognosis that at times depends on age. There are also differences in the etiology and biology of tumors in these 2 patient populations.

The goal of treatment for brain tumors is to improve survival rates, minimize long-term complications associated with the tumor and the treatments, and, when possible, preserve physical and neurologic function and intellectual ability. At M. D. Anderson, the multidisciplinary care of pediatric patients with brain tumors involves input from pediatric neuro-oncologists, neurosurgeons, neuroradiologists, radiotherapists, neuropathologists, pediatric nurses, pediatric intensive care unit specialists, psychologists, child-life specialists, social workers, teachers, rehabilitation therapists, endocrinologists, and ophthalmologists.

This chapter discusses the diagnostic, treatment, and supportive-care approaches used at M. D. Anderson in the management of children and adolescents with brain tumors.

DIAGNOSIS

Clinical Presentation

The clinical presentation of childhood brain tumors varies and often depends on the patient's age and developmental level before tumor diagnosis, the site of origin, and the specific tumor type. The most common presentations are related to the obstruction of the flow of cerebral spinal fluid (CSF), which results in hydrocephalus and the classic triad of symptoms associated with increased intracranial pressure: morning headaches, vomiting, and lethargy. This symptomatology occurs most commonly with rapidly growing tumors of the midline or posterior fossa. Signs of increased intracranial pressure in school-age children can be more subtle, such as a decline in academic performance, a personality change, and intermittent headaches that do not necessarily occur in the morning and that can wax and wane. When these symptoms occur and are accompanied by occasional morning vomiting, they are often initially attributed to school phobia.

In neonates, increasing head circumference or a persistently bulging fontanelle can be indicative of increased intracranial pressure from hydrocephalus. Expansion of the skull can sometimes compensate for the increase in pressure and can delay the onset of the more classic symptoms of the tumor. In very young children, irritability, anorexia, developmental delay, and regression of motor skills may also occur. For example, there is cause for concern if a young child who has begun to sit alone loses that ability. In addition, the "setting-sun" sign, a paralyzed upward gaze, is associated with severely increased intracranial pressure.

A tumor located infratentorially in the cerebellum or brainstem may produce symptoms such as imbalance, upper-extremity incoordination, gait instability, and a tendency to fall to one side. In addition, when the brainstem is involved, single or multiple cranial nerve palsies can occur. The most common cranial nerve involved in childhood brain tumors is cranial nerve VI (the abducens). When this nerve is involved, the young patient in not able to look laterally. A cranial nerve VI deficit can also occur nonspecifically with increased intracranial pressure. In the case of pontine gliomas, the cranial nerves most commonly affected are VI, VII (facial nerve), and VIII (auditory nerve).

Supratentorial tumors are commonly associated with focal disorders such as motor weakness, sensory changes, speech disorders, seizures, and reflex abnormalities. Infants with supratentorial tumors may exhibit a hand preference, which ordinarily is not established until children are 4 to 5 years old. Optic-pathway tumors can cause visual disturbances, such as decreased visual acuity, Marcus Gunn pupil (an afferent pupillary defect), nystagmus, visual-field defects, or combinations of these disorders. Tumors of the suprasellar and third ventricular regions may initially be associated with neuroendocrine deficits, such as diabetes insipidus and hypothyroidism. Infants with these tumors can also have "diencephalic syndrome," which is classically characterized by a failure to thrive, emaciation, increased appetite, and a euphoric affect. Parinaud's syndrome, a classic presentation of tumors of the pineal region, manifests as: (a) paresis of upward gaze, (b) dilated pupils that react to accommodation but not to light, (c) nystagmus to convergence or retraction, and (d) eyelid retraction.

Spinal cord tumors and spinal cord dissemination of brain tumors may manifest as long nerve-tract motor or sensory deficits (or both), bowel and bladder deficits, and back or radicular pain. Patients with meningeal metastatic disease from brain tumors or leukemia may present with signs and symptoms similar to those in patients with subtentorial tumors (Kuttesch and Ater, 2004).

Evaluation

Because of the myriad symptoms associated with brain tumors, the examining physician must approach the evaluation with a high degree of suspicion, especially with midline tumors. The evaluation of a patient suspected of having a brain tumor constitutes an emergency. The initial evaluation should include a complete history and physical examination and a neurologic assessment with neuroimaging. A computed tomography (CT) scan can detect approximately 95% of tumors and remains an appropriate screening tool. However, magnetic resonance imaging (MRI) is now considered to be the neuroimaging standard for detecting brain tumors and to be better than CT at determining the tumor's location. The characteristics detectable by MRI are also useful when making a differential diagnosis. The delineation of tumors in the pituitary or suprasellar region, the optic pathway, and the subtentorium is better with MRI than with CT. MRI also has better resolution and can detect nonenhancing, infiltrating tumors better than CT. When the results of a CT scan are positive for the presence of a tumor, the patient is usually required to undergo MRI so that physicians can appropriately plan a therapeutic intervention. If the tumor is located in the posterior fossa and the imaging characteristics are consistent with medulloblastoma or ependymoma, MRI of the entire spine is performed to rule out spinal metastases. However, the results of an MRI of the spine can be difficult to interpret for several weeks after surgical intervention because of the presence of blood and postsurgical changes. Because the MRI scan can be a critical resource for staging medulloblastomas and ependymomas, a preoperative MRI scan of the spine is recommended.

Patients with tumors of the midline and the pituitary, suprasellar, and optic chiasmal region should undergo evaluation for neuroendocrine dysfunction. A formal ophthalmologic examination is beneficial for patients with tumors of the optic-pathway region to document the effect of the disease on the patient's oculomotor function, visual acuity, and visual fields. Measurements of beta-human chorionic gonadotropin and alpha fetoprotein levels in serum and CSF can assist in the diagnosis of germ cell tumors, which are preferentially located in the suprasellar and pineal regions.

For patients with tumors that have a propensity to spread to the leptomeninges, such as medulloblastomas and primitive neuroectodermal tumors (PNETs), ependymomas, and germ cell tumors, lumbar puncture can be useful for obtaining a CSF specimen for cytologic analysis. However, lumbar puncture is contraindicated in patients with newly diagnosed hydrocephalus that is secondary to CSF flow obstruction and in patients with subtentorial tumors. Lumbar puncture in these patients may lead to downward brain herniation resulting in neurologic compromise and death.

Effect of Neurofibromatosis on Diagnosis

Within the Division of Pediatrics at M. D. Anderson, a comprehensive clinic has been established for children with neurofibromatosis (NF). NF type 1, which is caused by an autosomal dominant mutation on chromosome 17, is the most common subtype of NF. Children with NF type 1 have an increased risk for developing both benign and malignant tumors. NF type 1 is diagnosed in approximately 1 in 3,000 children on the basis of 2 or more of the following clinical findings: a family history of NF in a first-degree relative, an optic-pathway glioma, Lisch nodules in the iris, a plexiform neurofibroma, axillary freckling, café-au-lait spots, orthopedic malformations (e.g., scoliosis), or some combination of these features. More than 15% of children with NF type 1 are found to have an optic-pathway glioma on MRI. These optic-pathway gliomas may be asymptomatic and may remain stable requiring no treatment. As shown in Table 3–1, in children with NF, optic chiasmal or hypothalamic gliomas are less likely to progress and less likely to require therapy than in children who have these gliomas but do not have NF. Therefore, treatment for children who have NF and 1 of these gliomas is recommended only when objective signs of progression are present. Other low-grade or even anaplastic gliomas can also have an indolent course in children with NF.

Hyperintense areas on fluid-attenuated inversion recovery images or T_2-weighted images on MRI, especially in the brainstem, can be mistaken for brainstem gliomas. These areas are often called "unidentified bright objects," and they are associated with neuropsychologic alterations, especially if they occur in the thalamus (Moore et al, 1996). These unidentified bright objects are most likely hamartomas or developmental abnormalities that require no therapy. Children with NF type 1 are also at increased risk for developing neurofibrosarcomas, neurofibromas, rhabdomyosarcomas, and other tumors.

Table 3–1. Outcome of Optic Chiasmal or Hypothalamic Gliomas in Children With and Without Neurofibromatosis

Outcome	With NF (n = 15)	Without NF (n = 31)
Stable disease	12	8
Progressive disease	2	21
Postoperative death	0	1
Lifetime follow-up	1	1

Abbreviation: NF, neurofibromatosis. Source: Janss et al, 1995.

Table 3–2.   Frequency of Specific Tumor Types in Primary
             Central Nervous System Tumors of Childhood

Tumor Type	Frequency
• Supratentorial astrocytoma	25% to 40%
Low grade	15% to 25 %
High grade	10% to 15%
• Medulloblastoma and PNET	10% to 25%
• Cerebellar astrocytoma	10% to 20%
• Ependymoma	5% to 10%
• Brainstem glioma	10% to 20%
• Craniopharyngioma	6% to 9%

Abbreviation: PNET, primitive neuroectodermal tumor.

NF type 2, which is caused by an autosomal dominant mutation of chromosome 22, is much less common than NF type 1. Children with NF type 2 have a higher risk of developing meningiomas, ependymomas, bilateral acoustic neuromas, or gangliogliomas than do those with NF type 1.

The children we see in the Neurofibromatosis Clinic at M. D. Anderson are followed annually for signs and symptoms of brain or spinal cord tumors and for management of any related neuropsychologic conditions.

Neuropathology

The neuropathologists at M. D. Anderson are an important part of the pediatric brain cancer diagnostic team, because the final recommendations for treatment rest primarily on the pathologic diagnosis of the tumor. The types and incidence rates of common childhood brain tumors are shown in Table 3–2. Pathology specimens and neurologic images are presented for review at a weekly neuropathology conference. In addition to the standard hematoxylin and eosin–stained slides, immunohistochemical staining and determination of the MIB-1 proliferative index are frequently used to reach the final diagnosis. Consensus must be reached by all neuropathologists who review the tumors before a final diagnosis is made.

TREATMENT

Current proven therapies that are effective in treating many types of brain tumors in children include neurosurgery, radiotherapy, and chemotherapy (with both standard and novel agents). The following discussion describes the approach taken at M. D. Anderson in the delivery of these therapies. The survival rates of children with brain tumors treated with the best standard methods are shown in Table 3–3.

Neurosurgery

The neurosurgeon is frequently the first physician to be called on after a brain tumor has been diagnosed in a pediatric patient because these tumors

Table 3–3. Survival Rates of Children With Brain Tumors
            Treated With the Best Standards

Tumor Type	5-yr Overall Survival Rate
Low-grade astrocytoma	
Cerebellar	>95%
Supratentorial	60% to 90%
Medulloblastoma and PNET	
High risk	40% to 85%
Average risk	60% to 70%
Ependymoma	40% to 60%
Anaplastic astrocytoma	20% to 40%
Glioblastoma multiforme	5% to 20%
Brainstem glioma	10% to 20%

Abbreviations: PNET, primitive neuroectodermal tumor; yr, year.

are often found in a midline location and may obstruct the flow of CSF, resulting in obstructive or noncommunicating hydrocephalus. The intracranial pressure may rise acutely, and the associated neurologic deterioration provides the impetus to seek medical attention. Surgery can then be undertaken to relieve the hydrocephalus-related pressure, decrease the effect of the mass, obtain tissue for diagnostic testing, and remove the tumor. Recent advances in image-guided surgery have made surgical intervention a safer therapeutic option than it was previously.

Hydrocephalus

As stated, obstructive hydrocephalus commonly occurs in pediatric patients with brain tumors. Tumors located in the region of the third ventricle (e.g., optic-chiasmal or hypothalamic gliomas, craniopharyngiomas, pituitary tumors, and subependymal giant-cell astrocytomas of tuberous sclerosis) can directly obstruct the flow of CSF at the level of the foramen of Monro or just distal to that foramen in the body of the third ventricle. More distally, tumors in the posterior fossa (e.g., diffuse pontine gliomas, tectal gliomas, pineal region tumors, brainstem or fourth ventricular ependymomas, medulloblastomas, pilocytic astrocytomas, and choroid plexus tumors) may cause an obstruction at the level of the cerebral aqueduct, the fourth ventricle, or the foramina of Magendie or Luschka. Immediate relief of increased intracranial pressure secondary to obstructive hydrocephalus is of paramount importance.

The goal of treating obstructive hydrocephalus is to drain off excessive CSF, thus decreasing intracranial pressure. This can be accomplished by using 1 of 3 procedures. The procedure chosen depends on the patient's clinical presentation, the tumor pathology, and the anticipated outcome.

In the first procedure, rapid control of intracranial pressure can be obtained by placing an externalized ventricular drain, usually by a frontal burr hole. This procedure can be performed in an emergency room, intensive care unit, or operating room. With posterior fossa tumors, care must be taken not to drain CSF too rapidly for fear of a theoretical upward herniation.

In the second procedure, the externalized drain can be converted to a ventriculoperitoneal shunt at the outset if it seems likely that the patient will have chronic hydrocephalus after the tumor is removed. Alternatively, the shunt can be placed later if it becomes necessary.

Third, an endoscopic third ventriculostomy may be performed. This procedure involves puncturing a hole in the midline floor of the third ventricle just posterior to the mamillary bodies and using an endoscope to directly visualize the anatomy. The great advantage of this procedure is the ability to treat hydrocephalus without having to implant a permanent indwelling system. This procedure creates communication between the CSF of the third ventricle and that of the prepontine cistern (the subarachnoid space distal to the fourth ventricle) and essentially re-creates normal CSF flow by bypassing the region of the obstruction. Not all patients are candidates for this procedure; the obstruction must be distal to the foramen of Monro so that the endoscope may be passed transcortically to the lateral ventricle and then through the foramen of Monro to the third ventricle to visualize the floor. Another contraindication to this procedure is a posterior fossa tumor that causes the prepontine space to be obliterated (the pons and basilar artery will be pressed against the clivus). In this case, there is no room to pass the puncturing device, and the risk of injury to the basilar artery or brainstem is too high.

Tumor Resection

Direct tumor removal serves several functions: (a) relief of the direct effect of the mass on critical structures results in a decrease in symptoms, (b) tumor removal may reduce hydrocephalus, (c) the tissue removed can be analyzed to confirm the pathologic diagnosis, and (d) aggressive and complete resection often provides the best treatment for almost all brain tumors in the pediatric population.

Complete surgical resection is associated with improved prognosis. In fact, data suggest that the survival rates for children with low-grade astrocytomas, pilocytic astrocytomas, and ependymomas are improving as a result of surgical advancements, and cures may be effected by complete surgical resection. In addition, even children with malignant tumors such as medulloblastomas and high-grade gliomas (i.e., anaplastic astrocytomas and glioblastomas) have notably higher survival rates with a gross or near-total resection than do children with these tumors who undergo minimal or no surgical resection (Wisoff et al, 1998). Data also suggest that the efficacy of adjuvant treatments (i.e., chemotherapy and radiotherapy) is enhanced when a large percentage of the tumor is removed.

At M. D. Anderson, we rarely proceed with a biopsy at the time of diagnosis. Instead, we usually proceed with surgical resection. Exceptions to this rule occur when the risk of surgery is too high because of the tumor's location and in the case of tumors for which the results of imaging studies are characteristic. Tumors that fall into this category are certain optic-pathway tumors and pontine gliomas for which tissue sampling is not needed for diagnosis. In patients with pontine gliomas, biopsy does not improve the accuracy of diagnosis or provide a therapeutic benefit (Epstein and McCleary, 1986). However, a tumor of the brainstem that is not a typical pontine glioma or a focal brainstem tumor may be sampled by biopsy or removed, depending on location and imaging characteristics.

We also consider surgery, when possible, for patients with recurrent tumors. The use of repeat surgery often depends on the child's condition, the extent and location of the tumor, and other treatments that might be necessary. Surgery with additional therapy can provide long-term control of certain tumor types.

Surgical Adjuncts

A surgeon's armamentarium includes multiple adjuncts that aid in increasing the amount of tumor that can be resected while increasing the overall safety of the surgery. These adjuncts are used during both the preoperative and intraoperative phases of the surgical treatment.

Preoperatively, MRI plays a large role. Analysis of standard T_1-weighted, T_2-weighted, fluid-attenuated inversion recovery, diffusion-weighted, and gadolinium-enhanced images facilitates the diagnosis of the tumor with a certain degree of accuracy. Knowledge of standard cerebral anatomy allows the surgeon to judge the location of the tumor in relation to functional anatomic regions. The ability to locate functional anatomy is further enhanced by the use of functional MRI, which is a blood oxygen level–dependent imaging technique. While in the MRI scanner, the patient is administered a battery of simple intellectual tasks designed to activate the corresponding functional area of the cortex. During task activation, increased blood flow to the cortical region involved in generating metabolic activity results in increased oxygenated hemoglobin concentration because the amount of oxygen delivered is greater than the amount of oxygen extracted. Therefore, the net amount of regional deoxyhemoglobin decreases relative to that of oxyhemoglobin. The decrease in paramagnetic deoxyhemoglobin results in an increased MRI signal; overlaying this signal on a regular MRI scan allows the functional anatomy to be located.

Diffusion tensor imaging, or tractography, takes anatomic location a step further. Whereas functional MRI locates cortical functional anatomy and is useful for identifying the proximity of a tumor to this anatomic region, it does not allow location of the descending white-matter fibers or of their relationship to more deeply seated tumors. Tractography makes use of the diffusion of free-water protons along white-matter tracts. If the direction of the diffusion can be mapped, then maps of the white-matter fiber tracts can be generated and subsequently color coded. Thus, the location of the posterior limb of the internal capsule can be imaged and identified in relation to a deep-seated tumor. A surgeon who understands this anatomic relationship is better prepared to protect the tracts and preserve neurologic function.

Image-guided surgery is one of the most commonly used intraoperative adjuncts. A preoperative MRI scan of a patient is stored in a computer graphics workstation in the operating room. Then radiopaque markers (fiducial marks) placed on the patient's skin before MRI are registered 1 by 1 from the patient to the image. The computer can then construct a location map. A device can be used to identify a point on the patient's head or subsequently in the brain and to locate this point on the MRI scan stored in the computer, allowing accurate planning of the skin incision and generation of a trajectory to deep-seated tumors that spares eloquent cortex. During resection, image-guided surgery further aids the surgeon in differentiating normal brain tissue from tumor in cases when it is not apparent on direct visualization.

Sonography is another useful intraoperative adjunct. A transducer emits high-frequency sound waves, which are reflected differently by tissues of dissimilar densities. The echogenicity of the tumor as well as the differences in echogenicity at the tumor-brain interface are imaged on a screen, and updated real-time images assist the surgeon in planning the corticectomy at the beginning of the resection and in determining whether any tumor tissue remains at the anticipated end of the procedure. This technique is less useful in a postirradiated brain, which frequently appears as echogenic as the tumor itself.

The last intraoperative adjunct of critical importance is a smear preparation or frozen section stained with hematoxylin and eosin. A smear is an excellent and rapid technique that preserves the cytologic characteristics of the specimen and can be performed with a small amount of tissue. Frozen specimens are cut into 4-μm sections. This size substantially preserves the architecture of the specimen. During stereotactic biopsy, as performed at M. D. Anderson, a sample of tissue is prepared by using both of these techniques to confirm that the biopsy has obtained abnormal tissue. Other specimens are then saved permanently for pathologic examination. During resection, both smears and frozen specimens from the tumor tissue are analyzed again to help the surgeon determine how aggressive the surgery should be and to give the patient's family some information about the tumor.

Radiotherapy
Radiotherapy at M. D. Anderson involves state-of-the-art techniques for focal and craniospinal therapy.

New Techniques for Focal Therapy

Modern radiotherapy is defined as "conformal." Ideally, conformal radio-therapy delivers the prescribed dose to the target as designated by the radiation oncologist with minimal radiation to the surrounding normal tissues. Conformal radiotherapy results in less toxicity and fewer long-term side effects compared with conventional radiotherapy techniques. The use of conformal radiotherapy is of the utmost importance in treating pediatric brain tumors because such therapy is better suited than older techniques to sparing the normal brain and other tissues that are at a critical phase of development.

To achieve conformality, it is essential to know the exact anatomic location of the tumor and its relation to the surrounding normal structures. This goal cannot be achieved with conventional radiotherapy simulation and planning techniques, because these methods are based on plain radiographs, which are limited in their ability to demonstrate soft tissues. Only a few anatomic structures, such as the skeleton or locations that interface with air, can be reliably demonstrated with conventional simulation techniques. Brain tumors in particular are hard to locate precisely within the cranial cavity. In using older techniques, radiotherapy fields tended to be large and parallel-opposed to ensure that the tumor was not missed. Such techniques needlessly exposed a large volume of the brain and other cranial tissues to radiation.

The advent of CT in the 1970s revolutionized the field of radiation oncology. Not only could most tumors be reliably demonstrated, but by reconstructing the images in different three-dimensional (3D) planes, radiation oncologists could visualize and treat the tumor from any angle. This ability is called the "beam's eye view" function, and it has led to the current modern era of using image-based 3D planning and treatment radiotherapy (3DRT). At M. D. Anderson, all pediatric brain tumors are simulated on one of several available simulation devices (AcQSim; Philips Medical Systems, Cleveland, OH) of which the CT scan is an integral part. With the help of orthogonal lasers, the child is placed on a simulator table in the desired position, and the child's head is then immobilized with a thermoplastic mask. A CT scan with or without contrast is then obtained at 3-mm slices throughout the cranium. After a reference point is placed on the mask, the child can be taken off the table. The simulation process takes about 45 minutes. The actual designing of the beams and the blocks to be used is performed virtually on a treatment-planning computer to which the CT data are sent. On each CT slice, the radiation oncologist outlines the tumor and critical normal anatomic structures that are to be spared from the radiation as much as possible (e.g., the optic pathways or the cochleae). If the tumor is not visualized well on the CT scan, which frequently happens with brain tumors, higher-sensitivity MRI scans can be fused with the CT data to enhance our ability to localize the tumor.

The volume of tumor detectable by any imaging technique is defined as the gross tumor volume (GTV). Delivering radiotherapy to the GTV alone is an inadequate treatment approach for many malignant brain tumors because of radiographically undetectable microscopic extension of tumor cells surrounding the gross tumor. The additional volume to be treated because of likely undetected tumor cells is called the clinical target volume (CTV). The CTV varies from zero or minimal for noninvasive tumors to a few centimeters for highly malignant tumors. The planning computer can add a specified margin to the CTV automatically in all spatial directions. Usually, the radiation oncologist will prescribe a lower dose to the CTV than to the GTV because the former contains less tumor burden and more functioning neurologic tissue than does the GTV.

To account for some movement and day-to-day slight variations in the patient's position, a planning target volume (PTV) is also developed. The PTV in the brain is typically only a few millimeters because immobilization is excellent and there is no organ movement related to breathing. The radiation oncologist needs to outline the organs at risk and specify the maximal allowable dose to them, which is just as important as the PTV. The dosimetry-oncology team will then go through a process of virtual simulation and planning to find the best way to orient the radiation beams to achieve the goals of maximally treating the tumor while sparing the noninvolved organs at risk of radiation exposure. The computer also designs the exact position of the collimator leaves, which are now used in place of the conventional lead blocks to shape the beam. Treatment plans can be objectively evaluated and compared by using a dose-volume histogram for each tumor volume and normal structure. To achieve a satisfactory dose distribution, 3 to 5 beams are incorporated into most 3DRT plans.

Techniques developed for radiosurgery are occasionally used for fractionated stereotactic radiotherapy, in which a customized bite block achieves immobilization, and the target volumes are localized in a reference 3D frame attached to the immobilizing device. Multiple beams or arcs are designed to hit the tumor from many angles. This technique is suitable only for small volumes and achieves a high degree of conformality.

In the last 5 years, a growing number of patients at M. D. Anderson have received intensity-modulated radiotherapy (IMRT). With IMRT, the dose across every field of radiation is not homogeneous but is modulated by changing the collimator aperture multiple times for each field. The initial simulation process with IMRT is similar to that for 3DRT. The patient is immobilized and scanned on the CT simulator. GTV and CTV are outlined, and doses are prescribed. The ideal plan is produced by using specialized commercial software. The computer will usually assign many beams, in addition to modulating the intensity for each, to approach as nearly as possible the prescription determined by the radiation oncologist. IMRT usually achieves a greater conformality than does 3DRT. However, IMRT is more labor intensive and more costly than 3DRT. IMRT is best suited for irregularly shaped tumors or for tumors located next to a critical structure that would be difficult to spare with 3DRT.

Craniospinal Radiotherapy

Craniospinal radiotherapy (CSRT) was designed for tumors that may spread through the CSF. Because of the large volumes of tissue treated in CSRT, a child usually experiences more considerable side effects with CSRT than with treatments that require only partial brain irradiation. In addition to total epilation, possible short-term side effects are headaches, lethargy, nausea, vomiting, diarrhea, esophagitis, and pancytopenia. Managing side effects during the course of radiotherapy requires diligent supervision from the pediatric-radiation oncology team. Long-term side effects can be devastating. Radiotherapy to the whole brain may lead to cognitive deterioration, cataracts, pituitary deficiency, and hearing impairment. Radiotherapy to the entire spine can cause decreased height. Fortunately, the indications for delivering CSRT have decreased in recent years. The risk of CSF spread from an ependymoma of any grade or location is considered to be low. Therefore, all children with localized ependymomas who undergo radiotherapy receive radiation to the tumor bead only via conformal techniques. Likewise, germinomas are not currently treated with CSRT but rather with a combination of chemotherapy and local radiotherapy. However, CSRT is still used to treat ependymomas with proven CSF dissemination and in germinomas that recur after combined chemotherapy and radiotherapy.

Indications to deliver CSRT early after diagnosis are medulloblastomas, supratentorial PNETs, and aggressive embryonal tumors. The need to treat the entire craniospinal axis was first indicated by Cushing and Bailey in 1930. Attempts to give local therapy only resulted in almost uniform failure. Therefore, CSRT remains the standard of care in treating medulloblastomas in spite of the toxicity involved.

For standard-risk medulloblastomas, we offer 2 treatment alternatives. The first is a reduced dose of CRST: 23.4 Gy given at 1.8 Gy per fraction 13 times, followed by a boost to the posterior fossa of 54 Gy. This treatment is followed by chemotherapy. Because CSRT is the primary cause of long-term toxicity, the goal of this regimen is to reduce the dose of CSRT and to compensate for the reduction by adding chemotherapy. The second alternative is treatment with radiotherapy alone at a total of 30 Gy to the craniospinal fields followed by a boost of 54 Gy to the posterior fossa.

Patients with high-risk medulloblastomas who have evidence of tumor dissemination in the CSF, as determined by cytology or MRI, require high doses to the craniospinal axis (36 to 40 Gy). The dose to the posterior fossa remains 54 Gy.

Traditional treatment simulation for CSRT used to take approximately 90 minutes; a lot of cooperation was required from the child because the position for treatment (lying prone and immobile with the face in a special mask) is somewhat uncomfortable. The CT simulator has made the process much faster and easier for the patient; the time on the simulator table is now 45 minutes. After the child is immobilized in the required position, a CT scan of the entire head and spine is obtained. Reference points in the brain and spine are established, after which the child can be taken off the table. The fields for the brain and spine are then placed virtually by the treatment-planning computer using data obtained from the CT simulator. Designing the brain fields requires the expertise of the radiation oncologist and the dosimetrist. All the meninges at the base of the brain have to be treated without excessive irradiation to the eyes. Nonetheless, scattered radiation to the lenses is unavoidable and may lead to cataracts. The superior border of the posterior field needs to match the lower lateral brain fields, and treatment must be planned meticulously so that overdosage or underdosage of the junction does not occur.

In younger children or infants, the spinal cord field depth is less than 5 cm from the skin surface, so we prefer to treat the spinal field using high-energy electrons rather than photons. Using high-energy electrons minimizes the exit dose of the radiation beyond the spinal canal and greatly reduces short-term side effects (Chang et al, 2002). It should also reduce some of the late effects, but this is harder to quantify. An additional dose to the posterior fossa is also carefully planned with oblique fields in the attempt to reduce the dose to both cochleae. Reducing cochlear exposure is especially relevant in patients with medulloblastomas, because many of these patients also receive cisplatin, which can be ototoxic.

Chemotherapy

Chemotherapy and other investigational therapies are showing promise for the treatment of childhood brain tumors. The results of randomized phase II and III clinical trials over the last 15 to 20 years support the recommendation that chemotherapy should be considered an important and standard part of therapy for children with medulloblastomas, PNETs, CNS germ cell tumors, incompletely resected ependymomas, malignant gliomas, CNS rhabdomyosarcomas, and unresectable low-grade gliomas. For a specific discussion about chemotherapy and investigational therapy for certain childhood brain tumors, please see Chapter 4. For guidelines on the treatment of rare brain tumors, please refer to our previously published chapter (Ater and Rytting, 1997).

FOLLOW-UP AND SUPPORTIVE CARE

Follow-up examinations are done after initial therapy to monitor for tumor recurrence, and supportive care is provided as needed. Routine follow-up in the pediatric neuro-oncology clinic at M. D. Anderson includes physical and neurologic examinations, evaluation of growth and development, and MRI scans. The follow-up interval depends on the type of tumor, risk of recurrence, and potential treatment-associated problems. Children who have had cranial irradiation or who show growth delay receive annual endocrine screening tests and are referred to our pediatric endocrine clinic if any problems are suspected. The most common conditions detected during follow-up care of children with brain tumors are described below.

Neuropsychologic Evaluation

Children with brain tumors are at increased risk for general intellectual decline and specific neurocognitive impairments (Radcliffe et al, 1992; Ater et al, 1997b; Copeland et al, 1999). For that reason, children treated at M. D. Anderson for brain tumors undergo a battery of neuropsychologic evaluations at diagnosis, if possible, and annually thereafter. The assessment should include measures of intellect, academic achievement, memory, attention, language, executive skills (planning and organization), fine-motor and perceptual-motor skills, and behavioral/emotional status.

Long-term follow-up of neuropsychologic functioning is crucial because the side effects of treatment may increase over time. Declines in neurocognitive function occurring as many as 10 years postdiagnosis are not uncommon. Affected areas tend to be in nonverbal domains such as attention, spatial memory, and perceptual-motor skills. As a consequence, these children frequently have difficulties with mathematics in school. Younger children (5 years old and younger) are usually affected more than older children and adolescents and may have verbal and nonverbal disabilities.

Recently, cognitive remediation programs have been devised to help children with an attention deficit learn strategies to compensate for their difficulties at school. One successful program at M. D. Anderson and a number of other cancer centers involves teaching children exercises to increase focus and processing speed, strategies for approaching academic tasks, and cognitive-behavioral techniques to reinforce learning and improve self-confidence and self-esteem (Butler and Copeland, 2002).

In addition to neurocognitive evaluations, consultations with an affected child's home school are often required to apprise teachers and counselors about the effects of brain tumors and their treatment and provisions that may need to be instituted in the classroom to promote the child's learning. The results of the neuropsychologic assessment are given to the school by M. D. Anderson's education and psychology staffs along with recommendations about instructional modifications that might be beneficial for the child.

Children and adolescents with NF type 1 are at increased risk for learning, cognitive, and behavioral difficulties. This risk is further increased with the diagnosis of a brain tumor (Moore et al, 1994; DeWinter et al, 1999). Because approximately 40% to 50% of children with NF type 1 have a learning disability and a similar number suffer from behavioral problems, such as attention deficit/hyperactivity disorder, obsessive-compulsive disorder, or oppositional-defiant behavior, we place a strong emphasis on assessing these functions (North et al, 1997). Children with NF type 2 do not have an increased incidence of these problems, so neuropsychologic assessment is not done for them on a routine basis.

For children with NF type 1, our neuropsychologic assessment strategy is designed to determine a child's strengths and weaknesses in a variety of areas, with concentration on areas known to be at particularly high risk. Weaknesses known to exist in a high percentage of these children include deficits in visual-spatial abilities, reading, language, and attention. In addition to intellectual assessment, we also administer tests of academic achievement, language, memory, fine-motor skills, visual-spatial and construction skills, and attention. We also administer questionnaires to the child's parents and teachers to determine whether the child might have attention deficit/hyperactivity disorder as well as other behavioral and psychosocial disorders. All this information is conveyed to the parents in the form of a written report with verbal feedback either by telephone or in person.

Part of this evaluation process involves consulting with our educational liaison, a specialist in school psychology and learning disabilities. The educational liaison integrates the results of our neuropsychologic and behavioral assessment with the child's medical profile and works with the child's parents and school personnel to determine whether an educational need exists that is not being addressed satisfactorily. The educational liaison attends Admission, Retention, and Dismissal meetings and participates in the design of an Individual Educational Plan. A full battery of neurocognitive and behavioral evaluations is administered annually to track the patient's progress and to enable the educational liaison to make recommendations for remediation and school intervention.

Children with brain tumors also have a high incidence of acquired learning and cognitive difficulties resulting from the tumor, surgical resection, and therapy. Thus, each child newly diagnosed with a brain tumor is administered a comprehensive battery of neuropsychologic tests that assess the same general functional domains described above; ideally, these tests are administered before surgery or initiation of any therapy. If a child is medically unable to complete an evaluation, it is completed at the earliest possible time thereafter. This evaluation will be used as a baseline with which to gauge future changes, either positive or negative, that result from the therapy.

In some cases, surgery results in improved cognitive status because removing the tumor relieves cranial pressure. In other cases, surgery results in reduced cognitive status because the tumor has invaded critical brain areas or the surgical approach caused unavoidable damage to areas subserving higher-order cognitive skills. Cranial irradiation is associated with cognitive decline, especially in younger patients, and some chemotherapy regimens may place the child at increased risk for transient or permanent cognitive sequelae (Moore et al, 1992; Ater et al, 1997b; Copeland et al, 1999). For these reasons, we believe it is critical that evaluations are repeated annually.

Late Neurologic Effects

Aside from focal neurologic deficits, the most common neurologic problems that occur in children treated for brain tumors are seizures and headaches. Seizures can be a presenting sign of the tumor and may resolve after surgery. However, in many children with either residual tumor or surgical scarring, long-term use of an anticonvulsant is required. For long-term management of seizures, carbamazepine and phenytoin are the most commonly used agents. Valproic acid is efficacious for children who are allergic to other anticonvulsants. Children being treated with chemotherapy are being converted to non-p450 enzyme–inducing anticonvulsants, such as levetiracetam or gabapentin, to make the chemotherapy more effective and to reduce hypermetabolism. Some of our protocols for new agents now require the use of nonenzyme-inducing anticonvulsants. Occasionally, children who have not previously had seizures will begin having seizures several years after completing therapy. Although recurrent tumor is always a concern and must be excluded, late seizures may also occur in children without tumor recurrence and are possibly related to brain scarring or focal calcification.

Headaches occurring in children treated for brain tumors often raise concerns about tumor recurrence and may need to be evaluated in the pediatric neuro-oncology clinic. Children who have a ventriculoperitoneal shunt have a lifelong risk of shunt malfunction and potential for increased intracranial pressure. Therefore, even children who have not received therapy for many years can have an acute emergency caused by shunt malfunction. Finally, to complicate matters further, children who have received cranial irradiation also seem to have an increased incidence of true migraines and migraine-like headaches. Some of these are complicated migraines with transient neurologic deficits such as weakness or speech problems that resolve spontaneously. Our pediatric neurologist is consulted on many of these cases to ensure appropriate therapy.

Endocrine Evaluation

Endocrine deficits occur in many of our pediatric patients treated for brain tumors. In some, the deficit is related to the tumor being located in the hypothalamus. For example, children with germ cell tumors of the hypothalamic region present with diabetes insipidus and growth hormone deficiency and can progress to panhypopituitarism. Patients with other hypothalamic tumors, such as astrocytomas and craniopharyngiomas, are at increased risk for panhypopituitarism related to the tumor, surgical intervention, radiotherapy, or some combinations of these. These same patients also have an increased risk of osteoporosis in later life, most likely resulting from hormone imbalances. For these reasons, all of our patients with midline tumors are followed regularly in the pediatric endocrine clinic.

Children who receive whole-brain irradiation for embryonal tumors are also at increased risk for developing endocrine deficits such as growth hormone deficiency and thyroid-stimulating hormone deficiency. These children are screened annually and are often referred to the pediatric endocrine clinic. Hormone-replacement therapy, including growth-hormone replacement, is recommended for all our patients when it is clinically indicated (Vassilopoulou-Sellin et al, 1995).

Other Multidisciplinary Care

Audiologic and ophthalmologic follow-up is necessary in many children with brain tumors. Cranial irradiation and some chemotherapeutic agents (primarily cisplatin) can lead to hearing loss. Changes in vision or visual fields can be the first sign of growth of a centrally located tumor, especially in the optic pathway. Speech therapy and ongoing evaluation may be needed for children with cranial nerve deficits caused by tumors near the brainstem or for those who have cerebellar mutism. Finally, occupational therapy and physical therapy may be needed during the postoperative period and later. Some neurologic deficits, such as spastic hemiparesis, evolve over time and can improve with ongoing occupational and physical therapy. All these services are available for children at M. D. Anderson and can be coordinated with follow-up visits in the pediatric neuro-oncology clinic.

KEY PRACTICE POINTS

- Pediatric brain tumors have a diverse array of symptoms and signs at presentation.

- The diagnosis of neurofibromatosis is important when present in children with brain tumors because this genetic disease may affect prognosis and treatment.

- To ensure good neurologic status and long-term outcome, it is critical to remove the child's brain tumor as completely as possible without causing injury. When possible, for optimal outcome, neurosurgery for pediatric brain tumors should be performed at a major center with state-of-the-art operating-room equipment by a neurosurgeon skilled in removal of brain tumors.

- New radiotherapy techniques can improve the quality and duration of survival for children with brain tumors.

> • Children with CNS tumors have unique supportive-care needs that
> should be attended to by a multidisciplinary team familiar with the
> specific needs of these patients.

SUGGESTED READINGS

Ater JL, Rytting M. Rare malignant brain tumors. In: Black P, Loeffler JS, eds. *Cancers of the Nervous System*. Cambridge, MA: Blackwell Science, Inc; 1997a:1196–2222.

Ater JL, van Eys J, Woo SY, Moore B III, Copeland DR, Bruner J. MOPP chemotherapy without irradiation as primary postsurgical therapy for brain tumors in infants and young children. *J Neurooncol* 1997b;32:243–252.

Butler RW, Copeland DR. Attentional processes and their remediation in children treated for cancer: a literature review and the development of a therapeutic approach. *Journal of the International Neuropsychological Society* 2002;8:115–124.

Chang EL, Allen P, Wu C, Ater J, Kuttesch J, Maor MH. Acute toxicity and treatment interruption related to electron and photon craniospinal irradiation in pediatric patients treated at The University of Texas M. D. Anderson Cancer Center. *Int J Radiat Oncol Biol Phys* 2002;52:1008–1016.

Copeland DR, deMoor C, Moore BD, Ater JL. Neurocognitive development of children after a cerebellar tumor in infancy. *J Clin Oncol* 1999;17:3476–3486.

DeWinter AE, Moore BD III, Slopis JM, Ater JL, Copeland DR. Brain tumors in children with neurofibromatosis: additional neuropsychological morbidity? *Neurooncol* 1999;1:275–281.

Epstein F, McCleary EL. Intrinsic brain-stem tumors of childhood: surgical indications. *J Neurosurg* 1986;64:11–15.

Gurney JC, Smith MA, Bunin GR. In: Reis LAG, Smith MA, Gurney JC, et al, eds. *Cancer Survival and Incidence Among Children and Adolescents: United States SEER Program 1975–1995*. Bethesda, MD: National Cancer Institute SEER Program. NIH publication No. 99–4649; 1999:51–63.

Janss AJ, Grundy R, Cnaan A, et al. Optic pathway and hypothalamic/chiasmatic gliomas in children younger than age 5 years with a 6-year follow-up. *Cancer* 1995;75:1051–1059.

Kuttesch JF, Ater JL. Brain tumors in childhood. In: Behrman RE, Kliegman RM, Jenson HB, eds. *Nelson Textbook of Pediatrics*. Philadelphia, PA:WB Saunders; 2004:1702–1709.

Moore BD, Ater JL, Copeland DR. Improved neuropsychological outcome in children with brain tumors diagnosed during infancy and treated without cranial irradiation. *J Child Neurol* 1992;7:211–219.

Moore BD, Ater JL, Needle MN, Slopis J, Copeland DR. Neuropsychological profile of children with neurofibromatosis, brain tumor, or both. *J Child Neurol* 1994;9:368–377.

Moore BD, Slopis JM, Schomer D, Jackson E, Levy B. Neuropsychological significance of areas of high signal intensity on brain MRI in children with neurofibromatosis. *Neurology* 1996;46:1660–1668.

North KN, Riccardi V, Samango-Sprouse C, et al. Cognitive function and academic performance in Neurofibromatosis 1: consensus statement from the NF1 Cognitive Disorders Task Force. *Neurology* 1997;48:1121–1127.

Radcliffe J, Packer RJ, Atkins TE, et al. Three- and four-year cognitive outcome in children with non-cortical brain tumors treated with whole-brain radiotherapy. *Ann Neurol* 1992;32:551–554.

Vassilopoulou-Sellin R, Klein MJ, Moore III BD, Ried HL, et al. Efficacy of growth hormone replacement therapy in children with organic growth hormone deficiency due to intracranial tumors after irradiation. *Horm Res* 1995;43:188–193.

Wisoff JH, Boyett JM, Berger MS, et al. Current neurosurgical management and the impact of extent of resection in the treatment of malignant gliomas of childhood. A report of the Children's Cancer Group trial CCG-945. *J Neurosurg* 1998;89: 52–59.

4   Brain Tumors: Chemotherapy and Investigational Therapy

Joann L. Ater, Jeffrey S. Weinberg, Moshe H. Maor,
and Demetrios Petropoulos

CHAPTER OVERVIEW

This chapter covers the methods used in staging and treating the most common types of childhood brain tumors, with emphasis on the chemotherapy-radiotherapy programs and clinical trials of the Division of Pediatrics at M. D. Anderson Cancer Center. For tumor types such as medulloblastoma, in which the choice of chemotherapy and radiotherapy is interactive or concurrent, the radiation dose and timing are also discussed. The use of chemotherapy regimens to reduce or delay irradiation in young children is also addressed.

INTRODUCTION

The term "glioma" is used to refer collectively to all primary tumors of the brain and spinal cord or the central nervous system (CNS). Of more than 100 histologic subtypes of gliomas classified by the World Health Organization (WHO), 5 constitute 70% to 80% of all pediatric brain neoplasms: juvenile pilocytic astrocytoma, medulloblastoma and other primitive neuroectodermal tumors (PNETs), diffuse astrocytoma, glioblastoma multiforme, and ependymoma. This chapter discusses the approaches used in the treatment of these tumors and in the treatment of primary CNS germ-cell tumors.

LOW-GRADE ASTROCYTOMAS

Low-grade astrocytomas (LGAs) are the most common gliomas in children, accounting for 36% to 40% of childhood brain tumors. About 720 new cases of LGA are diagnosed each year in the United States. The WHO classifies these tumors as grades I or II. This group of tumors comprises a heterogeneous assortment of histologic subtypes that are located in multiple areas of the CNS and that have unique resectability, morbidity, and biologic behaviors.

WHO grade I LGAs include juvenile pilocytic astrocytoma, pleomorphic xanthoastrocytoma, and subependymal giant-cell astrocytoma. These tumors are well circumscribed, and malignant transformation is rare. WHO grade II LGAs include fibrillary, protoplasmic, gemistocytic, and mixed astrocytomas. Other WHO grade I/II gliomas—including infantile desmoplastic astrocytoma, infantile desmoplastic ganglioglioma, and oligodendroglioma—are rare in children but when found are treated similarly to LGAs.

The most common site of origin of LGAs is the cerebellum: 35% of astrocytomas, which are primarily juvenile pilocytic astrocytomas, arise in the cerebellum. Other common sites of origin are the cerebral hemisphere, hypothalamus, optic nerve/chiasm, brainstem, and spinal cord.

The goals of treatment for LGAs include improved survival, restoration of physical function, eradication of tumor, and preservation of cognition. Surgery alone can provide benefit in all of these areas if the tumor is accessible. When less than 1.5 cc of residual tumor volume remain after surgical resection, the 5-year progression-free survival (PFS) rate is greater than 90% for patients with a cerebellar or cerebral hemisphere LGA. For patients with an LGA in the brainstem or hypothalamic region, the 5-year PFS rate is approximately 50% with surgery. Therefore, adjuvant therapy is typically not offered to patients who receive gross total resection, but the patients are followed with neurologic examinations and magnetic resonance imaging (MRI) scans. Resection can also be considered for treatment of tumor recurrence, but only if surgery can be accomplished without risk of serious neurologic impairment; otherwise, alternative therapies must be considered.

For patients with residual tumor after surgery, the 5-year PFS rate is considerably lower than it is for patients without residual tumor. For patients with residual LGA in the cerebellum, cerebrum, optic pathway, and brainstem, the 5-year PFS rates are 40%, 30%, 75%, and 50%, respectively. For patients with residual tumor in the hypothalamic region, the PFS rate is lower, and the median time to progression is about 1 year. Therefore, for some patients with considerable amounts of LGA remaining after surgery, we recommend either postoperative radiotherapy or chemotherapy (Packer et al, 1993; Packer et al, 1997; Ater et al, 2002).

The most problematic LGAs are those that arise in the hypothalamic and optic nerve/chiasm regions (Ater et al, 2002). Gliomas occurring in this region are usually juvenile pilocytic astrocytomas. Because of the tumor location, surgery or radiotherapy can cause considerable morbidity. Without treatment, the tumor can cause long-term problems, including visual loss, emaciation or obesity, memory loss, hypopituitarism, and behavioral problems. The types of behavioral problems seen in children with midline brain tumors include rage attack, dysinhibition, tics, compulsivity, depression, and somnolence, all of which can be treated with appropriate medications, usually with required supervision of a psychiatrist, neurologist, or both. With panhypopituitarism, the most common problems are vasopressin-dependent diabetes insipidus; growth-hormone deficiency; and thyroid stimulating–hormone deficiency, which can lead to hypothyroidism.

Radiotherapy

The patient's age and the areas of the brain that require irradiation are the primary factors considered in determining the type of radiotherapy to be given. For example, a very small LGA in the brainstem of a very young child can be treated with stereotactic or focal radiotherapy with only a low risk of long-term complications. On the other hand, radiotherapy to a large hypothalamic or optic pathway glioma could lead to long-term vascular, endocrine, and intellectual problems in a very young child. See Chapter 3, "Brain Tumors: Diagnosis, Surgery and Radiotherapy, and

Table 4–1.   Results of Chemotherapy Trials for Progressive Low-grade Glioma

Chemotherapy	Reference	No. Pts	Mean Age (years)	NF (%)	OR (%)	Median TTP (months)	PD @ 12 wks (%)
Dactinomycin/VCR	Janss et al, 1995	29	3	20	7	27	3
VP-16/VCR	Pons et al, 1992	20		15	5	27	25
Cyclophosphamide	Kadota et al, 1999	15	3	33	7	NE	34
TPDCV	Prados et al, 1997	42	5	14	36	33	4.6
Carboplatin/VCR	Packer et al, 1997	78	3	19	33	44	6.6

Abbreviations: NE, not evaluated; NF, neurofibromatosis type 1; No. number; OR, odds ratio; PD, progressive disease; Pts, patients; TPDCV, thioguanine, procarbazine, dibromodulcitol (mitolactol), cyclohexylchloroethylnitrosourea, vincristine; TTP, time to progression; VCR, vincristine; VP-16, etoposide; wks, weeks.

Supportive Care," for a complete discussion of radiotherapy as treatment for brain tumors in pediatric patients.

Chemotherapy

For children younger than 10 years of age who have large hypothalamic or optic nerve/chiasmal LGAs, we usually recommend chemotherapy as first-line treatment. Two chemotherapy regimens have been reported to have activity against LGAs: cisplatin plus vincristine (Packer et al, 1993; Packer et al, 1997) and cyclohexylchloroethylnitrosourea (CCNU)-based regimens (Prados et al, 1997). M. D. Anderson is currently participating in the Children's Cancer Group (CCG) A9952 clinical trial, which is comparing these 2 regimens. The activities of 5 regimens investigated in phase II trials are reported in Table 4–1. Temozolomide and vinblastine are currently being investigated for their activity against recurrent LGA.

MEDULLOBLASTOMA AND OTHER
EMBRYONAL TUMORS

Embryonal tumors are the most common malignant CNS tumors in children, accounting for 20% to 25% of all pediatric CNS tumors. This group includes medulloblastomas, supratentorial PNETs, pineoblastomas, ependymoblastomas, medulloepitheliomas, and atypical teratoid/rhabdoid tumors. These tumors are histologically classified as WHO grade IV and have the potential to metastasize to the neuroaxis, with craniospinal fluid (CSF) seeding occurring in up to 30% to 40% of patients.

Medulloblastoma is the most common malignant CNS tumor in children, accounting for 20% to 25% of all brain tumors diagnosed in children younger than 15 years of age. Medulloblastomas can occur in adults, although less commonly. Because medulloblastoma is a cerebellar tumor, affected children usually present with symptoms of increased intracranial pressure, including acute onset of headaches, vomiting, diplopia, and occasional visual loss due to hydrocephalus, which is caused by obstruction of the fourth ventricle. Ataxia, dysmetria, and cranial nerve deficits can also be caused by the tumor's location in the cerebellum and because of pressure on or invasion of the brainstem. Patients with supratentorial PNETs present with symptoms of intracranial pressure or neurologic deficits related to the tumor's location within the cerebral hemisphere.

Preoperative Evaluation and Staging

Therapy for medulloblastoma, supratentorial PNET, and other embryonal tumors is determined on the basis of whether the patient is at average or high risk for recurrence. Average risk is defined as age older than 3 years and a diagnosis of medulloblastoma with no evidence of leptomeningeal involvement, less than 1.5 cc of residual tumor after surgery, and negative CSF cytology. High risk is defined as the presence of any of the following characteristics: 1.5 cc or more residual tumor after surgery, intracranial or spinal leptomeningeal disease, positive CSF cytology, or systemic metastasis. The prognoses for patients with other rare embryonal tumors (listed above) are poor, even without metastases; therefore, patients with these tumors are considered to be at high risk.

By the time of diagnosis, medulloblastoma has metastasized to the bone and bone marrow in about 1% of patients. Bone marrow evaluations are warranted only in patients at high risk who have extensive disease. A bone scan is necessary only if the patient is experiencing pain. Athough computed tomography (CT) is a useful detection tool, an enhanced MRI scan taken preoperatively is preferable because MRI can better define the characteristics of the tumor and the intra- and extracranial extent of disease. Also, if medulloblastoma is highly suspected, an MRI scan with contrast of the entire spine is helpful in determining whether spinal leptomeningeal tumor is present. A comparison of the preoperative and postoperative (obtained within 48 hours of surgery) MRI scans of the brain is necessary for determining the amount of residual tumor or the extent of surgical resection. An MRI scan of the spine done preoperatively, if the patient is stable, is helpful because postoperative evaluation of leptomeningeal disease can be obscured by blood resulting from the surgery. Thus, if not done preoperatively, an MRI scan of the spine should be delayed until 10 days after surgery.

Neurosurgery

For a posterior fossa tumor, surgical resection is the most important initial therapy to relieve hydrocephalus, pathologically confirm the diagnosis, and improve survival. Although extent of resection is an important prognostic factor and gross total resection is desirable, pursuing small amounts of tumor into the brainstem is not recommended. Overly aggressive surgery can cause long-term brainstem injury and mutism without improving survival.

Only about 30% of children with medulloblastoma are likely to require a permanent ventriculoperitoneal shunt. Therefore, an external ventricular drain is initially used to relieve hydrocephalus until normal CSF circulation is reestablished. Ventriculoperitoneal shunts are placed only in children who cannot be weaned from the ventricular drain or who develop delayed hydrocephalus after the drain is removed.

During the postoperative period, appropriate supportive care and rehabilitation are also needed. Ten to twenty percent of children with posterior fossa tumors develop transient mutism after surgery, with subsequent risk for persistent speech problems. Ataxia may initially be severe and may put the patient at risk for falls. Therefore, physical, occupational, and speech therapy should be incorporated into the multidisciplinary care of these children. Criteria for discharge after surgery include neurologic stability, adequate oral intake, and training to prepare the family to provide safe transfer and ambulation in the home.

Treatment of Average-Risk Medulloblastoma

After surgery, radiotherapy usually begins within 1 month; the risk for tumor recurrence increases with delay. Adequate information from the European and United States Children's Oncology Group (COG) trials indicate that, in patients whose tumors are carefully staged and who do not have residual tumor or metastasis, 24 Gy of craniospinal radiotherapy (CSRT) with 55 Gy to the posterior fossa followed by chemotherapy can result in 5-year survival rates of 70% to 80% (Ater and Bleyer, 2002b). This lower dose of CSRT with chemotherapy has been recommended because some of the long-term problems that have been noted in children with medulloblastoma are related to the CSRT dose. Higher-dose CSRT (35 Gy) was previously considered standard therapy for patients with average-risk medulloblastoma, and this dose yielded 5-year survival rates of about 70% in most trials. This higher-dose treatment is now usually reserved for patients older than 18 years of age for whom the risk for dose-related intellectual deterioration, growth problems, scoliosis, and endocrine deficits is less likely.

The most effective standard chemotherapy regimen for patients with average- and high-risk medulloblastoma is CCNU, vincristine, and cisplatin given for 6 to 8 cycles after completion of radiotherapy and weekly vincristine during radiotherapy. This regimen was originally reported by Packer et al (1994) and has also been compared with cisplatin, vincristine, and cyclophosphamide in a large COG randomized clinical trial. In that study, this regimen had superior results. At this point in treatment, if no phase III investigational study is open, the CCNU, vincristine, and cisplatin regimen is usually recommended; however, because we continue to strive to improve the outcome of these children with respect to both eradicating the tumor and lessening neurologic and intellectual deficits, we recommend participation in phase III studies.

The survival rate among children with medulloblastoma is now high enough that large clinical trials conducted by cooperative groups such as the COG are needed to further improve therapy. We strongly encourage newly diagnosed patients to participate in these trials. For a review of randomized clinical trials of medulloblastoma, see the report by Ater and Bleyer (2002b).

Treatment of High-Risk Medulloblastoma and PNET

More-aggressive therapy is required to achieve high rates of survival in children with high-risk embryonal tumors compared with children with average-risk medulloblastoma. The best results reported for patients with high-risk medulloblastoma or PNET are from Packer et al (1994), who treated patients with CCNU, vincristine, and cisplatin following 35-Gy CSRT and a total of 55 Gy to the posterior fossa. Vincristine was also given weekly during the radiotherapy. Chemotherapy was administered in 6 to 8 cycles at 6-week intervals. With this regimen, the 5-year event-free survival (EFS) rate was 85% for all patients and 63% for patients with leptomeningeal disease. Previous studies investigating the use of chemotherapy before radiotherapy, although theoretically appealing, have not yielded such good results (Prados et al, 1996). Therefore, unless a child is too debilitated to tolerate CSRT, we no longer recommend chemotherapy before radiotherapy for patients with a high-risk status. If the child qualifies for a phase II or III COG protocol for newly diagnosed, high-risk disease, we usually recommend participation so that answers might be provided to clinical questions through research that requires a large sample. For example, we are currently working with the COG to evaluate the role of concurrent carboplatin and radiotherapy followed by chemotherapy in patients at high risk. Standard therapy is offered as a nonprotocol alternative for patients who do not meet the eligibility criteria of the protocol.

Treatment of Young Children with Embryonal Brain Tumors

Treatment of young children with embryonal tumors is particularly difficult because of the risk for increased radiotherapy-related morbidity for this age group, particularly those younger than 3 years of age at diagnosis. With CSRT, young children are at high risk for short stature, decline in intellect, scoliosis and spinal deformity, endocrine deficits, and microcephaly. Also, in the past, standard radiotherapy resulted in only a 20% survival rate in children younger than 3 years. Therefore, in the mid-1970s, the Division of Pediatrics at M. D. Anderson began recommending surgery followed by chemotherapy upon diagnosis, with radiotherapy reserved for patients with tumor progression. The chemotherapy regimens that have been used are nitrogen mustard, vincristine, procarbazine, and prednisone (MOPP) (Ater et al, 1997); methotrexate, nitrogen mustard, vincristine, and procarbazine (MMOP); and more recently, the regimen investigated in COG protocols for infants. In addition, for young children whose tumors have a good initial response to induction chemotherapy (MMOP; ifosfamide, carboplatin, and etoposide [ICE]; or cyclophosphamide, vincristine, cisplatin, and etoposide), we more recently investigated the use of high-dose chemotherapy and stem cell rescue.

High-Grade Gliomas

The high-grade glioma category of brain tumors includes anaplastic astrocytoma, high-grade mixed glioma, anaplastic oligodendroglioma, high-grade glioma not otherwise specified, and glioblastoma multiforme. High-grade (malignant) gliomas are much less common in children and adolescents than in adults. Among pediatric patients, anaplastic astrocytoma (WHO grade III) is more common than glioblastoma multiforme (WHO grade IV). High-grade gliomas can occur in any location in the CNS, but occur most commonly in the cerebral hemispheres and brainstem. Fewer than 10% of gliomas that arise in or involve the optic pathway, hypothalamus, and cerebellum are high grade. Therefore, most studies that have addressed treatment of high-grade gliomas have focused primarily on either supratentorial tumors or brainstem gliomas (Ater and Bleyer, 2002a). Supratentorial high-grade gliomas account for only 10% of brain tumors treated in patients younger than 21 years of age, and intrinsic pontine gliomas make up another 8% to 10% of all pediatric brain tumors.

Surgery
The first mode of treatment in patients with high-grade glioma is surgery. Surgery is performed to confirm the diagnosis; relieve symptoms of increased intracranial pressure; and whenever possible, provide specific antitumor therapeutic benefit by decreasing the tumor burden. Although no prospective trial has assessed how extensive the resection needs to be to benefit pediatric patients with high-grade glioma, evidence from the CCG indicates that surgical removal of more than 90% of the tumor improves outcome (Wisoff et al, 1998). This group reported a significantly better 5-year PFS rate for children who have more than 90% of tumor resected compared with children who have less than 90% of tumor resected for both anaplastic astrocytoma (44% versus 22%, respectively; $P = 0.05$) and glioblastoma multiforme (26% versus 4%, respectively; $P = 0.046$) (Wisoff et al, 1998). Nonetheless, the CCG trial did not ascertain whether this benefit is a result of tumor biology and invasiveness or evidence that more aggressive tumor removal will improve survival. These findings also have been supported by studies at M. D. Anderson where the extent of resection was

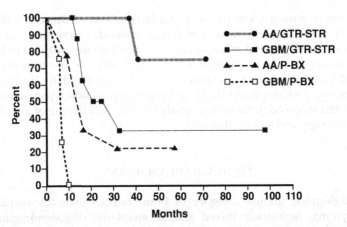

Figure 4–1. Progression-free survival rate related to extent of tumor resection. All patients were treated with radiotherapy and a chemotherapy regimen of thioguanine, procarbazine, cyclohexylchloroethylnitrosourea, and hydroxyurea at M. D. Anderson. Abbreviations: AA, anaplastic astrocytoma: GBM, glioblastoma multiforme; GTR-STR, gross total resection and subtotal resection; P-BX, partial resection or biopsy.

found to be associated with improved survival in patients who received surgery, radiotherapy, and chemotherapy (see Figure 4–1).

For diffuse brainstem glioma, surgery is not a useful treatment modality. Eighty-five to ninety percent of tumors that arise in the brainstem are diffuse intrinsic pontine anaplastic astrocytoma or glioblastoma multiforme, and 10% to 15% are focal LGA. Recognition of relatively favorable focal low-grade tumors is essential because of their comparatively indolent course and the fact that they should be managed in a distinctly different way from high-grade tumors, with surgery, observation, and radiotherapy or chemotherapy for progression typically resulting in a good outcome. Focal brainstem gliomas are now excluded from our clinical trials on intrinsic brainstem tumors. The diagnosis of intrinsic pontine glioma is made on the basis of MRI criteria, and patients with this tumor have a very poor prognosis. Biopsy and surgery are usually of no benefit (Epstein and McCleary, 1986); the risk seems to outweigh the benefit of an attempted resection. Current standard therapy for diffuse pontine glioma is radiotherapy. At M. D. Anderson, we favor the use of chemotherapy or other radiosensitizers during radiotherapy to increase its efficacy. We have previously investigated the use of oral etoposide (Kuttesch et al, 1999) and topotecan (Sanghavi et al, 2003) in combined chemotherapy-radiotherapy regimens. Currently, we are investigating the use of cyclooxygenase-2 inhibitors with radiotherapy as a way to increase the effectiveness of radiotherapy.

In summary, from the partial evidence we now have, it appears that high-grade gliomas should be completely resected when it can be done without inflicting life-threatening neurologic deficit. The CCG trial indicates that complete resection of high-grade gliomas can improve survival, especially when combined with other treatment. The one exception is diffuse pontine glioma. The diagnosis of this tumor type rarely needs to be established with tissue confirmation; the resection does not provide evidence-based benefit nor is it sufficiently safe.

Chemotherapy

The role of chemotherapy has been the subject of most cooperative group studies of high-grade glioma in children throughout the world. European groups, the CCG, and the Pediatric Oncology Group (POG) have all focused on this issue. The results of randomized clinical trials on the use of chemotherapy in treating supratentorial high-grade glioma in children are difficult to interpret because of small samples, changing neuropathologic classification systems, and discrepancies in the diagnoses of different neuropathology reviewers. The results of several studies assessing different regimens are shown in Table 4–2.

The efficacy of chemotherapy has been tested in patients with recurrent tumors and in phase II preirradiation window studies performed by the POG, CCG, and other groups worldwide. The POG and CCG trials have been completed but have not yet been reported in the literature. It is hopeful that they will provide further evidence as to which chemotherapy regimen is best for treating high-grade glioma. However, studies of adults with high-grade glioma have shown that response rate alone is adequate for choosing the best chemotherapy regimen. Therefore, the common approach is to evaluate both tumor response and time to progression. The general opinion is that while some agents provide a rapid response rate, the response is so short lived that it is not appreciably beneficial. Other agents may produce a slower response but one that is longer lasting and, consequently, more beneficial to the patient. The North American Brain Tumor Consortium is now evaluating chemotherapy trials of high-grade glioma in adults by using statistical methods that evaluate both response and time to progression.

At M. D. Anderson, our approach to treating children with high-grade glioma has focused on using the most extensive surgical removal of the tumor possible, followed by involved-field radiotherapy for all but the youngest children (younger than 3 years of age). For chemotherapy protocols, we have investigated regimens that used CCNU-based combinations (Levin et al, 2000; Eisenstat et al, in press) and pairs of chemotherapy agents given before radiotherapy. Currently, our therapeutic strategy includes administering radiotherapy either alone or with temozolomide followed by temozolomide combined with other promising agents, such as cis-retinoic acid, thalidomide, cyclooxygenase-2 inhibitors, or tamoxifen for glioblastoma multiforme. Because of dosing restraints for very young children, the combination therapy is reserved for children older than 10 years of age. Temozolomide given during radiotherapy and then monthly

Table 4-2. Results of Chemotherapy Trials for High-Grade Glioma

Treatment	Dates	No. Pts	Study No.	EFS Reg1	EFS Reg2	5-yr EFS	Refs
CVP + RT vs. RT	1976–1981	58	CCG-943	CVP* + RT 45%	RT 13%		Sposto et al, 1989
8-in-1 + RT vs. CVP+RT	1985–1990	172	CCG-945	8-in-1 33%	CVP 36%	AA 28% GBM 16%	Finlay et al, 1995
TPDCV + RT	1984–1992	42	UCSF	36%		AA 42% GBM 24%	Levin et al, 2000
TPCH + RT	1990–2000	28	MDACC	36% OS = 50%		AA 45% GBM 25%	Eisenstat et al (in press)

Abbreviations: 8-in-1, 8 drugs (cisplatin, cyclohexylchloroethylnitrosourea, vincristine, cytarabine, cyclophosphamide, etoposide, dexamethasone, mannitol) given in 1 day; AA, anaplastic astrocytoma; CCG, Children's Cancer Group; CVP, cyclohexylchloroethylnitrosourea, vincristine, prednisone; EFS, event-free survival; GBM, glioblastoma multiforme; MDACC, M. D. Anderson; No., number; Pts, patients; Refs, references; Reg, regimen; RT, radiotherapy; TPCH, thioguanine, procarbazine, cyclohexylchloroethylnitrosourea, hydroxyurea; TPDCV, thioguanine, procarbazine, dibromodulcitol (mitolactol), cyclohexylchloroethylnitrosourea, vincristine; OS, overall survival; UCSF, University of California at San Francisco; yr, year.

Table 4–3. Treatment of Ependymoma

Staging Category	1ˢᵗ Surgery	Chemotherapy	2ⁿᵈ Surgery	Conformal Radiotherapy
Supratentorial				
Total resection				
• Anaplastic	X			X
• Nonanaplastic	X			
Partial resection	X	X	X	X
Infratentorial				
Total resection	X			X
Partial resection	X	X	X	X

thereafter is often recommended for children with anaplastic astrocytoma and children younger than 10 years of age who have glioblastoma multiforme.

EPENDYMOMA

The most important prognostic factors for a child with ependymoma are extent of surgical resection, age (less favorable for children younger than 4 years of age), and treatment with radiotherapy (Chiu et al, 1992; Horn et al, 1999). Staging, such as that for medulloblastoma, should be performed before treatment initiation. Appropriate therapy is determined on the basis of tumor staging, primary tumor location, and amount of residual tumor. For children with posterior fossa and anaplastic supratentorial tumors of average risk (that is, the patient has negative CSF cytology, no evidence of metastases on an MRI scan of the brain and spine, and no macroscopic residual tumor), involved-field radiotherapy is recommended.

We have a new protocol that involves using surgery alone with close follow-up to treat completely resected nonanaplastic supratentorial ependymoma. This approach is based on a very small series from New York University that had good results with surgery alone in this patient group (Hukin et al, 1998). Complete resection with observation is still not considered the standard of care for ependymoma, so it is recommended that children who fit the eligibility criteria be enrolled in our protocol (see Table 4–3).

Chemotherapy is given only for children who have residual ependymoma after surgery or whose tumor has recurred. New evidence suggests that children with ependymoma who have residual tumor after surgery benefit from pre-radiotherapy chemotherapy. In a recent study by the CCG, children between the ages of 3 and 21 years of age who have residual ependymoma after surgery received 4 cycles of cisplatin, etoposide, cyclophosphamide, and vincristine before receiving involved-field radiotherapy. Of 33 evaluable patients receiving chemotherapy before receiving radiotherapy, 42% had a complete response, 18% had a partial response, 24% had a minor response/stable disease, and 15% had progressive disease. The 3-year EFS rate was 54%, which did not differ much from that of a group of children who did not have residual tumor and who were treated with radiotherapy without chemotherapy (Garvin et al, 2003). The children whose tumors responded to chemotherapy fared better than those whose tumors did not, with a 3-year EFS rate of 100% for patients with a complete response, 75% for a partial response, and less than 44% for a minor response/stable disease (Garvin et al, 2003).

Our new ependymoma protocol tests the hypothesis that, in patients with residual tumor, chemotherapy can make a second operation more feasible and facilitate subsequent tumor removal if the tumor does not respond completely to the chemotherapy. After the second procedure, children then receive involved-field radiotherapy.

Recurrent ependymomas can respond to other chemotherapeutic agents, including cisplatin, cyclophosphamide, and etoposide; ICE; CCNU combinations; and other regimens. After response is noted radiographically, a second resection can be attempted to provide palliation and prolong survival duration. At M. D. Anderson, we have some long-term (more than 5 years) survivors of recurrent ependymoma who received salvage therapy that included complete surgical resection.

Despite the evidence that ependymomas can respond to chemotherapy, no randomized clinical trial has shown a benefit with adjuvant chemotherapy for completely resected nonmetastatic ependymoma. Part of the problem is that to prove the efficacy of adjuvant chemotherapy, a large randomized clinical trial is needed. Even in cooperative groups, such a trial may not be feasible because of the rarity of this tumor. Therefore, our new protocol investigates the use of involved-field radiotherapy without chemotherapy for treating completely resected ependymomas. An outline of current ependymoma regimens is provided in Table 4–3.

CNS GERM-CELL TUMORS

Germ-cell tumors of the CNS are a heterogeneous group of tumors that occur primarily in children and arise predominantly in midline structures of the pineal gland and suprasellar regions. These tumors can disseminate along the CSF pathway. Germ-cell tumors of the CNS account for 1% to 2% of all pediatric brain tumors, and the peak incidence occurs in children between the ages of 10 and 12 years old. Overall, there is a male preponderance; however, there is a female preponderance for suprasellar tumors. Germ-cell tumors occur multifocally in 5% to 10% of cases, and they are much more prevalent in Asian populations than in European populations.

With regard to therapy, primary CNS germ-cell tumors are typically divided into 2 groups: the germinoma type and the nongerminomatous type (e.g., mixed germ-cell tumors, embryonal carcinoma, choriocarcinoma).

The nongerminomatous germ-cell tumors are also called secreting germ-cell tumors because most of them produce beta-human chorionic gonadotrophin, alpha-fetoprotein, or a combination of these. As with peripheral germ-cell tumors, analysis of these protein markers may be useful in establishing the diagnosis, monitoring treatment response, and monitoring post-therapy status. Surgical biopsy is recommended to establish the diagnosis of nongerminomatous germ-cell tumor, but diagnosis may be determined on the basis of the elevation of these proteins in CSF or serum. Distinguishing between germinomas and nongerminomatous tumors is important because germinomas have a much more favorable prognosis (greater than 90% 5-year survival rate) than nongerminomatous germ-cell tumors (40% to 70% 5-year survival rate); the latter requires more aggressive therapy (Diaz et al, 1999).

Treatment of Germinoma

The survival rate among patients with pure germinoma exceeds 90%. Post-surgical treatment of pure germinomas is somewhat controversial with regard to the relative roles of chemotherapy and radiotherapy. Excellent outcomes are reported in patients who have received local-field radiotherapy doses greater than 40 Gy and CSRT (see Chapter 3). Similarly, groups have reported excellent outcomes when chemotherapy has been incorporated into regimens that use reduced doses of radiotherapy (24 Gy to the local field alone). Over the past 12 years at M. D. Anderson, our treatment protocol for patients with germinomas has been carboplatin or cisplatin and etoposide for 2 to 4 cycles followed by ventricular or involved-field radiotherapy, and the survival rates have exceeded 90%. The dose of radiation is determined by tumor response to chemotherapy; lower-dose radiotherapy is given when there is a complete response to chemotherapy. In the future, we will be participating in a national study that will randomize patients to full-dose radiotherapy and chemotherapy followed by lower-dose radiotherapy. The goal of the study is to determine which regimen confers the best survival rate and the least toxicities.

Treatment of Nongerminomatous Germ-Cell Tumor

The therapeutic approach for nongerminomatous germ-cell tumors is more aggressive than that for germinomas, combining more intense chemotherapy regimens with CSRT. Five-year survival rates among patients with these tumors are markedly lower than those noted for patients with germinomas, ranging from 40% to 70%. At M. D. Anderson, we use an aggressive chemotherapy regimen that has been effective in treating systemic high-risk germ-cell tumors: cisplatin, vincristine, methotrexate, and bleomycin alternating with dactinomycin, cyclophosphamide, and vincristine and followed by CSRT (Kuttesch et al, 1996). In the near future, we will be evaluating the effect of carboplatin plus etoposide alternating with ifosfamide plus etoposide with radiotherapy. Future approaches may test the use of high-dose chemotherapy with dose-reduced radiotherapy (Diaz et al, 1999).

Recent trials have shown a benefit resulting from the use of high-dose chemotherapy with stem cell rescue. At M. D. Anderson, children with recurrent germ-cell tumors that are responsive to chemotherapy are eligible for our high-dose chemotherapy and stem-cell rescue protocol.

METASTATIC BRAIN TUMORS

In children, metastatic spread to the brain of nonbrain primary malignancies is uncommon. Childhood acute lymphoblastic leukemia and non-Hodgkin lymphoma can spread to the leptomeninges, causing symptoms of communicating hydrocephalus. Chloromas, or collections of myeloid leukemia cells, can occur throughout the neuroaxis. Rarely, brain parenchymal metastases from lymphoma, neuroblastoma, rhabdomyosarcoma, Ewing's sarcoma, and osteosarcoma occur. Therapeutic approaches are based on specific histologic diagnosis and may incorporate radiotherapy, intrathecal administration of chemotherapy, systemic administration of chemotherapy, or some combinations of these.

RECURRENT BRAIN TUMORS

As part of the M. D. Anderson Brain Tumor Center, the Division of Pediatrics participates in clinical trials aimed at improving treatment for current and future patients. As described above, treatment for a newly diagnosed brain tumor usually includes surgery and therapeutic protocols of radiotherapy combined with chemotherapy. When a brain tumor recurs, the child's chance for survival depends on several factors, including the pathology and location of the tumor, whether metastases are present, previous treatment, and the patient's clinical condition. Therefore, when a pediatric patient is referred to our center with recurrence of a brain tumor, we undertake a detailed reevaluation to determine the best treatment. We evaluate medical records to ascertain information about the previous treatment, such as type and dosage, response, and complications or toxicities. The MRI scans used to diagnose and confirm tumor progression are also reviewed. Occasionally, patients are referred to our center for tumor recurrence, and we find that the "recurrence" is actually radiation necrosis or an artifact of an MRI technique. If the MRI studies do not conclusively show recurrence, additional studies with dynamic MRI, magnetic resonance spectroscopy, and single-photon emission CT scans can help differentiate malignant tumors from postirradiation necrosis. For tumors that can disseminate with leptomeningeal spread, an MRI scan of the spine and lumbar puncture for CSF cytology may be required. Laboratory studies to evaluate organ toxicity from other therapies are also needed. A physical examination is important in determining current deficit and performance status. Finally, the pathology from the original diagnosis is reviewed to confirm or dispel the diagnosis of recurrent tumor.

For most patients, surgery is beneficial, even with tumor recurrence. Therefore, most children with recurrent tumors are initially evaluated for surgical resection of the tumor. If the tumor is still localized and can be resected, then surgery is usually part of the treatment. At times, chemotherapy is given before surgery to determine whether the tumor is sensitive to chemotherapy before its removal. The other focal treatment that may be considered is stereotactic radiotherapy or reirradiation. Reirradiation is usually an option only if the recurrence occurs more than 5 years after the previous radiotherapy. Stereotactic radiotherapy can be given only for small, localized tumors of certain types (such as ependymomas or LGAs) and is not considered for infiltrating high-grade gliomas. If a child has never received radiotherapy, surgery followed by radiotherapy may be the most appropriate treatment for tumor recurrence. For example, in our experience, radiotherapy can still be curative in the majority of children with recurrent LGAs after either surgery alone or surgery plus chemotherapy. Also, children younger than 3 years of age who are diagnosed with medulloblastoma and treated initially with chemotherapy without radiotherapy can be cured with salvage radiotherapy about 40% of the time (Ater et al, 1997).

If a child has already received radiotherapy and surgery is not feasible, the primary therapy for recurrent disease is usually chemotherapy, often with novel agents. The Division of Pediatrics at M. D. Anderson has an active New Agents Group that conducts phase I and II clinical trials for a variety of childhood tumors, including brain tumors. Therefore, for patients who are eligible for phase I or II protocols, these studies are carefully explained to parents and offered as therapy. These protocols generally consist of chemotherapy combinations, novel biologic therapies, or single new agents. Eligibility criteria for some protocols limits the number of previous chemotherapy regimens to 2. Therefore, new-agent studies are usually offered to patients with a first or second recurrence. Some of our most active agents (e.g., cisplatin, ifosfamide, and temozolomide) were initially evaluated in phase I and II studies such as these and were proven to be efficacious.

Treatment for children with recurrent or progressive embryonal tumors (i.e., medulloblastoma, PNET, atypical teratoid/rhabdoid tumor, pineoblastoma, ependymoblastoma, and CNS germ-cell tumors) usually involves either a new-agent or standard active combination chemotherapy, such as ICE, to determine whether the tumor is still chemotherapy sensitive. If the tumor responds to the chemotherapy, then the child may be a candidate for high-dose chemotherapy and stem cell rescue as potentially curative therapy. This aggressive approach is not appropriate for children who have tumors that are chemotherapy resistant.

For recurrent high-grade gliomas, we generally recommend a combination of surgery (when feasible) and chemotherapy with agents not previously used in the patient. For example, a child with recurrent glioblastoma previously treated with radiotherapy and a CCNU combination would be offered a combination of temozolomide, cis-retinoic acid, and celecoxib. We participate in protocols with our adult neuro-oncology group to test other temozolomide or irinotecan combinations.

Diffuse pontine glioma that progresses after radiotherapy is particularly difficult to treat; children with these tumors frequently have a poor performance status, intravenous chemotherapy is often poorly tolerated, and surgery is not feasible. Therefore, we generally recommend treatment with oral outpatient chemotherapy for palliation, unless a specific protocol for recurrent pontine glioma is available. If the family requests further therapy, the most commonly used nonprotocol regimens are temozolomide, low-dose oral etoposide, or CCNU-based combinations. At times, hospice care is more appropriate than further aggressive treatment, because these tumors often become rapidly fatal after progression. In that situation, our efforts in care are aimed at providing comfort for the child and support for the family.

With each recurrence, the possibility of surgery, alternative types of radiotherapy and chemotherapy, or other agents are considered. When the patient is not eligible for any study, recommendations for therapy are made on the basis of the child's previous treatment, performance status, and neurologic status as well as the patient's and the family's wishes. In children with a good performance status, commercially available chemotherapy regimens can control the tumor and prolong life.

ROLE OF HIGH-DOSE CHEMOTHERAPY AND AUTOLOGOUS STEM CELL RESCUE

Over the past 2 decades, high-dose chemotherapy with autologous stem cell rescue has been explored as a treatment option for patients with high-risk brain tumors (Dunkel and Finlay, 2002). The most encouraging outcomes have been reported for patients with embryonal tumors (medulloblastoma and cerebellar PNET) in a second complete or partial remission; germ-cell tumors that have recurred or progressed after initial treatment with chemotherapy, radiotherapy, or both; and miscellaneous tumors, such as atypical teratoid/rhabdoid tumor and anaplastic oligodendroganglioma.

With embryonal tumors, high-dose chemotherapy with autologous stem cell rescue is also recommended during the first remission if the patient has certain poor prognostic features such as presentation with metastases or incomplete tumor resection. It is also useful for children younger than 3 years old as a substitute for CSRT.

This approach has not been proven effective in other types of pediatric brain tumors, specifically ependymoma, brainstem glioma, and pineoblastoma. The usefulness of this approach for anaplastic astrocytoma, glioblastoma multiforme, and noncerebellar PNETs has not been defined. Patients treated with this approach appeared to develop substantial pulmonary, hepatic, and neurologic toxicities after the high-dose chemotherapy. Fortunately, children tend to tolerate this treatment better than adults.

The preparative regimen used in our department is tandem high-dose chemotherapy. Initially, patients receive intravenous cyclophosphamide at a dose of 7 g/m^2 followed 3 weeks later by intravenous triethylenethiophosphoramide (250 $mg/m^2/day$ for 3 days) and melphalan (60 $mg/m^2/day$ for 3 days). Both courses are supported with autologous stem cell rescue. We have found that leukopheresis can be successfully completed in most patients, even if the patient has received prior CSRT. On the other hand, previous exposure to nitrosourea and mechlorethamine has a considerable damaging effect on the stem cell pool and may limit the yield of stem cells.

COMPLICATIONS AND LONG-TERM CARE

Recent Surveillance, Epidemiology, and End Results data from the National Cancer Institute indicate that more than 70% of patients with childhood brain tumors will be long-term survivors. At least one half of these survivors will experience chronic problems as a direct result of their tumor, the treatment, or both. Potential problems include chronic neurologic deficits (e.g., focal motor and sensory abnormalities and seizure disorder), neurocognitive deficits (e.g., developmental delays and learning disabilities), and neuroendocrine deficiencies (e.g., hypothyroidism, growth failure, and delayed or absent puberty). Additionally, these patients are at considerable risk for secondary malignancies. The impact of these chronic complications on quality of life for these survivors of childhood brain tumors is only now being understood and appreciated. Therefore, at M. D. Anderson, we continue to perform interval evaluations on all children who have been diagnosed with a brain tumor to monitor for tumor recurrence and late effects of the tumor and its therapy.

KEY PRACTICE POINTS

- Chemotherapy is an effective treatment for obtaining response and control of incompletely resected progressive low-grade gliomas in children under 10 years old. Radiotherapy is an alternative treatment in older children.
- In medulloblastoma and cerebral PNET, regimens combining chemotherapy and radiotherapy have improved survival. In

average-risk patients, chemotherapy also lowers the long-term morbidity caused by radiation by allowing a lower radiation dose to the brain and spine.

· The combination of complete surgical resection, chemotherapy, and radiotherapy can improve survival for children with high-grade gliomas.

· Germ-cell tumors of the CNS are rare in children. When they occur, most types can be cured the majority of the time with radiotherapy and chemotherapy.

· Incompletely removed ependymomas can respond to pre-irradiation chemotherapy. This response to chemotherapy can facilitate more complete resection of the tumor at a second surgery or improve the outcome of radiotherapy.

Suggested Readings

Ater JL, Bleyer WA. Commentary on glioma during childhood. In: Pinkerton R, Philip T, Fervers B, eds. *Evidence Based Pediatric Oncology.* London, UK: BMJ Books; 2002a:171–188.

Ater JL, Bleyer WA. Commentary on medulloblastoma. In: Pinkerton R, Philip T, Fervers B, eds. *Evidence Based Pediatric Oncology.* London, UK: BMJ Books; 2002b:139–170.

Ater JL, Laws E, Bruner J, et al. Optic chiasmal/hypothalamic region tumors. In: Levin VA, ed. *Cancer in the Nervous System,* 2nd edition. New York, NY: Oxford University Press; 2002:158–170.

Ater JL, van Eys J, Woo SY, et al. MOPP chemotherapy without irradiation as primary postsurgical therapy for brain tumors in infants and young children. *J Neurooncol* 1997;32:243–252.

Chiu JK, Woo SY, Ater JL, et al. Intracranial ependymomas in children: analysis of prognostic factors. *J Neurooncol* 1992;13:283–290.

Diaz B, Balmadeda C, Matsutani M, et al. Germ cell tumors of the CNS in children: recent advances in therapy. *Childs Nerv Syst* 1999;15:578–585.

Dunkel IJ, Finlay JL. High-dose chemotherapy with autologous stem cell rescue for brain tumors. *Crit Rev Oncol Hematol* 2002;41:197–204.

Eisenstat DD, Kuttesch JF, Leeds N, et al. A phase II study of adjuvant 6-thioguanine, procarbazine, lomustine and hydroxyurea (TPCH) chemotherapy for high-grade gliomas in children and adolescents. *J Neurooncol.* In press.

Epstein F, McCleary EL. Intrinsic brain-stem tumors of childhood: surgical indications. *J Neurosurg* 1986;64:11–15.

Finlay JL, Boyett JM, Yates AJ, et al. Randomized phase III trial in childhood high-grade astrocytoma comparing vincristine, lomustine, and prednisone with the eight- drugs-in-1-day regimen. *J Clin Oncol* 1995;13:112–123.

Garvin J, Sposto R, Stanley I, et al. Childhood ependymomas: possible improved survival with the use of pre-radiation chemotherapy followed by radiotherapy. *Ann Neurol* 2003;54:109S.

Horn B, Heideman R, Geyer R, et al. A multi-institutional retrospective study of intracranial ependymoma in children: identification of risk factors. *J Pediatr Hematol Oncol* 1999;21:203–211.

Hukin J, Epstein F, Lefton D, et al. Treatment of intracranial ependymoma by surgery alone. *Pediatr Neurosurg* 1998;29:40–45.

Janss AJ, Grundy R, Cnaan A, et al. Optic pathway and hypothalamic/chiasmatic gliomas in children younger than age 5 years with a 6-year follow-up. *Cancer* 1995;75:1051–1059.

Kadota RP, Kun LE, Langston JW, et al. Cyclophosphamide for the treatment of progressive low-grade astrocytoma: a Pediatric Oncology Group phase II study. *J Pediatr Hematol Oncol* 1999;21:198–202.

Kuttesch JF, Ater JL, Lockhart S, et al. Activity of POMB/ACE in patients with mixed germ cell tumors of the CNS. Paper presented at the 7th International Symposium on Pediatric Neuro-Oncology; May 17, 1996; Washington, DC.

Kuttesch JF Jr, Foreman N, Ater JL, et al. Chemoradiotherapy for infiltrating pontine brain stem gliomas. *Med Pediatr Oncol* 1999;33:205.

Levin VA, Lamborn K, Wara W, et al. Phase II study of 6-thioguanine, procarbazine, dibromodulcitol, lomustine, and vincristine chemotherapy with radiotherapy for treating malignant glioma in children. *Neuro-oncol* 2000;2:22–28.

Packer RJ, Ater JL, Allen J, et al. Carboplatin and vincristine chemotherapy for children with newly-diagnosed progressive low-grade gliomas. *J Neurosurg* 1997;86:747–754.

Packer RJ, Lange B, Ater JL, et al. Carboplatin and vincristine for recurrent and newly diagnosed low-grade gliomas of childhood. *J Clin Oncol* 1993;11:850–856.

Packer RJ, Sutton LN, Elterman R, et al. Outcome of children with medulloblastoma treated with radiation, cisplatin, CCNU, and vincristine chemotherapy. *J Neurosurg* 1994;81:690–698.

Pons MA, Finlay JL, Walker RW, et al. Chemotherapy with vincristine and etoposide in children with low-grade astrocytoma. *J Neurooncol* 1992;14:151–158.

Prados MD, Edwards MS, Rabbitt J, et al. Treatment of pediatric low-grade gliomas with a nitrosourea-based multiagent chemotherapy regimen. *J Neurooncol* 1997;32:235–241.

Prados MD, Wara W, Edwards MSB, et al. Treatment of high-risk medulloblastoma and other primitive neuroectodermal tumors with reduced dose craniospinal radiotherapy and multi-agent nitrosourea-based chemotherapy. *Pediatr Neurosurg* 1996;25:174–181.

Sanghavi SN, Needle MN, Krailo MD, et al. A phase I study of topotecan as a radiosensitizer for brainstem glioma of childhood: first report of the Children's Cancer Group-0952. *Neuro-oncol* 2003;5:8–13.

Sposto R, Ertel IJ, Jenkin RDT, et al. The effectiveness of chemotherapy for treatment of high grade astrocytoma in children: results of a randomized trial. *J Neurooncol* 1989;7:165–177.

Wisoff JH, Boyett JM, Berger MS, et al. Current neurosurgical management and the impact of extent of resection in the treatment of malignant gliomas of childhood. A report of the Children's Cancer Group trial CCG-945. *J Neurosurg* 1998;89: 52–59.

5 WILMS' TUMOR

Norman Jaffe and Margaret G. Pearson

CHAPTER OVERVIEW

This chapter outlines the clinical manifestations, associated features, and methods used to investigate and establish a diagnosis of Wilms' tumor. Optimal therapy combines surgical extirpation of the tumor and chemotherapy. Occasionally, radiation therapy is also administered. Other conditions allied to or simulating Wilms' tumor are discussed. A follow-up schedule for use in evaluating patients successfully treated for Wilms' tumor is presented.

INTRODUCTION

Wilms' tumor is the most common malignant disease of the genitourinary tract in children, occurring in approximately 7.8 per 1 million children each year in the United States. Seventy-eight percent of the children are diagnosed between the ages of 1 and 5 years old, with a peak incidence at 3 to 4 years.

ETIOLOGY

The etiology of Wilms' tumor is unknown. Approximately 2% of tumors are possibly hereditary in origin. The disease may also arise in infants with congenital mesoblastic nephroma and persistent renal blastema-nephroblastomatosis complex, which is characterized by microscopic clusters of primitive renal epithelial cells with occasional tubular differentiation. If persistent renal blastema becomes massive and confluent, it is referred to as nephroblastomatosis. Extrarenal Wilms' tumor is a rare variant of classic Wilms' tumor and is located along the embryonic course of a metanephric blastema.

ASSOCIATED CONGENITAL ANOMALIES

In patients with Wilms' tumor, congenital anomalies may occur, including cryptorchidism, hypospadias, pseudohermaphroditism, duplications of the collecting system, hemihypertrophy, and aniridia. Wilms' tumor is also associated with several syndromes, such as neurofibromatosis and Beckwith-Wiedemann syndrome. Beckwith-Wiedemann syndrome is characterized by macroglossia and hyperplastic fetal visceromegaly involving the kidneys, adrenal cortex, pancreas, gonads, and liver. Hemihypertrophy may also be present. In addition to Wilms' tumor, children with Beckwith-Wiedemann syndrome are likely to develop neuroblastoma. WAGR syndrome is characterized by the presence of Wilms' tumor, aniridia, genitourinary malformation, and mental retardation. The features of Denys-Drash syndrome are male pseudohermaphroditism, early onset of renal failure, and an increased risk for Wilms' tumor.

Chromosomal anomalies associated with Wilms' tumor include trisomy 18, trisomy 8, 45,X Turner syndrome, pseudohermaphroditism, and deletion of chromosome 11. Chromosome 11p13 harbors the Wilms' tumor suppressor gene *WT1*, and chromosome 11p15 houses the putative Wilms' tumor gene *WT2*.

CLINICAL MANIFESTATIONS

Wilms' tumor is generally silent and is commonly detected as an abdominal mass during a well-baby clinic visit or by a parent while bathing or otherwise caring for the infant or child. The tumor lies deep in the flank and is frequently smooth and not tender. Palpation should be gentle and minimal to avoid rupturing the renal capsule and disseminating the disease. Pain is usually absent; however, when it occurs, it is often associated with hemorrhage in the tumor and, occasionally, hematuria. Unexplained fever, anorexia, and vomiting may occur, although rarely. Hypertension is present in approximately 25% of patients; the incidence of hematuria is similar. Wilms' tumor also occurs as bilateral disease in 3% to 5% of children, and it is occasionally reported in up to 10% of children.

INVESTIGATIONAL STUDIES

Any solid or semisolid mass within the abdomen should be regarded as malignant until proven otherwise. Once an intra-abdominal mass is detected, particularly in the flank, plain radiography of the abdomen should be performed. If the mass is suspected to be a Wilms' tumor or neuroblastoma (which is a more common intra-abdominal mass), ultrasonography and computed tomography (CT) of the abdomen with contrast should be considered for further delineation. Magnetic resonance imaging may be preferred over CT in some institutions. Also requested are chest radiography and radionuclide bone scan if the tumor appears to be a clear-cell sarcoma of the kidney. A combination of these studies may be required.

A plain radiograph showing a bulging flank mass and increased density with loss of renal outline displacing the intestines toward the opposite side of the abdomen may indicate the presence of a Wilms' tumor. Curvilinear and punctate calcifications are present on radiographs in approximately 10% of cases. The calcifications are subtle and never dense.

CT with intravenous contrast is the gold standard used to evaluate the extent of the abdominal tumor and the integrity of the contralateral kidney. Contrast examination may be helpful in assessing the necessity (or ability) to amputate 1 kidney in patients with bilateral Wilms' tumor. Enlargement of the pelvic calyceal system is encountered in approximately 40% of patients. Total loss of renal function is unusual in patients with Wilms' tumor.

Ultrasonography is useful in establishing the patency of the inferior vena cava. This may occasionally be involved by a tumor thrombus, which can extend to the right atrium. Rarely, angiography may also be required for complicated surgical procedures to delineate the extent of the tumor and involvement of adjacent structures. Angiography also defines the blood supply and reveals displacement of the renal pedicle and aberrant vessels.

DIFFERENTIAL DIAGNOSES

The primary clinical and radiologic differential diagnoses of Wilms' tumor are neuroblastoma, rhabdomyosarcoma, and hepatoblastoma. In addition, benign cystic lesions should be considered, including those of multicystic kidneys and hydronephrosis as well as mesenteric and duplication cysts.

HISTOLOGIC CLASSIFICATION

Wilms' tumor is generally categorized as being of either favorable or unfavorable cell type. Favorable cell types account for approximately 80% of Wilms' tumors, whereas unfavorable types account for approximately 15% to 20%. Categorization of the unfavorable type is further subdivided into diffuse anaplastic, clear-cell, and sarcomatous varieties. Scattered areas of anaplasia may also be present in favorable-type tumors (up to 10% of specimens).

STAGING

The following staging system was devised by the National Wilms' Tumor Study and has been generally adopted:

Stage I: The tumor is limited to the kidney and is completely excised without rupture before or during removal. The surface of the renal capsule is intact, and no residual tumor is present beyond the margins of the resection.

Stage II: The tumor extends beyond the kidney, penetrating through the outer surface of the renal capsule into the perirenal soft tissue, but is completely excised. No residual tumor is apparent beyond the margins of the excision.

Stage III: A residual nonhematogenous tumor is present but is confined to the abdomen. In addition, any of the following may occur:

a) Lymph nodes in the hilus, para-aortic chain, or beyond the abdominal para-aortic chain are identified.

b) Tumors undergoing biopsy may rupture before or during surgery. This may result in diffuse peritoneal contamination from spillage beyond the flank.

c) Implants may be found on peritoneal surfaces.
d) The tumor may extend beyond the surgical margins of the resection either microscopically or grossly.
e) The tumor may not be completely resectable because of local infiltration into vital structures.

Stage IV: Hematogenous metastases are present in the lungs, and the liver. Bones or brain may also be involved.
Stage V: Both kidneys are involved.

TREATMENT

Treatment of Wilms' tumor involves the 3 major modes of cancer therapy: surgery, chemotherapy, and radiotherapy.

Surgery
Surgical removal is attempted in all cases of Wilms' tumor. In the event that immediate surgical removal is not possible, percutaneous needle biopsy for diagnostic purposes may be considered. Alternatively, an open biopsy may be performed. Following surgical resection, pathologic examination is performed to determine the tumor's histologic subtype. Stage is established after surgical extirpation, with attention to the pathologic and radiographic studies described earlier.

Chemotherapy
The following chemotherapeutic agents have been shown to be effective in Wilms' tumor: vincristine, dactinomycin, doxorubicin, cyclophosphamide, and ifosfamide. Figures 5–1, 5–2, and 5–3 show 3 selected chemotherapy

Week	0	1	2	3	4	5	6	7	8	9	10	11	12	13	14	15	16	17	18

A   A   A   A   A   A   A

V V V V V VV V V V V   V*   V*   V*

Figure 5–1. National Wilms' Tumor Study 5 (regimen EE-4A). This regimen is administered to patients with stage I disease and favorable or anaplastic histology and stage II disease and favorable histology. Abbreviations: A, dactinomycin (45 mcg/kg intravenously); V, vincristine (0.05 mg/kg intravenously); V*, vincristine (0.067 mg/kg intravenously). Reprinted from Green DM, Breslow NE, Beckwith JB, et al. Comparison between single-dose and divided-dose administration of dactinomycin and doxorubicin for patients with Wilms' tumor: a report from the National Wilms' Tumor Study Group. *J Clin Oncol* 1998;16:237–245, with permission from ASCO.

Week	0	1	2	3	4	5	6	7	8	9	10	11	12	13	14	15	16	17	18	19	20	21	22	23	24
	A			D+		A			D+				A			D*			A			D*			A
			V	V	V	V	V	V	V	V	V		V*			V*			V*			V*			V*
XRT																									

Figure 5–2. National Wilms' Tumor Study 5 (regimen DD-4A). This regimen is administered to patients with stages III and IV disease and favorable histology and patients with stages II to IV disease and focal anaplasia. Abbreviations: A, dactinomycin (45 mcg/kg intravenously); D*, doxorubicin (1.0 mg/kg intravenously); D+, doxorubicin (1.5 mg/kg intravenously); V, vincristine (0.05 mg/kg intravenously); V*, vincristine (0.067 mg/kg intravenously); XRT, radiotherapy. Reprinted from Green DM, Breslow NE, Beckwith JB, et al. Comparison between single-dose and divided-dose administration of dactinomycin and doxorubicin for patients with Wilms' tumor: a report from the National Wilms' Tumor Study Group. *J Clin Oncol* 1998;16:237–245, with permission from ASCO.

Week	0	1	2	3	4	5	6	7	8	9	10	11	12	13	14	15	16	17	18	19	20	21	22	23	24
	D						D						D						D						D
		V	V	V	V	V	V	V	V		V	V	V*	V*					V*						V*
					C*					C			C*			C			C*			C			C*
										E						E						E			
XRT																									

Figure 5-3. National Wilms' Tumor Study 5 (regimen I). This regimen is administered to patients with stages II to IV diffuse anaplastic disease and patients with stages I to IV clear-cell sarcoma of the kidney. Abbreviations: C, cyclophosphamide (14.7 mg/kg/day × 5 intravenously); C*, cyclophosphamide (14.7 mg/kg/day × 3 intravenously); D+, doxorubicin (1.5 mg/kg intravenously); E, etoposide (3.3 mg/kg/day × 5 intravenously); V, vincristine (0.05 mg/kg intravenously); V*, vincristine (0.067 mg/kg intravenously); XRT, radiotherapy. Reprinted with permission from the Children's Oncology Group.

regimens published in National Wilms' Tumor Study V. These regimens are currently used at M. D. Anderson. They may be modified as dictated by the patient's clinical presentation and the tumor's response to therapy.

Radiotherapy

Radiotherapy is administered for Wilms' tumors that are stage III (confined to the abdomen) or IV (metastasized to the lungs). The dosage of radiotherapy varies according to patient age. Details are provided by the National Wilms' Tumor Study protocols and are available to members of the Children's Oncology Group.

SPECIAL TREATMENT CONSIDERATIONS

In the treatment of Wilms' tumors, some conditions require special treatment consideration. These conditions include inoperable and bilateral tumors; recurrent, progressive, and resistant tumors; rare metastases; rhabdoid tumors of the kidney; congenital mesoblastic nephromas; and nephroblastomatosis.

Inoperable and Bilateral Tumors

Inoperable and bilateral Wilms' tumors are generally treated with preoperative chemotherapy, which is administered to render the tumor resectable and, in the case of bilateral tumors, to conserve as much renal tissue as possible. Preoperative treatment usually comprises vincristine, dactinomycin, and doxorubicin (see Figure 5–1). Cyclophosphamide is occasionally added. Preoperative treatment is generally administered for 2 to 3 months. The extent and timing of the subsequent operation are determined on the basis of the tumor's response to treatment. Surgery is followed by completion of the chemotherapy protocol. Surgery may also be followed by postoperative radiotherapy, and chemotherapy is generally administered after completion of radiotherapy.

Recurrent, Progressive, and Resistant Tumors

Disease that recurs or progresses after treatment or that resists treatment is usually managed with a multidisciplinary approach that combines surgery and radiotherapy and occasionally investigational chemotherapy. Cyclophosphamide and ifosfamide are the mainstays of salvage treatment, particularly if these agents have not previously been used. A bone marrow transplant may also be considered. In the latter circumstance, multiple alkylating agents are used, including cyclophosphamide, triethylenethiophosphoramide (Thiotepa), and melphalan.

Rare Metastases

Cisplatin and radiotherapy are generally used for patients with clear-cell sarcoma of the kidney that has metastasized to the skeleton. Brain metastases are treated by surgical resection (if possible), radiotherapy, or both. Pretreatment with high doses of ifosfamide may also be considered. Although the prognosis is usually grave, several patients with brain, liver, and skeletal metastases have been cured.

Tumors Allied to or Previously Considered Wilms' Tumor

Three tumors known to be associated with Wilms' tumor are rhabdoid tumor of the kidney, at one time considered a subtype of Wilms' tumor; congenital mesoblastic nephroma, which is thought to eventually develop into Wilms' tumor; and nephroblastomatosis, which is called a precursor of Wilms' tumor. The treatment recommendations for these entities vary.

Rhabdoid Tumor of the Kidney

Rhabdoid tumor is no longer classified as a Wilms' tumor. Generally diagnosed after a nephrectomy, rhabdoid tumors are treated with vincristine, dactinomycin, doxorubicin, cisplatin, and ifosfamide. Although the prognosis for these tumors is grave, some patients survive. Radiotherapy may also be administered, particularly for suspected residual microscopic or recurrent disease.

Congenital Mesoblastic Nephroma

Congenital mesoblastic nephroma occurs in early childhood and is generally considered a benign entity. It is uncertain whether it eventually develops into Wilms' tumor. Congenital mesoblastic nephroma is generally diagnosed after a nephrectomy. Opinion is divided as to whether postoperative chemotherapy should be required; most treatment centers implement systematic monitoring and withhold chemotherapy.

Nephroblastomatosis

It is generally believed that nephroblatomatosis precedes Wilms' tumor, but opinion is divided as to whether chemotherapy should be administered. Most patients at M. D. Anderson with this condition are treated with the same regimens used for patients with stage I or II Wilms' tumor. Diligent follow-up is required.

SIDE EFFECTS OF THERAPY

The side effects of Wilms' tumor involve the gastrointestinal, hepatic, and cardiac systems; chest, uterus, and ovaries; and skeleton.

Gastrointestinal System

Antiemetics are usually administered with chemotherapy. Most of the chemotherapeutic agents used cause transient nausea and vomiting. Occasionally, vomiting may also occur after surgical resection of the tumor. Intestinal obstruction, particularly in the immediate postoperative period, should be suspected, but the vomiting may also be a result of adhesion, fibrosis, or intussusception. Rarely, radiotherapy enteritis or malabsorption may supervene later.

Hepatic System

Rarely, severe hepatic damage may occur from veno-occlusive disease. The damage is usually associated with dactinomycin and radiotherapy, especially when a portion of the liver was in the irradiated field.

Cardiac System

Congestive cardiac failure has been reported after treatment with doxorubicin, particularly when doxorubicin is administered in combination with radiotherapy to the lungs. The cumulative dose of doxorubicin is usually limited to 200 to 300 mg/m^2 to prevent cardiac damage. This dose limitation is particularly relevant for patients with pulmonary metastases who will subsequently receive pulmonary radiotherapy. We also recommend delivery of doxorubicin over a 24-hour period rather than as a pulse to minimize cardiotoxic effects.

Chest, Uterus, and Ovaries

Radiotherapy to the chest can affect breast maturation, and radiotherapy to the uterus may result in low-birth-weight babies. Radiotherapy to the ovaries may result in premature menopause and problems in reproductive function.

Skelton

Kyphoscoliosis may occur after radiotherapy is administered to the hemiabdomen, with only part of the vertebral column included in the irradiation portal. With the advent of modern techniques, kyphoscoliosis can generally be avoided.

FOLLOW-UP EVALUATION

Recurrent tumors, pulmonary metastases, or both are prone to occur within the first 3 years after diagnosis and initiation of treatment. At M. D. Anderson, patients are followed at monthly intervals for 2 years. At each visit, a clinical examination and chest radiograph are done. The interval between visits over the next 3 years is extended, and annual follow-up is

Table 5–1. Follow-up Schedule After Completion of Chemotherapy

	Years After Treatment						
Examination	2	2–2.5	2.5–3	3–3.5	3.5–4	4–5	5+
Chest radiograph	1 mo	1.5 mo	2 mo	3 mo	4 mo	6 mo	1 yr
Laboratory studies	1 mo	1.5 mo	2 mo	3 mo	4 yr	6 yr	1 yr
Physical examination	1 mo	1.5 mo	2 mo	3 mo	4 mo	6 mo	1 yr
Abdominal ultrasound	EOC and annually thereafter						

Abbreviations: EOC, end of chemotherapy; mo, month; yr, year.

implemented after 5 years. Ultrasonography of the abdomen is performed annually to detect the presence of a recurrent tumor within the tumor bed and to establish the integrity of the contralateral kidney. Table 5–1 outlines the M. D. Anderson post-treatment follow-up schedule.

PROGNOSIS

The overall cure rate for patients with all stages of Wilms' tumor combined is greater than 60%. Patients with stages I and II Wilms' tumor have a cure rate of 90%.

KEY PRACTICE POINTS

- Optimal management of Wilms' tumor includes chemotherapy, surgery, and radiotherapy.
- Side effects of treatment may involve the gastrointestinal, hepatic, cardiac, genital, and skeletal systems.
- A schema of the follow-up evaluation schedule is presented in Table 5-1.

SUGGESTED READINGS

Beckwith JP. National Wilms' Tumor Study: an update for pathologists. *Pediatr Dev Pathol* 1988;1:79–84.

Bracken RB, Sutow WW, Jaffe N, et al. Preoperative chemotherapy for Wilms' tumor. *Urology* 1982;19:55–60.

Coppes MD, de Krake J, van Dijken PJ. Bilateral Wilms' tumor: long-term survival and some epidemiological features. *J Clin Oncol* 1989;7:310–315.

Green DM, Breslow NE, Beckwith JB, et al. Effect of duration of treatment on treatment outcome and cost of treatment for Wilms' tumor: a report from the National Wilms' Tumor Study Group. *J Clin Oncol* 1998;16:3744–3751.

Huff DS. Nodular renal blastema, nephroblastomatosis and Wilms' tumor: a report of two cases. *Am J Pathol* 1973;70:23a–24b.

Jaffe N. The impact of chemotherapy on Wilms' tumor. In: Johnson DC, Logothetis CJ, von Eschenbach AC, eds. *Systemic Therapy for Genitourinary Cancer.* Chicago, IL: Year Book Medical Publishers, Inc.; 1989:143–157.

Jaffe N, McNeese M, Mayfield JK, et al. Childhood urologic cancer therapy-related sequelae and their impact on management. *Cancer* 1980;45:1815–1822.

National Wilms' Tumor Study Committee. Wilms' tumor: status report, 1990. *J Clin Oncol* 1991;9:877–887.

Paulino AC. Current issues in the diagnosis and management of Wilms' tumor. *Oncology* 1996;10:1553–1571.

Pritchard-Jones K. Controversies and advances in the management of Wilms' tumor. *Arch Dis Child* 2002;87:241–244.

Tournade MF, Com-Nougué C, de Kraker J, et al. Optimal duration of preoperative therapy in unilateral and non-metastatic Wilms' tumor in children older than six months: results of the Ninth International Society of Pediatric Oncology Wilms' Tumor Trial and Study. *J Clin Oncol* 2001;19:488–500.

6 NEUROBLASTOMA

Joann L. Ater and Laura L. Worth

CHAPTER OVERVIEW

Neuroblastoma has varying presentations and a survival rate that ranges from 0% to 100% depending on the tumor biology. The challenge in managing this tumor is determining which therapies can effectively yet safely produce cure. For patients with high-risk disease, aggressive and novel treatments are needed. For patients with low- and intermediate-risk disease, we continue to define, through prognostic indicators, minimal, least-toxic curative therapies. This chapter describes the recommendations of the Division of Pediatrics at M. D. Anderson Cancer Center for evaluating and treating children and adolescents with neuroblastoma.

INTRODUCTION

Neuroblastoma is an embryonal cancer of the peripheral sympathetic nervous system. It is the third most common pediatric cancer, accounting for about 8% of childhood malignancies. About 500 new cases of neuroblastoma are diagnosed each year in the United States. The median age of patients at diagnosis of neuroblastoma is 2 years. Ninety percent of cases are diagnosed before age 5 years, and 1 in 7,000 children younger than 5 years old have a diagnosis of neuroblastoma. It is also the most frequently diagnosed neoplasm in infants, accounting for 28% to 39% of neonatal malignancies. Although less commonly, neuroblastoma also occurs in adolescents and young adults.

Most children with neuroblastoma require coordinated care in a multidisciplinary setting involving pediatric oncologists and pediatric surgeons. Children with advanced-stage disease or unusual presentations may also require evaluation and treatment on the radiotherapy, pediatric neurology, and pediatric bone marrow transplant (BMT) services. Adult patients with neuroblastoma who present to M. D. Anderson are treated on the adult sarcoma service, often in collaboration with the Division of Pediatrics.

CLINICAL PRESENTATION

Neuroblastoma can mimic several other disorders and thus is sometimes difficult to diagnose. It may develop at any site of sympathetic nervous system tissue and can be accompanied by nonspecific systemic symptoms (Table 6–1). However, the signs and symptoms of neuroblastoma are usually characteristic of the tumor site and the extent of disease.

More than 70% of neuroblastomas arise in the abdomen, either in the adrenal gland or in retroperitoneal sympathetic ganglia. The primary tumor is usually a firm, nodular mass located in the flank or midline that causes abdominal discomfort. When the tumor is retroperitoneally located, it can be difficult to palpate, particularly in an uncooperative child, so a large mass can go unnoticed until symptoms associated with metastasis are

Table 6–1. Clinical Presentations of Neuroblastoma

Tumor Type	Signs and Symptoms
Mass	• Cervical or supraclavicular swelling or mass ± Horner's syndrome; may be thoracic extension of paraspinal mass or metastasis from abdomen • Nodular, firm midline abdominal, or flank mass • Posterior mediastinal mass found incidentally because of respiratory or other symptoms
Metastatic	Fever, irritability, failure to thrive, bone pain, anemia, bleeding, hepatomegaly, subcutaneous nodules, orbital proptosis ± periorbital ecchymoses
Neurologic	• Opsoclonus-myoclonus syndrome and ataxia due to paraneoplastic syndrome without brain metastasis • Weakness or paralysis due to spinal invasion of paraspinal tumor • Horner's syndrome due to tumor involvement of superior cervical ganglion
Catecholamine related	Hypertension, flushing, and increased sweating; secretory diarrhea due to vasoactive intestinal peptide

Table 6–2. Frequency (%) of Neuroblastoma By Primary Site and Stage of Disease

Sites	I $n = 62$	II $n = 63$	III $n = 165$	IV $n = 289$	IV-S $n = 62$	I to IV-S $n = 641$
Cervical	18	14	6	0	0	5
Thoracic	16	41	16	6	7	13
Abdominal						
Adrenal gland	42	27	36	59	69	49
Nonadrenal gland	23	17	40	29	8	28
Combination	—	—	1	2	3	2
Unknown	—	—	—	5	13	3
Totals	99	99	99	101	100	100

Source: Berthold, 1990.

noted. An ultrasound of the abdomen can be useful in screening an abdominal mass when neuroblastoma is suspected. On a plain radiograph or computed tomography (CT) scan, areas of calcification and hemorrhage may be noted. Wilms' tumor, another common flank mass occurring in young children, does not usually calcify and typically has a smooth, well-defined contour. Neuroblastoma originates from cervical, thoracic, or pelvic ganglia in about 30% of cases. Table 6–2 shows the frequency at which primary neuroblastoma tumors occur at different sites correlated with the stage of disease at presentation (Berthold, 1990).

A myriad of signs and symptoms accompany metastatic neuroblastoma, including fever, irritability, failure to thrive, bone pain, bluish subcutaneous nodules, orbital proptosis, and periorbital ecchymosis. Orbital proptosis and periorbital ecchymosis can be pathognomonic for neuroblastoma and, if present, may prompt the initiation of additional studies to confirm the diagnosis and determine the extent of disease. The most common sites of metastasis are the long bones and skull, bone marrow, liver, lymph nodes, and skin. Lung metastasis is rare, occurring in less than 3% of patients. Neurologic signs and symptoms at presentation are less common. Involvement of the superior cervical ganglion can result in Horner's syndrome. Paraspinal neuroblastoma can invade the neural foramina and produce symptoms of spinal cord and nerve root compression. Finally, neuroblastoma can present as a paraneoplastic syndrome of autoimmune origin manifesting as ataxia or opsoclonus-myoclonus syndrome ("dancing eyes and dancing feet"). In such cases, the primary tumor is in the chest or abdomen, and the brain is negative for tumor (Rudnick et al, 2001).

Some neuroblastomas produce catecholamines, which can cause increased sweating and hypertension, and some release vasoactive intestinal peptide, which causes secretory diarrhea. These unusual presentations, along with spinal cord compression, are found more commonly with thoracic neuroblastoma than with abdominal neuroblastoma. Some infants present with a unique stage of disease referred to as IV-S, which often includes subcutaneous tumor nodules, massive liver involvement, and a small stage I or II primary tumor with no bone involvement.

PATHOLOGY, PATHOGENESIS, AND PROGNOSIS

Neuroblastomas include a spectrum of tumors with varying degrees of neural differentiation, ranging from undifferentiated small round cells to tumors containing mature ganglion cells (ganglioneuroblastoma or ganglioneuroma). Prognosis has been shown to vary on the basis of the histologic definition of tissue pattern as determined by the Shimada classification system. A favorable prognosis is determined on the basis of the amount of stroma, degree of tumor cell differentiation, and number of tumor cell mitoses. Such tumors may resemble other small round-cell tumors, i.e., rhabdomyosarcoma, Ewing's sarcoma, and non-Hodgkin lymphoma.

The genetic event or events that trigger the formation of a neuroblastoma are not known; however, the pathogenesis of neuroblastoma is likely to be related to a succession of prenatal and perinatal mutational events. These mutations may be caused by environmental and genetic factors. For example, there is an increased incidence of neuroblastoma among children whose mothers or fathers experienced occupational exposure to certain chemicals, were farm workers, or worked in the field of electronics (DeRoos et al, 2001). There is a familial disposition for neuroblastoma in 1% to 2% of patients. Genetic characteristics of neuroblastoma that are of prognostic importance and that are currently used along with clinical factors to determine treatment include amplification of the N-MYC protooncogene (*mycn*) and hyperdiploidy of tumor-cell DNA content. The amplification of N-MYC is important prognostically, independent of stage and patient age, and is strongly predictive of poor outcome. Hyperdiploidy confers a better outcome if the child is younger than 1 year of age at diagnosis. Genetic abnormalities, including loss of heterozygosity of 1p, 11q, and 14q and gain of 17q, are commonly found in neuroblastoma tumor tissue. Other biologic factors associated with prognosis include level of nerve growth factor receptor (Trk-A) expression, presence of the multi-drug resistance-associated protein, and telomerase activity (Maris and Matthay, 1999). Clinical trials are currently underway to determine whether these factors can be used to further refine therapies on the basis of risk. Thus, therapy can be reduced for patients predicted to be at intermediate or low risk for relapse and intensified for those predicted to be at high risk for relapse.

Diagnosis and Staging

On plain radiographs, CT scans, or magnetic resonance imaging scans of the chest and abdomen, the primary neuroblastoma tumor is generally discovered as a mass or multiple masses. Tumor markers (i.e., homovanillic acid [HVA] and vanillylmandelic acid [VMA] in urine) are elevated in 95% of cases. Tests for these tumor markers help to confirm the diagnosis of neuroblastoma. A pathologic diagnosis is made using tumor tissue obtained by biopsy or tumor resection. For localized tumor that appears removable without risk for significant procedure-induced morbidity, the pediatric surgeons at M. D. Anderson recommend attempting a complete resection. However, if there is evidence of widespread metastasis, chemotherapy should not be delayed until the primary tumor is surgically resected.

Neuroblastoma can be diagnosed at presentation without a biopsy of the primary tumor if there are neuroblasts in the bone marrow and if the levels of VMA or HVA in the urine are elevated. Additionally, at M. D. Anderson, positivity for chromogranin and synaptophysin in the bone marrow on immunohistochemical analysis is useful in confirming the diagnosis of neuroblastoma and in distinguishing neuroblastoma from other small round-cell tumors that can metastasize to the bone marrow. Bone marrow neuroblasts can be evaluated to determine any cytogenetic changes associated with neuroblastoma, such as a 1p deletion, double minutes, and N-MYC oncogene amplification. The M. D. Anderson cytogenetics laboratory utilizes a fluorescence in situ hybridization (FISH) probe to determine N-MYC amplification. FISH is performed using a Vysis LSI N-MYC probe (Vysis, Downer's Grove, IL). This spectrum-orange probe contains DNA sequences specific to the N-MYC oncogene located in the 2p24.1 region and is useful in detecting amplification of N-MYC. Although less specific, 17q+ can also be detected in bone marrow utilizing FISH. In neuroblastoma, 17q+ is also associated with poor prognosis.

In less advanced cases of neuroblastoma in which there is no bone marrow involvement, tumor tissue is required for diagnosis and full evaluation of prognostic factors, such as the Shimada histologic classification system. In children with stage II or III disease, these prognostic factors can make an important difference in the intensity of therapy recommended. M. D. Anderson participates in investigational studies to determine the significance of other prognostic factors, and tumor tissue is necessary for these studies.

In Table 6–3, the tests used to evaluate neuroblastomas are described. An evaluation of metastatic disease should include a bone scan to detect cortical bone involvement and bilateral bone marrow aspirates and biopsies to detect marrow disease. In young children, plain radiographs of long bones may be necessary to identify bone metastases near joints. The joints are difficult to evaluate because growth plates are displayed brightly on the bone

Table 6–3. Descriptions of Tests Used to Stage Neuroblastoma Tumors

Test	Possible Findings	Comments
Physical examination	See Table 6–1.	Periorbital ecchymoses and abdominal mass, especially with bone pain, make stage IV neuroblastoma highly likely. Bone marrow aspiration and biopsy may provide tissue for diagnostic tests without surgery. For paraspinal tumors, check for signs of spinal cord compression. Elevated blood pressure could be caused by catecholamines or renal vascular compromise.
Laboratory tests: serum CBC d/p, electrolytes, calcium, BUN, creatinine, LFTs, LDH, PT, PTT, ferritin, 24-hour urine test for HVA and VMA, and creatinine	Anemia, thrombocytosis, or pancytopenia; high Cr ± hyperkalemia, hypercalcemia, prolonged PT, PTT, high LDH, and ferritin	Ferritin must be obtained before surgery to be prognostically significant. It is an acute-phase reactant that rises with stress. LDH may also be very high and could serve as tumor marker.
Abdominal ultrasound or x-ray of abdomen	Abdominal primary	Useful initial screening tests; x-ray may show calcified mass.
Bilateral bone marrow aspirations and biopsies	Tumor metastasis diagnostic of neuroblastoma	Obtain cytogenetics, immunohistochemistry for synaptophysin and chromogranin, and FISH for N-MYC and p17+.
Bone scan, CXR and CT chest CT abdomen and pelvis	Cortical bone mets; paraspinal mass, primary tumor, liver, lymph node mets	May also see primary tumor. Pulmonary metastases rare; Intravenous and oral contrast needed, but scan time is short.
MRI of abdomen and pelvis	Good evaluation of abdominal tumor	Requires longer sedation and is more expensive than CT. Use CT or MRI, but not both.
Skeletal survey	Bone metastases	Clarify results of bone scan.
PET	Full evaluation of tumor	Not yet used routinely. Not FDA approved for neuroblastoma evaluation and follow-up.
I^{123} MIBG scintigraphy	Identify sites of MIBG-positive tumor	If positive, MIBG can also be used therapeutically. Test takes several days to complete.

Abbreviations: BUN, blood urea nitrogen; CBC d/p, complete blood count with differential and platelets; Cr, creatinine; CT, computed tomography; CXR, chest x-ray; FDA, Food and Drug Administration; FISH, fluorescence in situ hybridization; HVA, homovanillic acid; I^{123}, iodine 123; LDH, lactose dehydrogenase; LFT, liver function test; mets, metastases; MIBG, meta-iodobenzylguanidine; MRI, magnetic resonance imaging; PET, positron emission tomography; PT, prothrombin time; PTT, partial thromboplastin time; VMA, vanillylmandelic acid.

Table 6–4. The International Neuroblastoma Staging System

Stage	Description
Stage I	Tumors confined to the organ or structure of origin
Stage II	Tumors that extend beyond the structure of origin but not across the midline, with (stage IIB) or without (stage IIA) ipsilateral regional lymph node involvement
Stage III	Tumors that extend beyond the midline, with (IIIB) or without (IIIA) bilateral lymph node involvement
Stage IV	Tumors that disseminate to distant sites (e.g., bone, bone marrow, liver, distant lymph nodes, and other organs)
Stage IV-S	Tumors in patients younger than 1 year, with dissemination to liver, skin, bone marrow, or to a combination of these sites without bone involvement and with a primary tumor that would otherwise be considered stage I or II

scan and can obscure sites of disease. A CT or magnetic resonance imaging scan that includes the abdomen and pelvis should always be obtained to fully evaluate the liver and paraspinal regions for metastasis, even if the primary appears to originate in the chest or neck. As with adult patients, a left supraclavicular mass may be the presenting sign of an abdominal tumor in children. A positron emission tomography scan can also help accurately determine the extent of tumor, but it is less readily available. Meta-iodobenzylguanidine (MIBG), which is taken up specifically by cells of sympathetic origin, provides a highly sensitive and specific indicator for the detection of neuroblastoma metastases. Scintigraphy using iodine-123 MIBG can be used to stage the tumor and to follow patients. The study takes several days to complete and thus is not always practical for use in evaluating newly diagnosed patients who are ill.

Clinical extent of disease and age, together with cytogenetics and molecular markers performed on the tumor tissue, are used to estimate prognosis and to determine risk-appropriate therapy. Although several staging systems have been used, the International Neuroblastoma Staging System (INSS) is the universal standard. The INSS categories are described in Table 6–4.

TREATMENT

Patients are classified by risk group when determining the best treatment approach. The most important clinical and biologic prognostic factors currently used to determine risk group are patient age at diagnosis, tumor stage (INSS), N-MYC status, Shimada histology, and ploidy in infants (see Table 6–5; note that ploidy is not included in this table). The prognoses shown are the best survival rates documented in recently published studies (see "Recent Studies" column on Table 6–5). The treatment

Table 6–5. Features of Neuroblastoma Risk Groups

Risk Group	INSS Stage	Age	N-MYC Status	Shimada Histology	Survival	Recent Studies
Low	I	All	Any	Any	90%–100%	DeRoos et al,
	II	<1 yr	Any	Any		2001; Maris
	II	>1 yr	Any	Favorable		and Matthay,
	IV-S	<1 yr	<10 copies	Favorable		1999; Murray
						et al, 1994
Intermediate	III	>1 yr	<10 copies	Favorable	75%–98%	DeRoos et al,
	III and IV	<1 yr	<10 copies	Any		2001; Murray
	IV-S	<1 yr	<10 copies	Unfavorable		et al, 1994
High	II	>1 yr	Any	Unfavorable	20%–60%	Chan et al, 1996;
	III	All	>10 copies	Any		Maris and
	IV	<1 yr	>10 copies	Any		Matthay,
	IV	>1 yr	Any	Any		1999; Murray
						et al, 1994

Abbreviation: INSS, International Neuroblastoma Staging System

recommendation for low-risk neuroblastoma for patients with stage I or II disease is usually surgical removal, and for patients with stage IV-S disease, the treatment recommendation is observation. Even in patients with stage II disease with small amounts of residual tumor, the survival rate after surgery is more than 90%, with no further therapy required. Furthermore, chemotherapy or radiotherapy for the rare case of local recurrence can still be curative. Children with spinal cord compression at diagnosis may require urgent chemotherapy, surgery, or radiotherapy to avoid neurologic damage. Patients with stage IV-S disease also have a favorable prognosis—a survival rate of nearly 100%, with supportive care required only if the tumor regresses spontaneously. Chemotherapy or resection of the primary does not improve survival. Infants younger than 2 months old with stage IV-S neuroblastoma are at higher risk if they have massive liver involvement and respiratory compromise. In this patient group, low-dose cyclophosphamide or very low-dose hepatic radiation may be recommended to alleviate symptoms. For children with IV-S neuroblastoma who require treatment for symptoms, the survival rate is 81%.

Treatment of intermediate-risk neuroblastoma (see Table 6–5) includes surgery, chemotherapy, and in some cases radiation. Chemotherapy for this risk group usually includes moderate doses of cisplatin or carboplatin, cyclophosphamide, etoposide, and doxorubicin given over 4 to 9 months. Radiotherapy is utilized when there is an incomplete response to chemotherapy. Children with stage III disease and infants younger than 12 months old with stage IV neuroblastoma and favorable characteristics have an excellent prognosis (greater than 90% survival rate) with this moderate treatment. In the intermediate-risk group, obtaining adequate diagnostic material for determination of the Shimada pathologic classification and of N-MYC amplification is critical so that children with unfavorable features can receive more aggressive treatment and those with favorable features can be spared excessive therapy.

Treatment of high-risk neuroblastoma (see Table 6–5) usually consists of induction chemotherapy followed by high-dose chemotherapy and autologous BMT or peripheral blood stem cell transplant (PBSCT).The results of a national randomized study showed a significantly improved survival rate for patients who underwent BMT as a follow-up to chemotherapy compared to those who did not (Matthay et al, 1999). The administration of cis-retinoic acid (CRA) for 1 year following BMT further increased the 5-year event-free survival rate for these patients to 50%; this survival advantage is clearly superior to the 20% survival rate for patients who received chemotherapy without BMT or CRA. However, better therapy is needed for the majority of patients with high-risk neuroblastoma. New therapies currently under investigation include new chemotherapeutic agents, high-dose chemotherapy with multiple stem cell rescues, monoclonal antibodies combined with growth factors, and antitumor vaccines. It is also hoped that biologic studies of neuroblastoma will eventually lead to new genetic targets for therapy.

Role of Bone Marrow Transplantation

Depending on the stage of disease, some patients with neuroblastoma may benefit from high-dose chemotherapy and radiotherapy followed by hematopoietic stem cell rescue. One such group is patients with stage IV disease in first complete or good partial remission (defined as greater than 90% reduction in the size of the primary tumor, metastatic disease limited to bone, and greater than 90% decrease in catecholamine excretion or absence of demonstrable disease except for residual radionuclide uptake in the bone scan). High-dose chemotherapy plus radiotherapy is also useful for patients with stage III disease with unfavorable histology or N-MYC amplification and for patients with stage I or II disease with disseminated relapse after systemic chemotherapy. The latter group undergoes transplantation during second complete or good partial remission.

At M. D. Anderson, all children with newly diagnosed, high-risk neuroblastoma are evaluated for eligibility for high-dose chemotherapy and stem cell rescue. In order to be considered for stem cell rescue, the child's tumor must be chemotherapy sensitive. Typically, the first re-evaluation takes place after 2 to 3 cycles of induction chemotherapy. If there is significant shrinkage of the tumor bulk and clearance of bone marrow metastasis, the patient is ready for stem cell collection. Because of the risk for tumor contamination, vigorous examination of the bone marrow, including a bilateral biopsy and immunohistochemical staining with synaptophysin and chromogranin, is done. If residual tumor is present, the procedure is repeated after each of 1 or 2 more cycles of chemotherapy until complete remission of bone marrow is obtained. Ideally, peripheral blood stem cells are best harvested during the recovery phase of the next cycle of chemotherapy.

At M. D. Anderson, we ensure that the efforts of the pediatric oncology team and the bone marrow transplant team are well coordinated to facilitate the placement of a central venous catheter, mobilization of granulocyte colony-stimulating factor (G-CSF), and leukaphereis. If there is good initial response to chemotherapy, stem cell harvest may take place before definitive tumor resection. After second-look surgery, the patient may receive 1 more cycle of chemotherapy before proceeding to PBSCT.

We use 2 preparative regimens: (a) total-body irradiation combined with melphalan, etoposide, topotecan, or cisplatin or (b) melphalan administered in combination with cyclophosphamide and topotecan or thiotepa. For patients who will undergo peripheral blood stem cell collection, stem cells are collected when the white cell count is recovering from chemotherapy. The dose of G-CSF is doubled to twice-daily administration. A peripheral blood CD34+ cell count may be obtained on the morning of the fourth day of G-CSF injection. A circulating CD34+ count of $15/\mu L$ or greater is predictive of good stem cell recovery. For patients who have received extensive chemotherapy, bone marrow recovery may be sluggish or inadequate. Multiple stem cell aphereses or even a direct bone marrow harvest may be necessary to collect an adequate number of progenitor cells.

We and others have demonstrated that even if the marrow appears microscopically clear of neuroblastoma cells, residual tumor cells can still be demonstrated by flow cytometry and FISH. CD34+ progenitor-cell selection is now routinely used at M. D. Anderson for patients with neuroblastoma who have a history of marrow infiltration. We have found this approach to be as effective as purging the bone marrow cells with a cocktail of monoclonal antibodies.

We occasionally encounter patients who have no evidence of disease elsewhere except for a small number of residual tumor foci in the bone marrow. These patients are not candidates for autologous PBSCT, but they may be eligible for an allogeneic PBSCT if a matched donor (related or nonrelated) is available. In addition to being free of tumor contamination, allogeneic stem cells may also facilitate the graft-versus-tumor effect.

Once hematologic reconstitution is achieved post-transplant and the patient is able to take medications by mouth, 13-CRA is administered as a differentiation/maturation agent to modulate the behavior of any residual tumor. CRA-administered post-transplant has been shown to improve the disease-free survival rate. CRA is administered orally at a dose of $80\,mg/m^2$ twice a day for 14 consecutive days on a 28-day cycle. This schedule improves the tolerability of CRA therapy. The potential side effects include dryness of mouth and skin, cheilitis, elevated liver enzyme and lipid levels, and increased intracranial pressure. Treatment is continued for 6 to 12 months. Irradiation to sites of prior bulky metastatic disease may be indicated in the post-transplant period.

Patients who do not achieve a complete or very good partial remission have a very high incidence of failure after PBSCT. The chemotherapy regimen may need to be changed to maximize tumor reduction before high-dose chemotherapy.

Therapy for Recurrence

With aggressive induction chemotherapy regimens that include cisplatin, 85% to 90% of children with neuroblastoma will have, at minimum, a very good partial response. However, with unfavorable stage III and stage IV disease, even after high-dose chemotherapy and PBSCT, 40% to 60% of patients will eventually have progressive tumor. Treatment of this recurrent neuroblastoma, especially after aggressive front-line therapy, is particularly difficult. If the child's blood counts have not fully recovered after high-dose chemotherapy and PBSCT, aggressive chemotherapy regimens may not be tolerated. In such a situation, if the parents wish to have further palliative chemotherapy, we typically prescribe low-dose oral etoposide at 50 mg/m^2 given for 3 weeks followed by 1 week of rest; this regimen can be repeated for up to 18 cycles. With some patients, we have observed objective responses lasting as long as a year. Because etoposide is well tolerated, children who receive it can maintain fairly normal activity during treatment. In addition, if a focal area of tumor in an area that has not previously been irradiated is involved in the recurrence, radiotherapy at 24 to 30 Gy can provide tumor control.

If the child has a recurrence after the transplant but also has normal blood counts with normal liver, kidney, and cardiac function and good performance status, we usually recommend aggressive chemotherapy. This chemotherapy may be administered either through participation in a phase I or II new-agent clinical trial or with a combination of agents with proven activity against neuroblastoma. Some children may meet the eligibility criteria for protocol therapies; however, excellent responses can be achieved with commercially available chemotherapy regimens that children may not have received previously. For all children referred for treatment of a recurrent tumor, we carefully evaluate the child's response to previous therapy, performance status, current organ function related to previous toxicity, and sites of recurrence to determine the therapy that will be most effective and least toxic. Some active second-line regimens are topotecan and cyclophosphamide; ifosfamide, carboplatin, and etoposide (ICE); and irinotecan. If the child has not yet received CRA, it can be included in a salvage regimen. Occasionally, patients may have an excellent response to first-line chemotherapy that allows administration of a second high-dose chemotherapy regimen and autologous or allogeneic stem cell rescue. A recently devised strategy is to administer an immunoablative but only a moderately myelosuppressive preparative regimen to facilitate the engraftment of donor cells. Subsequent withdrawal of graft-versus-host disease prophylaxis with or without the infusion of donor lymphocytes may confer antitumor activity. Only tumors that are not rapidly progressing are suitable for this investigative approach.

In addition to new agents, at M. D. Anderson, we previously investigated the use of anti-GD2 monoclonal antibodies and iodine-131 MIBG therapy, and some brief transient responses were achieved (Murray et al, 1994).

For any child receiving chemotherapy for treatment of a recurrent tumor, social work, child life, and other members of the mental health team provide supportive services for the child and his or her family. Because the treatment protocol for recurrent disease is usually palliative, the care provided by the mental health team is essential. After aggressive therapies, it is often difficult for parents to grasp the transition from treatment with curative intent to treatment with palliative intent.

NEUROBLASTOMA SCREENING

Opportunities and indications for prevention and early detection of childhood cancers are limited. Neuroblastoma is the most common extracranial solid tumor of early childhood, and its peak incidence occurs in early childhood. It is more common in young children than several other diseases for which screening of newborns is required by law. For example, neuroblastoma in children younger than 4 years old is twice as common as phenylketonuria and 5 to 10 times more common than galactosemia. In addition, neuroblastoma is the only childhood tumor for which a specific tumor marker is readily detectable. More than 90% of patients with neuroblastoma excrete HVA and VMA, which are easily measured in the urine by a number of quantitative and qualitative methods. Finally, as discussed earlier in this chapter, children older than 1 year with advanced-stage neuroblastoma have a dismal prognosis, even with intensive treatment, whereas children younger than 1 year old or with early-stage neuroblastoma have an excellent chance of survival with less-intensive treatment. Combined, these factors render neuroblastoma a good model for use in evaluating the feasibility of cancer screening in children. For these reasons, investigators in Japan, Europe, Canada, and the United States began mass screening programs for early detection of neuroblastoma in 6-month-old infants as a method of preventing advanced-stage, fatal neuroblastoma.

The Texas Outreach Program for Neuroblastoma Screening was initiated by M. D. Anderson to assess the feasibility of neuroblastoma screening in a United States population and to determine the best way to incorporate this or other future screening programs into the United States health system (Ater et al, 1998). The primary goal was to compare neuroblastoma screening methods for infants 5 to 10 months old, i.e., screenings administered by mail, in private physicians' offices, and in public health clinics. Texas was chosen as the ideal state in which to test the feasibility of neuroblastoma screening because of its diverse population, with respect to race, ethnicity, urban versus rural residence, and the availability of medical care.

Secondary goals were to determine the sensitivity, specificity, and positive predictive value of a monoclonal antibody enzyme-linked immunosorbent assay for HVA and VMA to detect neuroblastoma in a large population. This study was initiated in 1991 to test the methodology and feasibility of screening for neuroblastoma within the United States health care system.

Whereas we and others have been able to detect neuroblastoma in the early stages of development, follow-up data have shown that early detection does not decrease the number of advanced-stage (stage III or IV) neuroblastomas in older patients, even in countries where screening is mandatory and where participation is more than 80% (Woods, 2003). Therefore, neuroblastoma screening for infants is no longer recommended.

The biologic information gained from studying the tumors diagnosed by screening and the increased incidence of low-stage neuroblastoma at diagnosis provide further evidence that some infant neuroblastomas may spontaneously regress. We are currently working with other centers in the Children's Oncology Group on a study that prospectively follows infants diagnosed before age 3 months with a small adrenal primary and no metastatic disease who do not undergo surgery. It has been well documented that neuroblastoma in infants with stage IV-S disease regresses, thus removal of the primary is not required (Nickerson et al, 2000). Our work with the Children's Oncology Group will hopefully identify infants who do not require treatment for stage I or II neuroblastoma.

KEY PRACTICE POINTS

- Neuroblastoma can present with many different clinical signs and symptoms (Table 6-1).
- The most common primary locations are the abdominal sites in either the adrenal gland or paraspinal locations.
- Adequate staging of a child with neuroblastoma requires complete physical examination, laboratory evaluation, and radiographic studies (Table 6-3).
- Treatment and prognosis of neuroblastoma is determined on the basis of risk group; and patient age, tumor stage, and the histologic and genetic characteristics of the tumor are the most important determinants of risk group.

SUGGESTED READINGS

Ater JL, Gardner KL, Foxhall LE, Therrell BL, Bleyer WA. Neuroblastoma screening in the United States: results of the Texas Outreach Program for neuroblastoma screening. *Cancer* 1998;82:1593–1602.

Berthold F. Overview. Biology of neuroblastoma. In: Carl Pochedly, ed. *Neuroblastoma Tumor Biology and Therapy*. Boca Raton, FL: CRC Press Inc; 1990.

Chan KW, Petropoulos D, Choroszy M, et al. High-dose sequential chemotherapy and autologous stem cell reinfusion in advanced pediatric solid tumors. *Bone Marrow Transplant* 1997;20:1039–1043.

Chan LL, Ater J, Cangir A, et al. Fractionated high dose cyclophosphamide for advanced pediatric solid tumors. *J Pediatr Hematol Oncol* 1996;18:63–67.

De Roos AJ, Olshan AF, Teschke K, et al. Parental occupational exposures to chemicals and incidence of neuroblastoma in offspring. *Am J Epidemiol* 2001;154:106–114.

Maris JM, Matthay KK. Molecular biology of neuroblastoma. *J Clin Oncol* 1999;17:2264–2279.

Matthay KK, Villablanca JG, Seeger RC, et al. Treatment of high-risk neuroblastoma with intensive chemotherapy, radiotherapy, autologous bone marrow transplantation, and 13-cis-retinoic acid. *N Engl J Med* 1999;341:1165–1173.

Murray JL, Cunningham JE, Brewer H, et al. A phase I trial of murine monoclonal antibody 14G2A (Anti-GD2) given by prolonged intravenous infusion in patients with neuroectodermal tumors. *J Clin Oncol* 1994;12:184–193.

Nickerson HJ, Matthay KK, Seeger RC, et al. Favorable biology and outcome of stage IV-S neuroblastoma with supportive care or minimal therapy: a Children's Cancer Group Study. *J Clin Oncol* 2000;18:477–486.

Perez CA, Matthay KK, Atkinson JB, et al. Biological variables in the outcome of stages I and II neuroblastoma treated with surgery as primary therapy: a Children's Cancer Group Study. *J Clin Oncol* 2000;18:18–26.

Rudnick E, Khakoo Y, Antunes NL, et al. Opsoclonus-myoclonus-ataxia syndrome in neuroblastoma: clinical outcome and antineuronal antibodies—a report from the Children's Cancer Group Study. *Med Pediatr Oncol* 2001;36:612–622.

Schmidt ML, Lukens JN, Seeger RC, et al. Biologic factors determine prognosis in infants with stage IV neuroblastoma: a prospective Children's Cancer Group study. *J Clin Oncol* 2000;18:1260–1268.

Woods WG. Screening for neuroblastoma: the final chapters. *J Pediatr Hematol Oncol* 2003;25:3–4.

7   SOFT-TISSUE TUMORS

R. Beverly Raney, Richard J. Andrassy, Martin Blakely,
Tina V. Fanning, Moshe H. Maor, and John Stewart

CHAPTER OVERVIEW

Research has led to a better understanding of soft-tissue tumors and
to improvements in the multidisciplinary care of patients with rhabdomyosarcoma, nonrhabdomyosarcomatous soft-tissue sarcoma, aggressive fibromatosis, and neurofibromas. This chapter outlines the diagnostic and therapeutic strategies used at M. D. Anderson Cancer Center in
the treatment of children and adolescents with these 4 types of soft-tissue
tumors.

INTRODUCTION

The category "soft-tissue tumors" includes the malignant neoplasms rhabdomyosarcoma (RMS) and nonrhabdomyosarcomatous soft-tissue sarcoma (NRSTS) and 2 histologically benign tumor types: aggressive fibromatosis and neurofibroma. RMS and NRSTS are collectively called "sarcomas." These tumors have the propensity to metastasize to other parts of the body via lymphatic vessels, blood vessels, or both. The likelihood of metastasis varies on the basis of tumor-tissue type, which is determined microscopically and by immunohistochemical staining. The presence of abnormal chromosomes in tumor tissue can confirm or challenge a diagnosis of soft-tissue tumor and provides additional information about the likely biologic behavior of the disease.

INCIDENCE AND EPIDEMIOLOGY

Sarcoma of soft tissue is the fourth most commonly occurring malignant solid tumor in individuals younger than 20 years of age, following only brain tumors, lymphomas, and carcinomas (including melanomas) in incidence (Ries et al, 1999). RMS is the most frequently occurring soft-tissue sarcoma in the first decade of life. In the second decade of life, the incidences of RMS and NRSTS are about the same (Raney, 1987; Ries et al, 1999). The cause of cellular proliferation in soft tissue is generally unknown, although, occasionally, a patient who has undergone radiotherapy for some other condition may develop a soft-tissue or bone sarcoma in the irradiated volume (McClay, 1989). The cause of aggressive fibromatosis is also unknown. In young people, it can accompany an autosomal-dominant genetic abnormality that produces multiple gastrointestinal polyps known as familial adenomatous polyposis of the colon (Kinzler et al, 1991). Neurofibroma may occur as a single lesion in an otherwise healthy person or it may present as a single growth or multiple growths surrounding the nerves of patients with neurofibromatosis, an inheritable autosomal-dominant disorder. In pediatric practice, RMS is the most frequent soft-tissue sarcoma, followed by NRSTS; aggressive fibromatosis is uncommon. Neurofibromas are common in patients with neurofibromatosis, but the malignant neurosarcoma occurs relatively less frequently.

DISEASE HISTIOTYPES AND CHROMOSOMAL ABNORMALITIES

The ability to examine soft-tissue sarcomas for chromosomal abnormalities has broadened our knowledge of the diversity of this group of tumors and is occasionally helpful in making a specific diagnosis when microscopic and immunohistochemical results are inconclusive. The histiotype and chromosomal abnormalities of RMS and NRSTS are distinctly different.

RMS

There are 3 major subtypes of RMS. The most frequent, embryonal RMS (about 65% of cases of RMS), resembles embryonic muscle tissue on microscopic evaluation, and it occurs most commonly in young patients (from birth to 10 years of age) with the tumor arising in the head and neck and genitourinary tract. Botryoid RMS (7% to 10 % of cases of RMS) is a distinct morphologic subtype of embryonal RMS that arises in hollow organs or regions such as the bladder, vagina, or nasopharynx. Its name is derived from the Greek word for grapes, botrys, because the tumor resembles a cluster of grapes. It too occurs in young patients. The third major type of RMS is the alveolar subtype, so called because it resembles lung tissue. Alveolar RMS (about 20% of the cases of RMS) typically occurs in adolescents and appears in an extremity or on the trunk. Embryonal and botryoid RMS tumors do not have a characteristic chromosomal translocation but often show loss of heterozygosity or of imprinting in the short arm of chromosome 11. By contrast, most alveolar RMS tumors have a translocation involving chromosome 13 and either chromosome 2 or chromosome 1. Patients with the t(2;13) translocation tend to be older than 5 years of age and to have a worse prognosis than younger patients with the t(1;13) translocation (Kelly et al, 1997; Qualman et al, 1998). Many of these latter patients are younger than 5 years of age. A fourth type of RMS, pleomorphic RMS, is uncommon and occurs primarily in adults.

A common feature of all varieties of RMS is that they stain positive for vimentin and desmin on immunohistochemical studies and, although less often, for other muscle markers, such as actin, myosin, MyoD1, and myogenin. Some undifferentiated soft-tissue sarcomas (about 5% of cases of RMS) stain positive for vimentin only. Because these tumors are as aggressive as alveolar RMS, the treatment recommendations for these 2 subtypes are usually similar.

NRSTS

A large group of NRSTSs take their name from microscopically normal-appearing tissues to which they bear a similarity. In infants, the most common of these is fibrosarcoma, which is characterized by the presence of 1 or more of chromosomes 8, 11, 17, or 20 or some combination of these with or without a t(12;15) translocation. Hemangiopericytoma, another subtype of NRSTS, occasionally occurs in infants and young children. In older children and adolescents, synovial sarcoma is the most common form of NRSTS. Several translocations between the X chromosome and chromosome 18 have been described in this tumor. Other types of NRSTS typically occur more frequently in adults (21 years old or older) and include neurosarcoma, which can arise from a previous neurofibroma, especially in patients with neurofibromatosis.

Less frequently occurring NRSTSs are small round-cell tumors of the abdomen, liposarcoma, leiomyosarcoma, malignant fibrous histiocytoma, vascular sarcoma, alveolar soft-part sarcoma, clear-cell sarcoma, and epithelioid sarcoma. Abnormal chromosomes also occur frequently in these cancers.

CLINICAL PRESENTATION

Soft-tissue tumors have distinct clinical presentations with respect to age at diagnosis, site of occurrence, and other features.

RMS

The median age of children and adolescents with RMS is 6 years old. The most common sites of occurrence of RMS are the head and neck, including the orbit; genitourinary tract, including the prostate, testis, vulva, cervix, and uterus; extremities; trunk; and retroperitoneum/pelvis. Uncommon sites include the perineal/perianal region, thorax, and biliary tract. Patients with head and neck RMS usually present with a painless, enlarging mass that can obstruct a sinus, grow into the nasal cavity, cause proptosis, or simulate chronic otitis media. With more deep-seated tumors, signs and symptoms may result from compression of nerves, blocked vessels, or both; bleeding from or compression of the urinary tract or bowel; difficulty breathing; or a painless mass on the trunk or extremity. The initial suspicion of tumor should be confirmed as soon as possible by obtaining a magnetic resonance imaging (MRI) scan. As with all sarcomas, an open-incision or needle biopsy is necessary to establish a diagnosis, and tissue samples should be sent for chromosome analysis if frozen-section analyses suggest that the lesion is malignant.

NRSTS

NRSTSs are more likely than RMSs to occur in or on an extremity or the trunk, whereas internal structures are not primary sites for this tumor, and the head and neck region is not commonly involved. Patients with NRSTS are usually more than 9 years old at diagnosis. Synovial, clear-cell, and epithelioid sarcomas are often located in an extremity near joints and tendons.

Aggressive Fibromatosis and Neurofibroma

Most common among patients older than 5 years, aggressive fibromatosis and neurofibromas usually appear as isolated lesions on an extremity or the trunk. However, some infants have aggressive fibromatosis that arises in the head and neck, especially in muscles of mastication. Infants are also more likely to have multiple lesions (Chung and Enzinger, 1981).

STAGING AND DIAGNOSTIC EVALUATION

The processes used to stage and diagnose RMS, NRSTS, and aggressive fibromatosis and neurofibroma differ. Following is a description of how these tumors are evaluated.

RMS

RMS is typically a systemic disease, and it is more likely than other soft-tissue sarcomas to spread to regional lymph nodes, bone marrow, bones, distant soft tissues, and pleural or peritoneal spaces adjacent to the primary site. Common to all soft-tissue sarcomas is the propensity to spread to lung parenchyma. Therefore, the diagnostic workup for determining extent of disease includes obtaining a posteroanterior and lateral chest roentgenogram, a computed tomography (CT) scan of the chest, bone marrow aspirates, a biopsy, a total-body bone scan, and samples of cerebrospinal fluid in patients with orbital or other parameningeal tumors (such as tumors of the nasopharynx, paranasal sinuses, pterygoid/infratemporal fossa, and middle-ear/mastoid region). MRI scans of patients with craniofacial tumors should include images of the base of the brain and intracranial structures, because parameningeal RMS can grow through the base of the skull. MRI or CT scans of the abdomen and pelvis should be obtained for all patients with tumors located at or below the diaphragm to examine the liver and the retroperitoneal and pelvic lymph nodes. If fluid is seen on films or encountered at the time of biopsy in patients with intrathoracic or intra-abdominal tumors, a sample should be sent for cytologic examination. Regional lymph node sampling should be performed when possible, especially in patients with extremity, paratesticular, perineal, and truncal tumors, because there is a relatively high likelihood of nodal spread. At M. D. Anderson, the preferred approach is to use the scintigraphic sentinel lymph node mapping technique, wherein a radionuclide tracer is injected around the tumor site 1 day before the scheduled excision or re-excision, followed on the day of operation by peritumoral injection of a vital dye. The surgeon then makes an incision over the regional lymph node bed with the most radionuclide emittance and removes the node or nodes that are stained with the vital dye (Neville et al, 2000). These tests are done to determine the location of disease so that radiotherapy fields can be planned. Other examinations should include a complete blood count; a white blood cell differential analysis; liver- and renal-function tests; measurements of lactate dehydrogenase and alkaline phosphatase levels; and a urinalysis. Screening for prior exposure to varicella and cytomegalovirus (CMV) is also recommended to assess the need

Table 7–1. Intergroup Rhabdomyosarcoma Study Surgico-Pathologic
Grouping System

Group	Definition
I	Localized tumor, completely removed with pathologically clear margins and no regional lymph node involvement
II	Localized tumor, grossly removed with microscopically involved margins (subgroup A); involved, grossly resected regional lymph nodes (subgroup B); or both (subgroup C)
III	Localized, gross residual disease after incomplete removal or biopsy only
IV	Distant metastases present at initial diagnosis

Table 7–2. Intergroup Rhabdomyosarcoma Study Staging System

Stage	Primary Tumor Sites*	Tumor Size†	Regional Lymph Node Involvement	Distant Metastases
1	Orbit, non-PM, head/neck, GU nonbladder/prostate, biliary tract	Any size	N0	M0
2	All other sites	≤ 5 cm	N0	M0
3	All other sites	≤ 5 cm	N1	M0
		> 5 cm	N0 or N1	
4	Any site	Any size	N0 or N1	M1

Abbreviations: GU, genitourinary; M0, no distant metastases; M1, distant metastases at diagnosis; N0, regional nodes not clinically involved by tumor; N1, regional nodes clinically involved by tumor; PM, parameningeal.

* Favorable sites are head and neck, nonparameningeal, and orbital sites; genitourinary sites other than the bladder and prostate; and biliary tract. All other sites are considered nonfavorable.

†Widest dimension.

for varicella-zoster (VZ) immunoglobulin in nonimmune children exposed to the VZ virus and for CMV-negative blood for a transfusion.

RMSs are categorized according to the Intergroup Rhabdomyosarcoma Study (IRS) Surgico-Pathologic Grouping System and the IRS Staging System (Tables 7–1 and 7–2, respectively) to ascertain whether the patient has a low, intermediate, or high risk of tumor recurrence. Treatment is then tailored to the appropriate risk level. It is standard practice to repeat imaging studies at 2- to 4-month intervals during and after therapy and to obtain blood samples and chemistries before each course of multiple-agent chemotherapy.

NRSTS

NRSTSs may spread to regional lymph nodes, but lymphatic invasion is uncommon, except in cases of synovial and epithelioid sarcomas. The lungs are the primary sites of metastasis, whereas bone marrow disease is unusual. A bone scan is usually obtained at diagnosis but is not repeated unless there is clinical suspicion of bone disease.

Aggressive Fibromatosis and Neurofibroma
We obtain chest radiographs on initial examination. The radiographs are
occasionally repeated along with an MRI or other imaging studies of the
primary tumor region at 4- to 12-month intervals.

TREATMENT

The treatments for RMS, NRSTS, and aggressive fibromatosis and neurofibroma differ based on the distinct features of these tumors. The treatments
found most effective at M. D. Anderson are described here.

RMS
Before the widespread use of multiple-agent chemotherapy protocols for
treatment of RMS, recurrent disease developed in 70% to 80% of patients
treated with surgery, radiotherapy, or both and was often accompanied by
metastatic deposits in the lungs. Patients eventually died of the disease.
In 1972, the National Cancer Institute approved the first of 5 major IRS
protocols (IRS-I through -V) for children and adolescents younger than
21 years of age who were newly diagnosed with RMS or undifferentiated
soft-tissue sarcoma. Since then, nearly 5,000 patients have been enrolled in
these studies and followed for assessment of response, event-free survival,
and overall survival. Several important lessons regarding the biology and
treatment of these diseases have been learned and documented (Raney
et al, 2001). This body of information is the largest available systematically collected documentation of experience managing young people with
RMS and undifferentiated soft-tissue sarcoma. At M. D. Anderson, we
follow the guidelines outlined in these protocols and continue to enroll
patients in studies whenever possible to facilitate further treatment improvements.
    The multidisciplinary RMS team at M. D. Anderson consists of pedi-
atric oncologists, pediatric and other surgeons (orthopedists, neurosurgeons, otolaryngologists, urologists, and plastic and reconstructive surgeons), dentists, diagnostic and interventional radiologists, pathologists,
radiation oncologists, other medical subspecialists, nurses, nurse practitioners, physician assistants, psychiatrists, psychologists, child-life workers, school teachers, and others as appropriate. Each member of the team
plays an important role in ensuring the best outcome for a patient and in
providing the best environment in which the patient can receive appropriate treatment and the family can receive support.
    Because multimodal treatment has produced the best results, we will
summarize our approach to managing patients with soft-tissue tumors
using RMS as the model. General principles will be reviewed first,

followed by specifics of the current protocols with respect to risk groups and prognosis.

Surgery

Table 7–1 shows the Surgico-Pathologic Grouping System that has been used since its initiation during the IRS trials, which began in 1972. The extent of disease at the time of initiation of chemotherapy is important in predicting outcome (Raney et al, 2001). Thus, when it is possible to remove a localized primary tumor completely (Group I) or grossly with only microscopic residual disease remaining (Group II), the patient has a better prognosis than when a gross tumor is left in place (Group III) or when there is distant metastatic disease in lungs, bone marrow, bones, or elsewhere (Group IV) (Crist et al, 1995; Crist et al, 2001). When cancer has not been suspected initially and the primary site is situated such that a wide local excision can be done, it is wise to remove the residual tumor, which will reduce the likelihood of local recurrence and decrease the amount of radiation that may be needed. However, in many situations, it is unwise or unacceptable functionally or cosmetically to attempt complete removal of the tumor at diagnosis. This is particularly true for tumors of the head and neck, where the usual approach is to obtain a biopsy for diagnosis and for other studies (e.g., chromosome and molecular biologic assays) followed by chemotherapy and radiotherapy.

Detailed surgical guidelines for treating tumors at the major primary sites are available in the current protocols. In general, surgical removal, if feasible before beginning chemotherapy, is recommended, along with sentinel lymph node biopsy for lesions arising in the extremities, trunk, and perineum. Large, deep-seated tumors arising in the chest, retroperitoneum, and pelvis are often so invasive of vital structures, such as major vessels and nerves, that biopsy is the preferred initial surgical procedure. The surgeon may then consider performing a delayed primary excision after the tumor has shrunk following several weeks of chemotherapy. The usual approach for patients with tumors of the orbit and bladder-prostate region is also biopsy followed by chemotherapy and radiotherapy in order to preserve the organs. Functional impairments, such as cataracts or diminished bladder capacity, can often be alleviated later. Boys with paratesticular sarcoma have a relatively high likelihood of regional spread of tumor to the draining lymph nodes in the ipsilateral renal hilum and along the para-aortic–caval chains and iliac nodes, especially if they are 10 years of age or older. Imaging studies are not reliable in distinguishing node-positive disease from node-negative disease, because small nodes may contain tumor cells and large ones may be reactive following the orchidectomy. Currently, an ipsilateral, nerve-sparing retroperitoneal lymph node dissection is recommended for boys 10 years old and older. If no nodal disease is found on pathologic examination, radiotherapy is withheld (Wiener et al, 2001).

Radiotherapy

Radiotherapy should be given to patients who have residual disease when chemotherapy is started. An exception is made for patients who have a completely resected Group I tumor in which the histologic subtype is alveolar RMS or undifferentiated soft-tissue sarcoma. These patients have a decreased incidence of local recurrence when postoperative radiotherapy alone is given to the tumor bed (Wolden et al, 1999). The radiotherapy dose is graduated according to the amount of tumor remaining and may be modified according to the volume of involvement. For example, a large volume, such as the whole abdomen or pleural space, will not tolerate the daily doses (usually 1.8 Gy per dose) that can be given to smaller volumes. The radiation oncologist will also treat a 2-cm margin of surrounding normal tissue to cover microscopic extension from the borders of the tumor, as determined by preoperative imaging studies, by the surgeon, or by both when gross tumor resection has been accomplished. Typically, for patients with gross residual disease, radiotherapy is delayed until chemotherapy has been given for 12 weeks, unless there is spinal cord compression or meningeal involvement by tumor at a cranial parameningeal site. In such a case, radiotherapy should be started within 2 weeks after initiation of chemotherapy (Raney et al, 2002). Patients who have microscopic residual disease may begin radiotherapy earlier; there is no advantage to delaying it. A recently completed IRS randomized trial of conventional, once-daily radiotherapy versus twice-daily, hyperfractionated radiotherapy for patients with gross residual disease showed no advantage of the twice-daily regimen (Donaldson et al, 2001); thus, patients are now being treated by conventional methods. At M. D. Anderson, we use conformal radiotherapy to optimize dose to the tumor volume and reduce dose to normal tissues (Michalski et al, 1995).

Chemotherapy

The efficacy of multiple-agent chemotherapy for patients with RMS was established nearly 30 years ago by investigators with the Children's Cancer Group (Heyn et al, 1974). Since then, several combinations of agents have been added to the generally accepted VAC regimen (vincristine, actinomycin D, and cyclophosphamide) in an attempt to increase disease control and survival (Crist et al, 1995; Crist et al, 2001). However, VAC remains the gold standard for patients with intermediate or high risk of disease recurrence. Injections of granulocyte colony- stimulating factor (G-CSF or filgrastim) or pegfilgrastim are given subcutaneously to support the white blood cell count and reduce the risk of neutropenic fever. Patients with a low risk of disease recurrence are usually treated with vincristine and actinomycin D without cyclophosphamide to avoid the risks of myelosuppression, bladder damage, and infertility, all of which are associated with cyclophosphamide.

Data from the IRS-III and -IV protocols (Crist et al, 1995; Crist et al, 2001) have indicated that categorizing patients on the basis of tumor histologic type, surgico-pathologic group, and stage could produce risk groups with nonoverlapping predictors of failure-free survival (FFS) rate and overall survival rate. As shown in Table 7–2, tumor stage is determined by site (favorable versus unfavorable), widest diameter (5 cm or smaller versus larger than 5 cm) of the primary tumor, and presence or absence of metastases. Regional lymph node spread is designated as N1 disease, and distant metastases are designated as M1 disease.

The IRS-V protocol is led by members of the Soft-Tissue Sarcoma Committee of the Children's Oncology Group (COG), which succeeded the IRS. Patients in the low-risk category are estimated to have an FFS rate of 88% at 3 years. These patients have localized, embryonal histologic tumors of any size at favorable sites (head and neck, nonparameningeal, and orbital sites; genitourinary sites other than the bladder and prostate; and biliary tract tumors) or localized and grossly resected (Groups I and II) embryonal tumors at unfavorable sites (all other sites). In patients with intermediate-risk disease, the FFS rate ranges from 55% to 76% at 3 years. This includes patients with any histology and localized tumors at unfavorable sites with gross residual disease (Group III) as well as all patients with localized tumors (Groups I, II, and III) of alveolar RMS or undifferentiated soft-tissue sarcoma. The intermediate-risk group also includes children younger than 10 years old with embryonal RMS and distant metastases. Patients in the high-risk group have an FFS rate of less than 30% at 3 years. This group includes all patients from birth to 50 years of age with distant metastases and alveolar RMS or undifferentiated soft-tissue sarcoma in addition to all patients with embryonal RMS and metastases who are 10 to 50 years of age.

The patients at lowest risk, those in subgroup A, receive vincristine and actinomycin D with or without radiotherapy, depending on the presence or absence of residual tumor. Patients at low risk (subgroup B) have somewhat more advanced disease and are treated with VAC and radiotherapy. Patients in subgroups A and B have been entered on the recently closed COG D9602 protocol. Patients in the intermediate-risk group may be entered on the ongoing COG D9803 protocol in which they may receive topotecan by random assignment in addition to VAC and radiotherapy. Topotecan was selected in an attempt to increase the FFS rate and the overall survival rate of these patients on the basis of its efficacy in a previous IRS trial (Pappo et al, 2001). Patients on that protocol had distant metastases at diagnosis and initially received topotecan as a single agent; this was called the "up-front window" approach. The drug was active and produced more tumor shrinkage in patients with alveolar RMS than in patients with embryonal RMS or undifferentiated soft-tissue sarcoma (Pappo et al, 2001). For patients with high-risk disease, the COG has been studying, in the D9802 protocol, the efficacy of an up-front window approach using irinotecan plus vincristine, because irinotecan may be more active in patients with the aggressive forms of the disease (Cosetti et al, 2002). The efficacy of the chemotherapeutic up-front window approach is assessed at week 5 after 2 cycles of treatment. Patients who have at least 50% shrinkage of tumor at that time will continue to receive irinotecan plus vincristine alternated with VAC, whereas those with an inferior response to irinotecan plus vincristine receive further cycles of VAC without irinotecan. Radiotherapy is also given to all patients with intermediate-risk and high-risk disease.

NRSTS

As a group, NRSTSs are considered less sensitive to chemotherapy and radiotherapy than RMSs. Surgical removal is the mainstay of treatment, especially for local control. The general principles outlined above for RMS apply for NRSTS with regard to wide local re-excision, assessing regional lymph node spread, and determining whether there is distant metastatic disease at diagnosis. Perhaps the best-studied NRSTS in young people is synovial sarcoma, which is relatively common in the second decade of life and has recently been reviewed by several researchers. Results from our own series of 44 patients (Okçu et al, 2001) and from a meta-analysis of 219 previously untreated patients younger than 21 years of age at diagnosis treated at M. D. Anderson, St. Jude Children's Research Hospital (Memphis, TN), and research hospitals in Germany and Italy (Okçu et al, 2003) suggest that chemotherapy is not very useful in preventing distant metastases in patients with apparently localized disease. On the other hand, radiotherapy for patients who appear to have no microscopic residual tumor after re-excision may improve the likelihood of local control (Okçu et al, 2001; Okçu et al, 2003). Thus, our current approach is to first remove gross disease whenever possible without major cosmetic or functional limitations; decide whether to apply radiotherapy to the local site, especially if the tumor is larger than 5 cm at widest dimension; and then watch closely for the appearance of local recurrence or distant metastases in the lungs.

We often present the clinical, radiologic, surgical, and pathological details of our soft-tissue sarcoma patients at our weekly Pediatric Tumor Conference, which is attended by all members of the multidisciplinary team. The goal of the meeting is to determine the best plan of treatment for patients and to review previous experience with a unique disease presentation. We also commonly present pertinent details of our NRSTS patients at the M. D. Anderson multidisciplinary Adult Sarcoma Conference, because such tumors are more common in older patients, and oncologists who care for older patients have more experience in following the evolution of this patient group. Currently, the preferred chemotherapeutic approach for treatment of NRSTS is a combination of doxorubicin and ifosfamide with mesna and G-CSF support, with the addition of radiotherapy as indicated.

Aggressive Fibromatosis and Neurofibroma

A locally infiltrative disease, aggressive fibromatosis has a tendency to recur despite multiple surgical attempts to cure it; however, it can often be controlled locally with moderately large doses of radiotherapy (in the range of 55 Gy). The difficulty is that many pediatric patients have not achieved adult size, and multiple operations, radiotherapy treatments, or a combination of these may produce a deformity that is not concealable. Thus, standard chemotherapy regimens, such as VAC, dacarbazine and doxorubicin or vinblastine and methotrexate, have been used over the years (Ayala et al, 1986; Raney et al, 1987; Skapek et al, 1998). Other approaches include antiestrogen agents such as tamoxifen and cyclo-oxygenase inhibitors such as sulindac (Izes et al, 1996). In about 50% of cases, 1 or more of these combinations can cause cessation of tumor growth while allowing the child to grow, eventually reducing the amount of tissue that must be removed relative to surrounding structures. Treatment options should be individualized according to the clinical situation, taking into account any prior attempts to achieve local control.

Unfortunately, there is no evidence that chemotherapeutic agents or radiotherapy can shrink neurofibromas, which are often large and occur in multiples in patients with neurofibromatosis. Thus, therapy for neurofibroma is currently limited to surgical removal. Advances in gene therapy may eventually give us better tools to combat neurofibromatosis and the accompanying neoplasms.

MANAGEMENT OF RELAPSE

For patients with chemotherapy-sensitive tumors, there are alternatives to standard VAC therapy for RMS and to standard doxorubicin plus ifosfamide for NRSTS. We typically perform a biopsy to confirm the presence of recurrent disease and initiate chemotherapy with the current COG protocol or with a combination of ifosfamide, doxorubicin, and etoposide for children with recurrent RMS. For patients with recurrent NRSTS, gemcitabine plus docetaxel may be useful. Another agent being studied at M. D. Anderson is lipo-vincristine, which is a new formulation of a known active drug that can sometimes retard the growth of recurrent soft-tissue sarcomas in young patients. We also have access to other new agents as a member of the COG, which is investigating a variety of chemical and biologic agents under the auspices of the National Cancer Institute. As these trials mature, numerous new drug combinations and therapeutic strategies will be introduced, such as gene therapy and targeted agents, including antiangiogenesis factors and biologic response modifiers.

Although the prognosis for young patients with recurrent cancer is generally poor, there is always hope for prolonging life in a meaningful and humane manner by attempting other forms of therapy, provided the patient and family agree to trying methods of controlling the disease that are still under investigation. When active interventions with drugs, biologic agents, radiotherapy, and surgery are no longer possible, our objectives change to providing palliative care to keep the patient comfortable for as long as possible and providing support for family members.

KEY PRACTICE POINTS

- Chemotherapy and often radiotherapy are necessary for successful treatment of RMS.
- Surgery to remove the gross disease and often radiotherapy are necessary for successful treatment of NRSTS. The role of chemotherapy is being explored.
- Surgical removal is also the mainstay of therapy for patients with aggressive fibromatosis. Sometimes neurofibromas need to be excised. Chemotherapy, radiotherapy, or both may benefit patients with aggressive fibromatosis, but these treatments are ineffective in patients with neurofibromas.

SUGGESTED READINGS

Ayala AG, Ro JY, Goepfert H, et al. Desmoid fibromatosis: a clinicopathologic study of 25 children. *Semin Diagn Pathol* 1986;3:138–150.

Chung EB, Enzinger FM. Infantile myofibromatosis. *Cancer* 1981;48:1807–1818.

Cosetti M, Wexler LH, Calleja E, et al. Irinotecan for pediatric solid tumors: The Memorial Sloan-Kettering experience. *J Pediatr Hematol Oncol* 2002;24:101–105.

Crist W, Gehan EA, Ragab AH, et al. The Third Intergroup Rhabdomyosarcoma Study. *J Clin Oncol* 1995;13:610–630.

Crist WM, Anderson JR, Meza JL, et al. Intergroup Rhabdomyosarcoma Study-IV: results for patients with nonmetastatic disease. *J Clin Oncol* 2001;19:3091–3102.

Donaldson SS, Meza J, Breneman JC, et al. Results from the IRS-IV randomized trial of hyperfractionated radiotherapy in children with rhabdomyosarcoma—A report from the IRSG. *Int J Radiat Oncol Biol Phys* 2001;51:718–728.

Heyn RM, Holland R, Newton WA, Jr, et al. The role of combined chemotherapy in the treatment of rhabdomyosarcoma in children. *Cancer* 1974;34:2128–2142.

Izes JK, Zinman LN, Larsen CR. Regression of large pelvic desmoid tumor by tamoxifen and sulindac. *Urology* 1996;47:756–759.

Kelly KM, Womer RB, Sorensen PHB, et al. Common and variant gene fusions predict distinct clinical phenotypes in rhabdomyosarcoma. *J Clin Oncol* 1997;15:1831–1836.

Kinzler KW, Nilbert MC, Su LK, et al. Identification of FAP locus genes from chromosome 5q21. *Science* 1991;253:661–665.

McClay EF. Epidemiology of bone and soft tissue sarcomas. *Semin Oncol* 1989;16:264–272.

Michalski JM, Sur RK, Harms WB, et al. Three-dimensional conformal radiation therapy in pediatric parameningeal rhabdomyosarcomas. *Int J Radiat Oncol Biol Phys* 1995;33:985–991.

Neville HL, Andrassy RJ, Lally KP, et al. Lymphatic mapping with sentinel node biopsy in pediatric patients. *J Pediatr Surg* 2000;35:961–964.

Okçu MF, Despa S, Choroszy M, et al. Synovial sarcoma in children and adolescents: thirty three years of experience with multimodal therapy. *Med Pediatr Oncol* 2001;37:90–96.

Okçu MF, Munsell M, Treuner J, et al. Synovial sarcoma of childhood and adolescence: a multicenter, multivariate analysis of outcome. *J Clin Oncol* 2003; 21:1602–1611.

Pappo AS, Lyden E, Breneman J, et al. Up-front window trial of topotecan in previously untreated children and adolescents with metastatic rhabdomyosarcoma: An Intergroup Rhabdomyosarcoma Study. *J Clin Oncol* 2001;19:213–219.

Qualman SJ, Coffin CM, Newton WA, et al. Intergroup Rhabdomyosarcoma Study: Update for pathologists. *Pediatr Dev Pathol* 1998;1:463–474.

Raney B. Soft-tissue sarcoma in adolescents. In: Tebbi CK, ed. *Major Topics in Adolescent Oncology.* Mount Kisco, NY: Futura Publishing Company, Inc; 1987: 221–240.

Raney B, Evans A, Granowetter L, et al. Nonsurgical management of children with recurrent or unresectable fibromatosis. *Pediatrics* 1987;79:394–398.

Raney RB, Maurer HM, Anderson JR, et al. The Intergroup Rhabdomyosarcoma Study Group (IRSG): major lessons from the IRS-I through IRS-IV studies as background for the current IRS-V treatment protocols. *Sarcoma* 2001;5:9–15.

Raney RB, Meza J, Anderson JR, et al. Treatment of children and adolescents with localized parameningeal sarcoma: experience of the Intergroup Rhabdomyosarcoma Study Group Protocols IRS-II through -IV, 1978–1997. *Med Pediatr Oncol* 2002;38:22–32.

Ries LAG, Smith MA, Gurney JG, et al. Cancer Incidence and Survival Among Children and Adolescents. Bethesda, MD: National Institutes of Health, National Cancer Institute; 1999. Report No.: NIH-NCI-99–4649.

Skapek SX, Hawk BJ, Hoffer FA, et al. Combination chemotherapy using vinblastine and methotrexate for the treatment of progressive desmoid tumor in children. *J Clin Oncol* 1998;16:3021–3027.

Wiener ES, Anderson JR, Ojimba JI, et al. Controversies in the management of paratesticular rhabdomyosarcoma: is staging retroperitoneal lymph node dissection necessary for adolescents with resected paratesticular rhabdomyosarcoma? *Semin Pediatr Surg* 2001;10:146–152.

Wolden SL, Anderson JR, Crist WM, et al. Indications for radiotherapy and chemotherapy after complete resection in rhabdomyosarcoma: a report from the Intergroup Rhabdomyosarcoma Studies I to III. *J Clin Oncol* 1999;17:3468–3475.

8   OSTEOSARCOMA

Norman Jaffe and Margaret G. Pearson

CHAPTER OVERVIEW

At M. D. Anderson Cancer Center, intra-arterial cisplatin, intravenous doxorubicin, high-dose methotrexate, and ifosfamide constitute the mainstay of treatment for children with osteosarcoma. Limb salvage or amputation is performed to extirpate the primary tumor. To achieve cure in patients with pulmonary metastases, surgical intervention is required in addition to chemotherapy.

INTRODUCTION

Malignant bone tumors are relatively rare in the pediatric age groups. Each year in the United States, these tumors constitute approximately 2% to 4%

of all malignancies in children 14 years old and younger and approximately 6.6% of all malignancies in adolescents 15 to 19 years old. Osteosarcoma is the most common type of bone tumor in these patients, and Ewing's sarcoma is the second most common.

ETIOLOGY

The etiology of osteosarcoma is unknown, but a relationship to growth may exist, because the tumor is encountered more commonly in preteens and teenagers than in younger children. The boy-to-girl ratio for this disease is 2 to 1. Osteosarcoma has been known to occur as a late complication of radiotherapy and in older patients with Paget's disease of the bone. It has also been associated with fibrous dysplasia, bone infarction, osteochondroma, and osteoblastoma. In patients with the hereditary form of retinoblastoma, osteosarcoma occurs much more frequently than in the general population and may occur in previously irradiated bone as well as at sites remote from the irradiated area.

Osteosarcoma occurs most often in the distal femur, followed by the proximal tibia and then the humerus. Less common sites of involvement include the fibula, iliac bone, vertebrae, and the bones of the hands and feet. Osteosarcoma of the jaw occurs more commonly in adults than in children and carries a more favorable prognosis than do such tumors at other sites.

CLINICAL MANIFESTATIONS

Most patients with bone tumors experience pain at the site of the lesion. The pain is usually accompanied by local swelling and a localized increase in temperature. Generally, the affected joint has reduced range of motion. Occasionally, patients and their parents attribute the cause to trauma. However, in almost every case, the tumor occurred first, and the traumatic incident drew attention to it.

HISTOLOGIC VARIETIES

The predominant histologic varieties of osteosarcoma are the conventional and the surface types. Within these categories, additional subtypes have been identified.

Conventional Osteosarcoma

Three primary subtypes of conventional osteosarcoma have been described on the basis of the predominant differentiation of tumor cells. Osteoblastic osteosarcoma is characterized by an abundant production of osteoid and accounts for approximately 50% of all cases of conventional osteosarcoma. Chondroblastic and fibroblastic osteosarcoma each account for approximately 25% of cases. The presence of osteoid in the latter 2 subtypes distinguishes them from chondrosarcoma and fibrosarcoma. Telangiectatic osteosarcoma is a rare variant of conventional osteosarcoma. Less common varieties include small- or round-cell types and a related condition called malignant fibrous histiocytoma.

Surface Osteosarcoma

Two types of surface osteosarcoma are commonly recognized: periosteal and parosteal. The periosteal form usually has a fair amount of cartilage. Many of the surface osteosarcomas have a slow growth rate, and they can usually be treated by wide local excision without additional adjuvant chemotherapy. The burden of diagnosis and of determining whether characteristics of tumor proliferation are present (which will influence therapy) usually rest with the pathologist. Occasionally, a more aggressive tumor may be encountered. In this circumstance, pre- and postoperative chemotherapy is administered. Surface osteosarcomas may occasionally be confused with traumatic periostitis and myositis ossificans.

BIOLOGIC BEHAVIOR

The biologic behavior of osteosarcoma is consistent with the premise that pulmonary micrometastases are present in at least 80% to 90% of patients at diagnosis. In the past, treatment of osteosarcoma generally involved amputation, which was performed in the absence of overt radiologic evidence of pulmonary metastases; however, metastases invariably surfaced 6 to 9 months later and thus were obviously preexistent. In the absence of effective treatment for metastases (chemotherapy, surgery, or a combination of these treatments is currently used), metastatic disease was usually the cause of the patient's death. These findings form the basis for current investigations and treatment of osteosarcoma.

DIAGNOSTIC INVESTIGATIONS

On suspicion of a malignant bone tumor, several investigations should be conducted. The primary lesion should be examined radiographically with anteroposterior, posteroanterior, medial, and lateral views taken. In osteosarcoma, radiography is able to demonstrate osteoblastic and lytic lesions, involvement of the cortex, and elevation of the periosteum (Codman's triangle). In addition, infiltration into the soft tissue with an osteoid matrix may be observed. Occasionally, a pathologic fracture may be present. Once osteosarcoma of the bone is established, additional studies are required, including a computed tomography (CT) scan of the chest and a radionuclide bone scan to search for pulmonary and bone metastases, respectively. To assess whether the patient is a candidate for a limb-salvage procedure, nuclear magnetic resonance imaging and, occasionally, a CT scan of the primary tumor will be requested. The entire bone must be visualized to rule out a skipped metastasis. Positron emission tomography is now being investigated as a tool for use in evaluating tumor response to chemotherapy before surgery.

Definitive Diagnosis

Pathologic examination of the tumor is required to establish a diagnosis. At M. D. Anderson, needle biopsy is used to help diagnose the tumor. With cytologic examination, the diagnosis may be revealed immediately after the biopsy. However, pathologic core biopsies are usually obtained concurrently to confirm the diagnosis and characterize the tumor's exact histologic variety, which may be osteoblastic, telangiectatic, chondroblastic, fibroblastic, small- or round-cell type, periosteal or parosteal, or malignant fibrous histiocytoma. It is not unusual to see an osteosarcoma with a mixed histology.

Treatment for Primary Disease

After the diagnosis and extent of disease have been established, a treatment strategy is developed and presented to the patient and the family in a meeting attended by medical and paramedical team members. The patient and the family are advised that optimum treatment involves an integrated multidisciplinary approach. Patients are usually treated with curative intent. The strategy involves the use of preoperative chemotherapy followed by surgical extirpation of the tumor and postoperative chemotherapy. When lung metastases are present, additional surgical procedures, generally a median sternotomy or bilateral thoracotomies, will be performed to extirpate overt disease after preoperative chemotherapy.

Chemotherapy

The following chemotherapeutic agents have shown activity in osteosarcoma: high-dose methotrexate with folinic acid (known as "leucovorin rescue"), doxorubicin, cisplatin, ifosfamide, and cyclophosphamide. These agents, when used in combination, have produced response rates between 80% and 100% in many primary tumors. These chemotherapy

Doxorubicin and Cisplatin

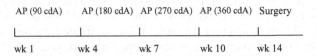

Figure 8–1. Initial therapeutic regimen. Doxorubicin (90 mg/m^2 intravenously over 48 hours) and cisplatin (120 mg/m^2 intra-arterially over 4 hours) are administered at 3- to 4-week intervals, with each course commencing on day 1. After the fourth course (cumulative dose of doxorubicin = 360 mg/m^2), surgical extirpation of the tumor is performed (week 14 to 16). Pathologic evaluation of the tumor is performed, and further treatment is determined on the basis of extent of tumor necrosis. See Figures 8–2 and 8–3. Abbreviations: A, doxorubicin; cdA, cumulative dose of doxorubicin; P, cisplatin.

combinations are currently used as pre- and postoperative (adjuvant) therapy to destroy macroscopic and microscopic disease. Preoperative chemotherapy is also referred to as "neoadjuvant" or "primary" chemotherapy.

Preoperative Intra-Arterial Chemotherapy

Intra-arterial administration of cisplatin has been shown to be highly effective in treating primary osteosarcoma at M. D. Anderson. Such treatment also provides systemic tumoricidal concentrations of cisplatin that can destroy pulmonary micrometastases. On the basis of this observation, our current treatment approach is to administer intra-arterial cisplatin at a dose of 120 mg/m^2 over 4 hours accompanied by intravenous doxorubicin at a dose of 90 mg/m^2 over 48 hours. Four such courses are administered at 3- to 4-week intervals (Figure 8–1). It is anticipated that more than 90% of tumors treated with this regimen will respond, facilitating optimum surgical extirpation of the tumor, which may involve amputation or a limb-salvage procedure.

Postoperative Chemotherapy

After surgical resection of the tumor, pathologic examination of the resected specimen is performed. In patients in whom more than 95% tumor destruction has been attained (called "good responders"), the outlook is considered favorable, and 2 courses of postoperative cisplatin plus doxorubicin are administered intravenously (using the same dose and schedule as for preoperative chemotherapy) (Figure 8–2). Alternatively, if there is 95% or less tumor destruction, the possibility for the development of pulmonary metastases increases. Therefore, postoperative treatment will comprise ifosfamide plus high-dose methotrexate. This regimen involves 3 courses of ifosfamide (14 g/m^2/course) administered at 3- to 4-week intervals

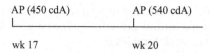

wk 17   wk 20

Figure 8–2. Therapeutic regimen for good responders (greater than 95% tumor necrosis). Postoperatively, good responders (patients in whom 95% tumor necrosis is achieved) receive 2 courses of doxorubicin (90 mg/m² /course) intravenously over 48 hours with 2 courses of cisplatin (120 mg/m² /course) intravenously over 4 hours. The first dose is administered at approximately week 17 and the second at approximately week 20. No further therapy is given. Observation is then implemented as outlined in Table 8–1. Abbreviations: A, doxorubicin; cdA, cumulative dose of doxorubicin; P, cisplatin.

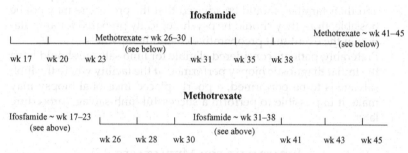

Figure 8–3. Therapeutic regimen for poor responders (95% or less tumor necrosis). Patients in whom a good response to initial therapy is not achieved receive ifosfamide (2 mg/m² intravenously every 12 hours for 7 doses) and high-dose methotrexate (12.5 mg/m² intravenously over 4 hours) with folinic acid rescue to commence at 24 hours until the methotrexate level is 0.3 μmol/L or less. Ifosfamide is administered every 3 weeks. High-dose methotrexate is administered every 10 to 14 days.

followed by 3 courses of high-dose methotrexate (12.5 g/m² /course) at 10- to 14-day intervals (Figure 8–3). The ifosfamide-methotrexate regimen is then repeated for a total of 6 courses each.

Surgery

All patients are candidates for amputation; however, with the success of adjuvant chemotherapy, particularly as administered in the preoperative phase, 60% to 80% of patients are generally rendered eligible for limb salvage. Limb salvage usually involves en-bloc resection of the tumor and the insertion of an internal metal prosthesis. Alternatively, an allograft or autograft (generally from the fibula) may be used.

The following criteria are used to determine eligibility for limb salvage.

- The procedure must be surgically feasible; the most important vessels and nerves must be preserved.

- A patient with a lower-extremity tumor should have reached maximum or near-maximum growth to avoid a limb discrepancy with
  growth in the contralateral limb.
- For patients who have not achieved maximum or near-maximum
  growth, an expandable internal prosthesis may be considered. In
  such a circumstance, lengthening procedures will be performed at
  periodic intervals.
- If the surgery is feasible, patients with upper-extremity lesions are
  usually considered eligible; however, an expandable prosthesis will
  probably be necessary for patients who have not reached maximum
  or near-maximum growth.
- During the administration of preoperative chemotherapy, patients
  and their families should be advised that the procedure may not be
  possible; thus, they should be psychologically prepared for amputation in the event that preoperative chemotherapy fails.
- Preferably, patients considered eligible for limb salvage should have
  the initial diagnostic biopsy performed at the facility where the limb
  salvage is to be performed; a poorly placed incisional biopsy may
  make it impossible to perform a successful limb-salvage procedure
  later.

TREATMENT FOR METASTASES

The treatment of pulmonary metastases and of resistant and recurrent disease requires special considerations and treatment options that differentiate their management from that of primary osteosarcomas.

Pulmonary Metastases

Postoperative ifosfamide alternated with high-dose methotrexate is administered to patients in whom overt pulmonary metastases develop after initial treatment with cisplatin and doxorubicin. Interposed between
the postoperative adjuvant therapies, surgical resection of the pulmonary
metastases is performed. The surgical procedure may involve a median
sternotomy or bilateral thoracotomies. The timing of the surgical procedures and chemotherapy is dictated by how well the metastases respond
to treatment; response is determined by conventional chest radiography
and CT.

Resistant or Recurrent Metastases

Patients who have recurrent or resistant pulmonary metastases generally
require surgical resection for cure; however, before the surgical procedure,
investigational or higher-dose conventional therapy is usually administered. Surgical resection is performed only if there is no evidence of extra-
pulmonary disease. The goal is always to conserve as much healthy lung
tissue as possible.

Investigational Therapies

Liposomal muramyl tripeptide phosphatidylethanolamine has been investigated at M. D. Anderson and appears to be somewhat successful. The approach was further explored in a nationwide trial. The results of the investigation are currently being analyzed. In the interim, the agent is no longer available for investigation or treatment.

Investigations in animals are also being conducted to determine whether inhalation techniques may prevent or eradicate pulmonary metastases. Clinical studies with this approach have recently been initiated.

SIDE EFFECTS AND COMPLICATIONS
OF CHEMOTHERAPY

Most chemotherapeutic agents cause nausea, vomiting, and a reduction in blood-cell count. Antiemetics are provided to prevent nausea and vomiting during chemotherapy, but patients may need to continue using antiemetics after being discharged from the hospital, especially following therapy with cisplatin, which is associated with prolonged nausea and vomiting. Patients may also need to be evaluated for dehydration after completion of chemotherapy if they are not taking adequate oral hydration secondary to nausea or if they continue vomiting. Adequate hydration is critical in patients receiving nephrotoxic chemotherapy (e.g., cisplatin, methotrexate, or ifosfamide). When the nausea and vomiting are not well controlled, intravenous hydration may be required, and it can frequently be implemented in an outpatient setting.

Inadequate nutrition is another hazard associated with prolonged nausea, vomiting, and mucositis, and all of these conditions are associated primarily with doxorubicin and cisplatin. For a few patients, treatment for inadequate nutrition requires support from a dietician. Frequently, the first step is to add a dieitary supplement (e.g., Boost) or to explore methods of adding calories and protein to the patient's preferred diet. Occasionally, patients require temporary placement of a gastrostomy tube to attain adequate nutritional support.

After each course of therapy (particularly cisplatin, doxorubicin, and ifosfamide), granulocyte colony-stimulating factor is generally administered to prevent depression of the white blood-cell count. Sulfamethoxazole or another antibiotic is prescribed to prevent infection. These measures may not be successful, and on occasion, patients are admitted to the hospital for fever and neutropenia, which usually occur 10 to 14 days after administration of the chemotherapy. Blood and platelet support may also be required. Patients and parents are advised that they should report to the hospital if a complication is suspected or if the patient's temperature is in the vicinity of 101.5°F degrees or 38.3°C.

Loss of hearing, especially in the high-frequency range, occurs in nearly all children treated with cisplatin. It is our practice to perform baseline audiography before starting treatment and to repeat the study after completion of cisplatin therapy. At any point, if the child or a parent reports significant changes in the child's hearing, a reevaluation should be performed. Some children require hearing aids. In our experience, young children whose speech and language skills are at an early stage of development at the time of treatment benefit more from hearing aids than do older children. Older patients seem to prefer using other strategies to compensate for hearing loss, e.g., lip reading.

Cardiomyopathy leading to cardiac failure is a potential risk after treatment with anthracyclines. Using safeguards during the administration of anthracyclines—such as monitoring cardiac function on a regular basis during and after treatment, administering cardiotoxic drugs over a period of more than 24 hours, and limiting the lifetime cumulative dose—has become routine for minimizing the risk of cardiomyopathy and cardiac failure. In some centers, cardioprotective agents are also administered. Because this side effect may occur many years after completion of therapy, patients and their primary physicians need to be aware of its risk.

Renal toxicity resulting from treatment with cisplatin, methotrexate, and ifosfamide is well known. Careful monitoring of renal function, adequate hydration, and alkalization of urine are used to prevent renal failure. We routinely prescribe calcium and magnesium supplements when cisplatin therapy is initiated. Later, as the therapy progresses, many patients also require potassium and phosphorus supplements, particularly after treatment with ifosfamide.

Reproductive functioning can also be adversely affected by chemotherapy. Both cyclophosphamide and ifosfamide have a high probability of inducing sterility in boys. It is unclear whether the risk is reduced in prepubescent boys compared with older boys. In teenage boys and young men, we suggest that the patient consider sperm conservation. Unfortunately, at this time, health insurance does not cover the cost of this procedure.

FOLLOW-UP

Pulmonary metastases and local recurrence may occur during or after completion of therapy. The follow-up schedule used at M. D. Anderson is outlined in Table 8–1. Pre- and postoperative chemotherapy and surgical extirpation of the primary tumor yield an actuarial disease-free survival rate of 60% to 65% in patients in whom pulmonary metastases do not develop. This survival rate is promising when compared with that of historical controls for whom the survival rate rarely exceeded 20%. Approximately 60% to 80% of patients are also considered for or rendered eligible to undergo a limb-salvage procedure. The survival rate of patients in whom metastasis is present or in whom it develops ranges from 15% to 25%.

Table 8–1. Frequency of Follow-up Examinations Starting 2 Years after Chemotherapy

Examination	Years After Chemotherapy						
	2	2–2.5	2.5–3	3–3.5	3.5–4	4–5	5+
Chest x-ray	1 mo	6 wk	2 mo	3 mo	4 mo	6 mo	1 yr
Primary tumor-site x-ray	3 mo	3 mo	6 mo	6 mo	1 yr	1 yr	1 yr
Physical exam	1 mo	6 wk	2 mo	3 mo	4 mo	6 mo	1 yr
Lab studies	1 mo	6 wk	2 mo	3 mo	4 mo	6 mo	1 yr
Chest CT	6 mo	6 mo	6 mo	6 mo	—	—	—
Bone scan	6 mo	6 mo	6 mo	6 mo	—	—	—
ECHO/EKG	1 yr	1 yr	1 yr	1 yr	1 yr	1 yr	1 yr
Audiography	1 yr	1 yr	1 yr	1 yr	1 yr	1 yr	1 yr

Abbreviations: CT, computed tomography; ECHO, echocardiogram; EKG, electrocardiogram; mo, month; wk, week; yr, year.

KEY PRACTICE POINTS

- Optimum treatment for primary tumors is chemotherapy and surgical extirpation.
- Pulmonary metastases should also be treated with chemotherapy and surgical extirpation.
- Specific diagnostic procedures are required to determine the characteristics and extent of tumor
- At M. D. Anderson, we administer intra-arterial cisplatin and intravenous doxorubicin as treatment for pulmonary tumors.
- Cure is achieved in approximately 65% of patients with nonmetastatic disease and in 15% to 25% of patients with metastatic disease.

Suggested Readings

Benjamin RS, Chawla SP, Murray J, et al. Preoperative chemotherapy for osteosarcoma: a treatment approach facilitating limb salvage with major prognostic indications. In: Jones SF, Salmon SE, eds. Adjuvant Therapy of Cancer IV. Philadelphia, PA: Grune and Stratton; 1984:601–610.

Hudson M, Jaffe MR, Jaffe N, et al. Pediatric osteosarcoma: therapeutic strategies, results and prognostic factors derived from a 10-year experience. J Clin Oncol 1990;8:1988–1997.

Jaffe N. Chemotherapy in osteosarcoma: advances and controversies. In: Muggia FM, ed. Experimental and Clinical Progress in Cancer Chemotherapy. Boston, MA: Martinus Nijholl; 1985:223–233.

Jaffe N, Carrasco H, Raymond K, et al. Can cure in patients with osteosarcoma be achieved exclusively with chemotherapy and abrogation of surgery? Cancer 2002;95:2202–2210.

Jaffe N, Knapp J, Chuang VP, et al. Osteosarcoma: intra-arterial treatment of the primary tumor with cis-diammine-dichloroplatinum II (CDP). Angiographic, pathologic, and pharmacologic studies. *Cancer* 1983;51:402–407.

Jaffe N, Smith E, Abelson HT, Frei S. Osteogenic sarcoma: adjuvant chemotherapy. *J Clin Oncol* 1983;1:251–254.

Meyers PA, Heller G, Healey J, et al. Chemotherapy for nonmetastatic osteogenic sarcoma: the Memorial Sloan-Kettering Experience. *J Clin Oncol* 1992;10:5–13.

Rosen G, Caparros B, Huvos AG, et al. Preoperative chemotherapy for osteogenic sarcoma. Selection of post-operative adjuvant chemotherapy based on the response of the primary tumor to preoperative chemotherapy. *Cancer* 1983;49:1221–1230.

Sutow WW, Gehan EA, Kijmert PA, et al. Multidrug adjuvant chemotherapy for osteosarcoma: interim report of the Southwest Oncology Group Studies. *Cancer Treat Rep* 1978;62:265–270.

Winkler K, Beron G, Dellinger G, et al. Neoadjuvant chemotherapy of osteosarcoma: results of a randomized cooperative trial (COSS-82) with salvage chemotherapy varied on histological tumor response. *J Clin Oncol* 1988;6:329–337.

9   EWING'S SARCOMA

Cynthia E. Herzog, Anita Mahajan, and Valerae O. Lewis

CHAPTER OVERVIEW

Optimal management of Ewing's sarcoma requires the comprehensive efforts of a multidisciplinary team of clinicians who understand the potential benefits and consequences of each treatment modality. Every effort should be made to enroll patients in prospective clinical trials to ensure appropriate quality assurance and standards of care. With current improvements in overall survival rates and the increasing number of patients living to adulthood, the need for long-term follow-up and surveillance for potential adverse effects must be emphasized. Although surgery is the preferred method of achieving local control, radiotherapy remains an integral component of the Ewing's sarcoma treatment plan, and as new technology becomes available, ongoing research efforts will focus on reducing acute and long-term toxic effects and improving tumor control.

INTRODUCTION

Ewing's sarcoma is the second most common primary tumor of bone. About 400 new cases are diagnosed each year in the United States, the majority of which occur in teens. Although most of these tumors arise in bone, there is often a large soft-tissue component, and strictly extraosseous tumors account for about 15% of cases. The Ewing's sarcoma family of neoplasms is composed of a spectrum of tumors. At one end of the spectrum is classic Ewing's sarcoma, an undifferentiated, small, round, blue-cell tumor. At the other end is primitive neuroectodermal tumor with neuronal differentiation (presence of Homer-Wright rosettes, neuronal markers, or both). Although historically considered to be distinct entities, Ewing's sarcoma and primitive neuroectodermal tumor have similar chromosomal translocations. In this chapter, this spectrum of tumors is collectively referred to as Ewing's sarcoma.

ETIOLOGY AND EPIDEMIOLOGY

Although the cell of origin remains unknown, Ewing's sarcoma is distinguished from other tumors by chromosomal translocations involving the *EWS* gene on chromosome 22q12. The other gene involved in the translocations is a member of the *ETS* family of transcription factors: *FLI* on 11q24 (83%), *ERG* on 21q22 (13%), or another *ETS* gene (rarely). The *EWS* gene is involved in translocations with non-*ETS* genes in several other sarcomas, including *WT1* in desmoplastic small round-cell tumors, *CHOP* in liposarcoma, and *ATF-1* in clear-cell sarcomas.

Although Ewing's sarcoma arises most commonly in bone, it is likely a neural crest tumor originating outside the central nervous system and sympathetic nervous system. The tumors typically occur in limbs, the chest wall, the paraspinal region, and the pelvis, and they metastasize to bone, bone marrow, and lungs. Ewing's sarcomas occur predominantly in the second decade of life. There is a slight male predominance, and these tumors are uncommon in African Americans.

Presenting Signs, Clinical Features, and Diagnostic Work-Up

The presenting signs and symptoms of Ewing's sarcoma are related to its location of origin. Patients typically present with bone pain or symptoms related to an enlarging mass. They may also have fever. If bone marrow metastases are present, there may be evidence of bone marrow suppression with anemia or pancytopenia. Serum lactate dehydrogenase is frequently elevated in patients with Ewing's sarcoma, especially when a large soft-tissue mass is present.

The diagnostic work-up for Ewing's sarcoma should include a plain radiograph and a magnetic resonance imaging scan of the primary lesion. The MRI scan should include the entire bone involved with the primary tumor so that noncontiguous sites of involvement can be identified. The evaluation should also include a bone scan, chest radiograph, computed tomography scan of the chest, and bone marrow biopsy and aspirate to look for metastases.

Pathology and Genetics

By light microscopy, Ewing's sarcoma is shown to have primitive monomorphic cells with scant cytoplasm and finely dispersed nuclear chromatin with a small, if any, nucleus. In about 50% of cases, there is some degree of rosette formation. Ewing's sarcoma is difficult to differentiate from other small round-cell tumors, especially if it lacks rosettes. For many years, Ewing's sarcoma was a diagnosis of exclusion; immunostaining was done to eliminate diagnoses of other small round-cell tumors, such as rhabdomyosarcoma and neuroblastoma. Currently, immunostaining for CD99 (MIC-2) is used to support the diagnosis of Ewing's sarcoma although this marker is not specific for this tumor. About 50% of Ewing's sarcomas stain with neuron-specific enolase. Electron microscopy findings include evidence of neural differentiation, neural secretory granules, and cytoplasmic processes.

The most specific marker for Ewing's sarcoma is the chromosomal translocation that is detected in 95% of these tumors (discussed above). Chromosome studies should be obtained on all small, round, blue-cell tumors to aid in the diagnosis of Ewing's sarcoma and because the specific chromosomal abnormalities might be related to prognosis.

Prognostic Factors

The prognosis for patients with Ewing's sarcoma is determined on the basis of stage of disease, tumor location, tumor size, chromosomal location, surgical margins, and response to chemotherapy.

Stage of Disease

The worst prognostic factor for patients with Ewing's sarcoma is the presence of metastatic disease at diagnosis or development of metastases a short time after diagnosis. Bone or bone marrow metastasis confers a worse prognosis than does lung metastasis.

Tumor Location

It became apparent in early studies of Ewing's sarcoma that the location of the tumor affects overall survival and local control. In Pediatric Oncology Group study #8346, the 5-year local control rates were found to be 44% for patients with sacral and pelvic tumors, 69% for proximal-extremity tumors, 80% for distal-extremity tumors, and 82% for central axis tumors ($P = 0.023$ by log rank analysis). In other studies, patients with pelvic primary tumors had less favorable median survival durations than patients with primary tumors at other sites (2 years versus up to 4.5 years, respectively). Because pelvic and proximal-limb tumors tend to be larger at diagnosis than tumors at other sites and because the size of the primary tumor at presentation is related to risk for metastatic disease, location appears to be an important factor in consideration of local control and overall survival.

Tumor Size

The size of the primary tumor also affects local control and thus prognosis. In the German Cooperative Ewing's Sarcoma Study (CESS) 86, a primary tumor volume exceeding 200 cc was associated with a worse outcome. A tumor volume of 100 cc or greater was associated with metastatic disease, and such tumors were more likely to arise in the pelvis.

Chromosomal Translocation

Only minimal data have been published on the prognostic significance of specific chromosomal translocations in Ewing's sarcoma. However, the specific translocation may be of prognostic significance, as has been found for specific translocations in rhabdomyosarcoma and synovial sarcoma.

Surgical Margins

The risk of local recurrence or progression of Ewing's sarcoma increases if residual disease remains after tumor resection. Positive microscopic margins or gross residual tumor are indications for postoperative radiotherapy. An intralesional resection increases the risk for local progression. Careful pathologic evaluation to identify both bone and soft-tissue surgical margins is required to locate residual disease when planning for radiotherapy. In the European Intergroup/Cooperative Ewing's Sarcoma Study (EICESS) and the CESS investigations, radiotherapy was shown to improve local control after intralesional surgical excision.

Response to Chemotherapy

As shown by Picci et al (1997), tumor response to chemotherapy provides useful prognostic information. In a group of 68 patients to whom radiotherapy was not administered, those without viable tumor in the resected specimen after chemotherapy had a better 5-year disease-free survival (DFS) rate than patients with pathologically proven microscopic disease (90% versus 53%, respectively; $P = 0.023$). In patients with macroscopic disease, the DFS rates were 90% versus 32%, respectively ($P = 0.0003$). The presence of an increased percentage of necrosis compared with the initial specimen also correlated with an improved survival rate (53% versus 32%, respectively; $P = 0.074$).

TREATMENT

Treatment of Ewing's sarcoma consists of a combination of systemic and local therapies. The effectiveness of radiotherapy in this disease was noted shortly after the tumor was initially described by James Ewing in 1921. In the 1950s and 1960s, limb preservation with radiotherapy was described. With radiotherapy, the 5-year survival rates were about 20%, with local control rates of approximately 70%. However, despite achieving local control, the majority of patients died of metastatic disease in this era.

In the 1970s, multiagent chemotherapy was found to reduce the frequency of metastasis, and the overall survival rate began to improve. This finding demonstrated the relative importance of chemotherapy and redefined the role of radiotherapy. Although radiotherapy was the standard of care for local control of Ewing's sarcoma in the early chemotherapy era, with the evolution of surgical techniques and the potential of limb-sparing surgery, the trend shifted toward surgery as the preferred local-control treatment option.

Studies show a survival advantage for patients who are able to undergo surgical resection alone or subtotal resection combined with radiotherapy compared with those treated locally with radiotherapy only. Systemic chemotherapy treats both local disease and known or presumed microscopic metastases, whereas local therapy targets the known local tumor. At M. D. Anderson Cancer Center, systemic therapy involves the use of immunotherapy in some patients, and local therapy involves surgery, radiotherapy, or a combination of the 2. Currently, patients with newly diagnosed nonmetastatic Ewing's sarcoma of the extremity have a 60% to 65% long-term survival rate. About 20% of patients present with metastatic disease at the time of initial diagnosis, and the long-term survival rate of these patients is 20% at best. Patients with localized Ewing's sarcoma with a primary tumor in the pelvis or proximal extremity and those with a bulky primary tumor are at high risk for treatment failure. These patients often respond initially to a combination of chemotherapy and local therapy (surgery, radiotherapy, or both); however, these treatments fail to produce a durable response.

A number of different regimens, including the use of total-body irradiation and autologous bone marrow transplantation, have been unsuccessful in improving the systemic control of Ewing's sarcoma. Although nearly 90% of patients who present with localized disease are disease-free at the end of therapy, the relapse curve is very steep in high-risk patients.

Chemotherapy

Since 1972, several Intergroup Ewing's Sarcoma Studies (IESS) have compared combination chemotherapy regimens in the United States. IESS I enrolled 331 eligible patients with localized, nonpelvic Ewing's sarcoma of bone between 1973 and 1978. This study compared vincristine, actinomycin D, and cyclophosphamide (VAC) alone with VAC plus either doxorubicin (VACA) or VAC plus pulmonary radiotherapy. The 5-year relapse-free survival rates for VAC alone, VACA, and VAC plus radiotherapy were 24%, 60%, and 44%, respectively. These results established the importance of doxorubicin in the treatment of Ewing's sarcoma. IESS II and subsequent studies have demonstrated that improved outcome is related to the dose intensity of doxorubicin.

The high response rate to ifosfamide and etoposide (IE) among patients with relapsed Ewing's sarcoma (16 of 17 patients or 94%) resulted in the incorporation of these drugs into frontline therapy in the third intergroup study, INT-0091. In this study, VACA alone was compared with VACA alternated with IE. Of the 2 regimens, VACA/IE was found to be superior, with a 5-year event-free survival (EFS) rate of 68% versus 54% for VACA alone. As a result, IE was incorporated into subsequent frontline therapies for Ewing's sarcoma. Other studies, however, have not shown a benefit of ifosfamide in the treatment of Ewing's sarcoma.

The current recommendation of the Children's Oncology Group for frontline therapy for Ewing's sarcoma is a combination of vincristine, doxorubicin, and cyclophosphamide alternated with IE in a dose-intensive manner using growth factor support and interval compression in an attempt to safely deliver chemotherapy in 14-day intervals rather than standard 21-day intervals.

In the German CESS 86 trial, patients with localized, high-risk tumors 100 mL or larger; central axis tumors; or both were treated with vincristine, actinomycin D, ifosfamide, and doxorubicin (VAIA). Those classified as low-risk were treated with VACA. The 10-year EFS rate was 52%, and there was no difference in outcome between the low-risk and high-risk groups, suggesting a benefit from substituting ifosfamide (6,000 mg/m^2/course) for cyclophosphamide (1,200 mg/m^2/course). Because both cyclophosphamide and ifosfamide are known to have a steep dose-response curve, in comparisons of the 2 drugs, an equitoxic dose should be used to determine superiority of 1 drug over the other with respect to efficacy. In this trial, 1,500 mg/m^2/course of cyclophosphamide would have been approximately equivalent to the 6,000 mg/m^2/course of ifosfamide used and may have produced the same results in the high-risk group.

The German CESS group subsequently collaborated with the British CESS group in the EICESS 92 trial. In that study, low-risk patients were treated with 4 courses of induction VACA and were then randomly assigned to either 8 additional courses of VACA or 8 courses of VAIA. High-risk patients received 14 courses of VAIA with or without etoposide. Preliminary results showed estimated 5-year EFS rates of 59% for the overall group, 66% for the low-risk group (n = 150), and 56% for the high-risk group (n = 329). At the time of the report in 2002, no statistically significant difference had been noted between the treatment arms.

Immunotherapy

ImmTher is a lipophilic disaccharide tripeptide derivative of muramyl dipeptide that is encapsulated into liposomes. ImmTher activates monocyte-mediated tumor cell killing in vitro and increases plasma tumor necrosis factor and neopterin levels in patients following intravenous infusion. In a phase I study, ImmTher induced regression of lung and liver metastases in 3 patients with metastatic colon carcinoma.

At M. D. Anderson, our goal is to exploit the chemosensitivity of Ewing's sarcoma by using a dose-intensive chemotherapy regimen with surgery, radiotherapy, or both for local control and to test the feasibility and effectiveness of combining this regimen with ImmTher. We use vincristine in combination with high doses of cyclophosphamide and doxorubicin without IE. Doxorubicin is given at a dose-intensive schedule of 90 mg/m^2/course with the cardioprotective agent. Dexrazoxane Etoposide is not used because of the proven risk of secondary leukemia and the lack of substantial data showing that it improves outcome in Ewing's sarcoma. We have chosen to maximize the dose of cyclophosphamide rather than use ifosfamide, because these 2 drugs have similar cytotoxic mechanisms and because ifosfamide causes greater nonhematologic toxicity, primarily renal. As has been indicated, the therapeutic advantage of ifosfamide is questionable, and we feel the same potential benefit may be gained by using higher doses of cyclophosphamide. The ifosfamide dose of 9,000 mg/m^2/course used in intergroup trial INT-0091 is equivalent to a cyclophosphamide dose of 2,300 mg/m^2/course. We administer 6 courses of an intensive cyclophosphamide regimen (4,000 mg/m^2/course).

Because the lung is a common site of metastasis, ImmTher is given to activate pulmonary macrophages that destroy residual tumor cells that are not eliminated by systemic chemotherapy. We initiate ImmTher after completion of primary therapy (i.e., chemotherapy plus surgery, radiotherapy, or both local treatments). We anticipate that ImmTher will decrease the rate of relapse during the first 2 years and improve both the 2-year DFS rate and the 3-year overall survival rate. On this protocol, patients are randomly assigned to receive or not receive ImmTher.

Therapy for Local Control

Several prospective studies have compared the role of radiotherapy with that of surgery for local control of Ewing's sarcoma, but no prospective, randomization trial of radiotherapy and surgery in patients with tumors of similar prognosis has been conducted. In general, over the last 30 years, it has been recommended that surgery be performed on expendable bones, such as fibulas or ribs, but that radiotherapy be considered in cases in which complete resection is not feasible or would be mutilating. The majority of studies have concluded that surgery produces superior local control compared to radiotherapy. Table 9–1 summarizes the largest trials

Table 9–1. Prospective Studies of Ewing's Sarcoma

Study	Modality	N	5-yr EFS (%)	5-yr LC (%)	5-yr OS (%)
CESS 81	S	242	60	96	
CESS 86	S + postop XRT	304	60	90	
EICESS 92	Preop XRT + S	246	60	95	45
	XRT	266	45	74	
POG 8346	S +/– XRT	37	80	88	88
	XRT	104	41	65	52
ET1	S +/– XRT	34		90	
	XRT	108		67	
ET2	S	114		90	
	S + postop XRT	20		100	
	XRT	56		88	
SSG IX	Amputation	8		100	
	WLE	35		89	
	S + XRT	17		94	
	XRT	28		87	
IESS I	S	3		100	
(pelvis)	S + postop XRT	7		71	
	XRT	57		70	
IESS II	S	11	73	91	
(pelvis)	S + postop XRT	8	62	100	
	XRT	39	59	85	
SJCRH	S	17	75	0	
	XRT	43	53	58	

Abbreviations: CESS, Cooperative Ewing's Sarcoma Study; EFS, event-free survival; EICESS, European Intergroup/Cooperative Ewing's Sarcoma Study; ET, Ewing's Trial (British Medical Research Council); IESS, International Ewing's Sarcoma Study; LC, local control; N, number of patients; OS, overall survival; POG, Pediatric Oncology Group; postop, postoperative; S, surgery; SJCRH, St. Jude Children's Reseach Hospital; SSG, Swedish Sarcoma Group; WLE, wide local excision; XRT, radiotherapy; yr, year.

conducted over the past 3 decades. There is an unavoidable bias, however, because higher-risk patients in whom surgery is not possible or in whom surgery results in incomplete resection were placed on the radiotherapy arm.

In the CESS 81 and 86 trials and the EICESS 92 trial, which accrued a combined total of 1,058 patients, surgery was performed when possible. In patients with high-risk disease, as outlined above, radiotherapy was recommended either before or after the surgical procedure at the discretion of the treating physician. The rate of local failure was 7.5% after surgery with or without postoperative radiotherapy, 5.3% after preoperative radiotherapy, and 26.3% after definitive radiotherapy alone ($P = 0.001$). In the radiotherapy-only group, 12% of 266 patients had distal extremity primary sites compared with 28% of 792 patients who underwent surgery with or without radiotherapy. In contrast, 34% of the radiotherapy-only group had pelvic primary sites versus 18% of the surgery groups. Of note, 80% of patients with pelvic primaries who had surgery also had radiotherapy. Definitive radiotherapy produced local control rates comparable with those of postoperative radiotherapy after intralesional resections; therefore, intralesional resection (or a debulking procedure) is not recommended. Patients with poor histologic response who were treated with postoperative radiotherapy after wide resection had improved local control compared with patients who underwent surgery alone. Patients who had marginal resections with or without postoperative radiotherapy had comparable rates of local control, yet the number of patients with good histologic response after initial chemotherapy was higher among those who did not receive postoperative radiotherapy (72.2% versus 38.5%, respectively).

Surgery

It is standard practice at M. D. Anderson to use neoadjuvant chemotherapy to decrease the size of the tumor prior to performing a wide resection. Five general principles are considered when creating the treatment plan.

- The treatment plan is formulated by a multidisciplinary team consisting of a medical oncologist, a radiation oncologist, and a surgical or orthopedic oncologist.
- The treatment is individualized on the basis of tumor location, tumor size, disease stage, and patient age.
- Surgical resection does not take precedence over systemic therapy.
- Surgical resection is performed in all cases in which the surgeon believes that the primary tumor can be removed completely.
- Radiation therapy is used adjuvantly if adequate margins (1 cm or greater) are not achieved.

Limb-Salvage Surgery: Endoprostheses and Allografts

Ewing's sarcoma is commonly found in skeletally immature patients, and resection of the tumor can often create growth discrepancy or abnormality. Amputation was historically the procedure of choice; however, improved oncologic outcome and technical advances in limb-salvage procedures have made limb salvage a feasible and valuable treatment option. However, in the growing child, limb-salvage procedures that rely on endoprostheses or allografts present unique concerns, such as the small size of the pediatric skeleton, the growth potential of the patient, the projected final length of the unaffected limb, and the need for correcting the ensuing limb-length discrepancy. Several variables contribute to the overall limb-length discrepancy, including systemic chemotherapy, overgrowth of the contralateral limb, slowing of the preserved growth plate in the adjacent affected joint, muscle atrophy, and muscle loss. Each of these variables can alter the expected growth of an extremity and must be considered when estimating the final height of the patient and hence the patient's final limb-length discrepancy. In their series of 15 children who underwent tumor resection and endoprosthetic reconstruction with extendable prostheses, Dominikus et al (1997) found that they underestimated the elongation needed to achieve equal leg lengths. The mean elongation exceeded the predicted growth by 24.3%. They attributed their underestimation to the reduced growth of the physis across the joint and to overgrowth of the contralateral limb.

There are several methods of estimating final height at skeletal maturity. The Green-Anderson Growth-Remaining Charts, the Moseley Straight-Line Graph, and the Menelaus Chronologic Age-Growth Remaining Method are all reliable tools for determining a child's final height. Using these methods, the length of the unaffected limb and hence the projected leg-length discrepancy can be estimated. Limb-length discrepancies less than 2 cm rarely have functional or clinical significance and can be easily corrected with shoe lifts, if necessary. Discrepancies of 1 to 2 cm after limb-salvage surgery are often purposeful. This size discrepancy allows for clearance of the foot if, during reconstruction, the extensor mechanism becomes compromised or nerve palsy creates a foot drop. However, discrepancies greater than 2 cm do not offer the same benefit. Functional gait analysis has shown that with discrepancies greater than 2 cm, patients develop gait abnormalities. Thus, for discrepancies greater than 2 cm, surgical intervention and alternative reconstructive methods are recommended.

If a child has growth remaining, discrepancies greater than 2 cm but less than 4 cm can be addressed by epiphysiodesis. If the contralateral physis lacks growth potential, distraction osteogenesis can be used to lengthen the shorter limb. However, in a young child who has undergone resection of a long-bone sarcoma, the estimated limb-length discrepancy can be quite large, and epiphysiodesis of the contralateral limb or limb lengthening of the ipsilateral limb often cannot achieve the length correction needed. Thus, several surgical and reconstructive procedures have been developed to reconstruct large skeletal defects and address ensuing leg-length discrepancies. Each reconstructive option has its advantages and disadvantages, and these conditions in addition to patient age, location of the sarcoma, resection level, lesion size, and disease stage need to be taken into account before a reconstructive procedure is chosen.

Ewing's sarcoma is commonly found in the diaphysis of a long bone, often sparing the physis. Sarcomas in this location can be resected, and the ensuing intercalary bone defects can be reconstructed with allografts, vascularized bone grafts, or both. Intercalary allograft reconstruction offers a biologic reconstruction option that preserves the growth plate. The risks involved in intercalary allograft reconstruction include late fracture, infection, and nonunion. These risks are more pronounced in patients receiving chemotherapeutic agents. This factor was reiterated by Hornicek et al (2001), who found that patients with intercalary allografts had a high rate of nonunion and that the incidence of nonunion increased when chemotherapy was given after the allograft. This fact has led many surgeons to immediately apply a vascularized fibula to osteosynthesis sites in patients who will receive postoperative chemotherapy, thus affording better healing at these osteosynthesis junctions.

Endoprosthetic reconstruction of skeletal defects is an excellent option for the adult sarcoma patient. However, reconstruction with the standard prosthesis is neither a practical nor a functional option in the skeletally immature patient. To address this issue, Scales and colleagues in 1976 designed the MARK I, the first extendable prosthesis. Many modifications of this prosthesis have been developed, and several investigators and companies have designed new versions of the device. At M. D. Anderson, we use a modular prosthesis (Biomet, Inc., Warsaw, IN and Stryker Orthopaedics, Mahwah, NJ) and a self-expanding prosthesis (REPIPHYSIS; Wright Technology, Inc., Arlington, TN).

The modular prosthesis consists of 4 segments: an articular segment, an intercalary expandable segment, lengthening segments, and an intramedullary segment. These expandable prostheses can be adapted for the distal femur, proximal femur, and proximal humerus by altering the articular components. Expansion takes place in the central intercalary segment. This telescoping segment expands with a jack-like device that is inserted perpendicular to the prosthesis and lengthens via a ratchet-like mechanism. Once the ratchet device has expanded the prosthesis to the desired length (1 to 2 cm), a spacer is inserted. A locking clip is then secured into the spacer, thereby preventing disassociation and collapse. Once the intercalary segment is maximally expanded, it can be exchanged for another intercalary segment in which the length that has already been achieved is incorporated into the new segment. This modularity affords the prosthesis infinite expansion capabilities. The spacer and the locking clip provide potentially stable elongation; however, fracture of the locking clip can lead to disassociation of the spacer.

Each expansion of the various prostheses requires a surgical procedure and a general anesthetic. Generally, components are lengthened in 1- to 2-cm increments. The limiting factor in the lengthening process is the soft tissue. If the surrounding muscles become taut, knee flexion or extension becomes restricted. Thus, expansion of the prosthesis is stopped before the neurovascular structures and surrounding muscles become taut. The patient generally remains in the hospital 2 to 4 days postoperatively. Physical therapy and continuous passive motion are initiated immediately. The patient is allowed to bear weight as tolerated with an assistive device.

The REPIPHYSIS prosthesis was developed to circumvent the mechanical and surgical difficulties encountered with standard expandable prostheses. After the component is implanted, future expansions are noninvasive. This prosthesis consists of 3 segments. The expandable body has a titanium tube that fits inside a polymeric tube. The polymeric tube (exterior body) is made of polyethylene ketone with a polyethylene tubular insert secured by a bolt. The expandable portion is connected to a titanium intramedullary component. A spring is compressed between the cylinders. When the inner coil is heated selectively by exposure to an external magnetic field, the locking mechanism of the spring is released, and the spring expands. The polyethylene heated by the electromagnetic field melts, and the prosthesis expands under the force of the expanding spring. These expansions can occur often and in small increments. The REPIPHYSIS most commonly used in the distal femur can also be adapted for the proximal tibia, proximal humerus, and proximal femur.

The complication rate associated with expandable prostheses remains high. The most common complications are related to failure of the expansion mechanism, aseptic loosening, stem migration, and infection. In 1993, Eckardt and associates reported a complication rate of 67% among patients using a Lewis Expandable and Adjustable Prosthesis (LEAP). The authors attributed the failures to collapse of the prosthesis, Jacobs chuck failure, rotation of the limb, excessive wear, debris, and various surgery-related complications. In this series, 7 of the 12 patients underwent revision of their prostheses. In a review of 32 patients with expandable prostheses, Eckardt et al (2000) reported that only 50% of their patients underwent expansion and that there had been a 50% complication rate. In 1997, Dominikus and colleagues reported on 23 patients with expandable prostheses. Of 6 patients followed long term, 3 had deep infections. The authors attributed the infection rate to the multiple operations needed for expansion.

The total number of operations required for expansion depends not only on the age and size of the patient (needed length) but also on the number of interval complications. Kenan and associates (1998) estimated that 10 to 15 surgeries per patient would be required during the expansion period. The experience of Schiller et al (1995) confirmed this estimation. They reported an average of 11 operations (range, 7 to 18 operations) among 6 patients who were between 9 and 11 years old when they first received an expandable prosthesis. The benefit of a noninvasive expanding prosthesis is that it eliminates the need for operative intervention and thus eliminates the risk for infection, which is imminent with each surgical procedure.

Careful patient selection is very important when considering an expandable prosthesis. Regardless of which component is used, an expandable prosthesis is a large responsibility for the surgeon, the patient, and the family. Diligent and close follow-up is necessary. Both the patient and his or her family must be committed to the decision and to the long rehabilitation process. Failure to participate in rehabilitation can lead to fixed flexion contractures and poor functionality. Although excellent flexion may be achieved in the immediate postoperative period, flexion contractures of up to 20 to 30 degrees can develop in as little as 2 weeks if aggressive physical therapy is not pursued. Correction of the flexion contractures often requires surgical intervention. Physical therapy can cause the patient discomfort, but it is necessary to achieve good functional outcome and to prevent additional surgery. It is very important for the family to be supportive of the patient during the rehabilitation process.

Growth potential is another consideration when a patient is a candidate for an expandable prosthesis. It may be more difficult to obtain equal leg lengths in a very young child (younger than 6 years old) whose parents are tall than in a young child whose parents are short. If the growth potential is so extreme that it cannot be corrected, an alternative means of surgical resection and reconstruction must be used.

Amputation or Rotationplasty

It has been proposed that a child not be considered a candidate for an expandable prosthesis if the limb-length discrepancy will be greater than 10 cm or if the femur is too small to accommodate the prosthesis. For these patients, amputation or rotationplasty are valuable alternatives. Rotationplasty was popularized by Van Nes for proximal femoral focal deficiency. This procedure and its variations have been used for resection of sarcomas of the proximal femur, distal femur, and proximal tibia.

Although the type of rotationplasty used varies depending on the type of resection performed, segments of the distal femur and proximal tibia are generally excised while the neurovascular bundle is left intact. The remaining distal part of the limb is externally rotated 180 degrees and attached to the proximal portion. Fixation of the proximal and distal segments has been performed with plate and screws or an intramedullary rod. The ankle can then function as a knee. Rotationplasties create below-knee amputations from above-knee resections. As time progresses, ankle motion increases, and the toes atrophy. The presence of a "knee joint" adds power, stability, and control to the patient's gait.

Although a prosthesis is required for bipedal ambulation, patients with rotationplasties have both functional and psychological advantages over amputees. A rotationplasty provides a functional knee joint and a longer lever arm for the prosthesis; the foot tolerates the socket load better than an above-knee-amputation stump. Patients with rotationplasties perform significantly better than patients with above-knee amputations. They are able to walk for longer periods of time, and they are able to participate in vigorous sports activities. Despite the shortened length and unusual appearance of the limb, patients with rotationplasties do quite well psychologically. They tend to adjust quickly to the limb appearance and tend not to view themselves as amputees. On the other hand, patients with endoprostheses are dissuaded from participating in high-impact activities. These children do not return to their pre-resection activity level. Rotationplasties also preserve the distal physis, allowing continued physiologic growth of the limb, and they create a more durable limb, so patients with rotationplasties can pursue athletic activities, including high-impact sports. Utilizing quality-of-life questionnaires, it was found that patients who had undergone rotationplasties could participate in daily weight-bearing activities and sports activities to a significantly greater degree than patients who had undergone limb-salvage surgery. However, rotationplasties are rarely first-choice procedures because of cultural stigmas, the evolution of limb-salvage surgery, and expandable endoprosthetic components.

Surgical Aspects of Pelvic and Spinal Ewing's Sarcomas

Ewing's sarcoma in the pelvis is difficult to manage because of the large tumor size, the complex anatomy, and the difficulty of achieving negative margins. However, complete surgical resection of the tumor improves local control, increases DFS, and eliminates the possibility of post-irradiation sarcoma in young patients. As with the long bones, surgical reconstruction depends on the location of the lesion within the pelvis and on the type of resection performed. Autograft or allograft fibula or both can often be used to reconstruct the pelvic ring, providing stability and improved functional outcome.

Solitary lesions in the mobile and immobile spine are treated with a combination of systemic chemotherapy, surgical resection, and reconstruction. These lesions have historically been managed with chemotherapy and radiotherapy; however, recurrences and late onset of neurologic compromise were noted. Combined anterior and posterior procedures have gained favor in the last decade, because they provide complete tumor resection and combat the late kyphosis seen following conventional radiotherapy.

Radiotherapy

Radiotherapy is used to enhance local control and preserve function in patients in whom there is a high risk for local recurrence in a postoperative setting, such as in patients who have residual disease, poor response to chemotherapy, or large tumors. Radiotherapy also appears to be beneficial in the preoperative setting where resectability is questioned because of anatomic considerations. Historically, primary tumors involving the pelvis, vertebrae, chest wall, or neurovascular structures usually require radiotherapy because of relative unresectability.

The factors to consider when determining the radiotherapy treatment plan are timing of treatment, tumor volume, critical structures in the irradiated volume, radiation dose, radiation fractionation, and toxicity.

Timing of Treatment

Whether radiotherapy is given preoperatively or postoperatively does not appear to have an impact on local control or survival. There is some evidence that the outcome of preoperative radiotherapy is inferior to that of postoperative radiotherapy, but this finding may have been the result of selection bias, that is, the preoperative radiotherapy group included patients with higher-risk disease or those with marginally resectable tumors who received radiotherapy prior to surgery to increase resectability. The current recommendation is to proceed to surgery or radiotherapy after 3 to 4 cycles of induction chemotherapy (given over 9 to 12 weeks), at which time response is also evaluated. In studies where radiotherapy is delayed (e.g., CESS 81, in which radiotherapy was administered in week 18) versus those in which radiotherapy occurs early (e.g., Swedish Sarcoma Group IX in which radiotherapy was administered in weeks 6 to 8 and CESS 86 in which radiotherapy was administered in weeks 9 to 10), the overall survival rates appeared inferior (40% versus 60%, respectively) in patients who had radiotherapy without surgery. Tables 9–1 and 9–2 show details and outcomes of pertinent studies.

Tumor Volume

External-beam radiotherapy should be designed to treat areas of macroscopic and microscopic local disease. The gross tumor volume (GTV), clinical target volume (CTV), and planning target volume (PTV) are defined before administration of radiotherapy. The GTV is defined as the presence of any visible palpable disease (or both) noted by clinical examination or radiographic studies. The CTV is defined as the GTV with an added margin that represents an area of possible occult disease. The PTV is an additional margin added to account for the movement of the patient and the inaccuracies caused by patient-beam positioning, and it is related to the therapy equipment and institutional standards.

In earlier studies, it was felt that the whole bone needed to be treated. Recent studies have shown that a smaller volume can be treated without compromising local control (Table 9–2). When delineating CTVs, one must respect anatomic boundaries, such as fascial planes and bony compartments, because these anatomic "walls" are not likely to be traversed by

Table 9–2. Prospective Studies of Ewing's Sarcoma With Details of Local Treatments and Radiotherapy Parameters

Trial	N	Years of accrual	Timing of local post-Tx	Volume of XRT	Definitive XRT (Gy)	Postop XRT (Gy)	Fractionation
CESS 81	45	1981–1985	Wk 18	WB 36 Gy; boost pre-Tx GTV + 5 cm	46–60	36	1.8–2 Gy/d
CESS 86	382	1986–1991	Wk 9	Pre-Tx GTV + 5 cm; boost 2 cm after 44 Gy	60	44	1.6 Gy BID split vs 2 Gy/d
EICESS 92	531	1992–1997	Wk 12		54	44 or 54 same for pre-op	1.6 Gy BID split vs 2 Gy/d
POG 8346	178	1983–1988	Wk 12	WB 39.6 Gy; boost vs IF	55.8		1.5–1.8 Gy/d
ET 1	142	1978–1986	Wk 3–6	25 to 45 Gy WB; boost 10 to 15 Gy		physician preference	15 fractions for primary fields
ET2	191	1987–1993	Wk 12		40–60	35–55	1.6 Gy BID split vs 2 Gy/d
SSG IX	88	1990–1999	Wk 9		42–60	42–60	1.5 Gy BID
IESS I	342	1973–1978		Local XRT with randomized WLI (15 Gy/10 d)	45–65		1.8–2 Gy/d
IESS II	214	1978–1982		45 Gy WB; boost GTV + 5 cm and 1 cm	45–65		1.8–2 Gy/d
SJCRH	43	1978–1988		Post-Tx soft tissue, pre-Tx bone	Response based 30–60		

Abbreviations: BID, twice a day; CESS, Cooperative Ewing's Sarcoma Study; d, day; EICESS, European Intergroup/Cooperative Ewing's Sarcoma Study; ET, Ewing's Trial (British Medical Research Council); GTV, gross tumor volume; Gy, gray; IESS, International Ewing's Sarcoma Study; IF, involved field; N, number of patients; POG, Pediatric Oncology Group; postop, post-operative; pre-Tx, pre-treatment; SJCRH, St. Jude Children's Research Hospital; SSG, Swedish Sarcoma Group; vs, versus; WB, whole bone; Wk, week; WLI, whole-lung irradiation; XRT, radiotherapy.

direct tumor extension. The CTV is generated by adding a 1.5- to 2-cm margin to the GTV. Field reductions can be performed after sufficient dose is delivered for microscopic disease (40 to 45 Gy). The final boost can be delivered to the site of residual disease (GTV2) with a 1- to 1.5-cm margin for CTV2. As noted above, the PTV margin depends on many factors that are specific to the patient and the treatment facility. Generally, the required margin is on the order of 0.5 cm.

Technology has improved such that conformal treatment with the use of all available diagnostic imaging information will allow for the reduction of the volume of irradiated tissue. New technologies, such as intensity-modulated radiotherapy or proton radiotherapy, can be used to further minimize dose to uninvolved surrounding tissue, thereby decreasing potential morbidities.

Critical Structures in the Irradiated Volume

The radiation tolerance of critical structures within the irradiated volume should always be taken into consideration. Acute and late morbidity are related to the volume of normal tissue irradiated and the dose that it receives as well as the other treatments that the patient has received and the patient's age. Particularly with young children, care must be taken to identify epiphyseal plates in growing bones and, if possible, to exclude them from the radiotherapy volumes to minimize the impact on the child's growth.

Radiation Dose

The optimal radiation dose will maximize tumor control and minimize normal-tissue toxicity. Local control has been correlated with response to induction chemotherapy, primary-tumor size, and dose of radiation used and currently recommended doses take these factors into consideration. If the patient has no residual disease after a good resection and a good histologic response, radiotherapy is not given. If the patient has gross residual disease, a final dose of 50 to 55 Gy is recommended with field reduction performed at 45 Gy. If the patient has had a resection and residual microscopic disease is suspected, then the recommended radiotherapy dose is 45 Gy. Care must be taken to identify critical structures in the irradiated field and to consider their tolerance in the final treatment plan. In general, with primary sites involving the vertebra, the final dose may be reduced to 45 to 50 Gy to minimize the possibility of unacceptable morbidity to the spinal cord.

Radiation Fractionation

In the CESS 86 and EICESS 92 studies, hyperfractionation at 1.6 Gy twice a day was evaluated with the goals of increasing the dose per day, shortening overall treatment time, and possibly minimizing long-term toxicity by reducing fraction size. The results have been found to be equivalent to conventional fractionation of 1.8 to 2.0 Gy per day. A confounding factor in the hyperfractionation studies is that a break was given every 2 weeks to allow for the administration of chemotherapy and to minimize acute toxicity. These planned breaks may have affected the final outcome. In other studies, the daily dose of radiation was 1.8 to 2.0 Gy with similar local control and morbidities. For large fields, such as the whole abdomen or the whole lung, it is recommended that the daily dose be reduced to 1.5 Gy to minimize acute and late treatment sequelae.

Toxicity

Acute and chronic toxicities vary greatly between patients because of the variability of the sites of irradiation. In general, all organs within the irradiated field are at risk, in a dose- and volume-dependent manner, for loss of function. Acute toxicity should be monitored carefully because of the potential cumulative effect of all treatment interventions. Permanent loss of function, impaired health status, decreased fertility, and general poor quality of life have been noted in some long-term survivors of Ewing's sarcoma.

The incidence of secondary malignant neoplasms (SMNs) has been noted to be higher in survivors of childhood malignancies than in the general population of people with no history of childhood malignancy. Whether this phenomenon is due to an underlying predisposition remains unclear; however, treatment interventions have been shown to increase the SMN rate. In long-term follow-up of Ewing's sarcoma patients, a 5% to 7% risk for development of an SMN has been noted. There is an apparent risk for development of a secondary hematopoietic malignancy within the first 5 years of follow-up. The risk for development of a solid SMN appears to increase after 10 years and then to increase indefinitely. Patients need to be advised of the risks for late side effects. Appropriate surveillance is recommended.

Treatment of Metastasis

Before the advent of effective systemic chemotherapy, prophylactic whole-lung irradiation (WLI) was used to reduce the incidence of pulmonary metastasis, on the basis of observations in small groups of patients where irradiated lung appeared to be protected from the subsequent development of metastatic disease. Since then, chemotherapy has been found to reduce pulmonary metastasis, and the role of prophylactic WLI has diminished due to the potential for causing pneumonitis. The use of WLI in advanced disease has been recommended in many studies, but no randomized trials have been performed. In a retrospective review of the experience of the EICESS in patients with advanced-stage Ewing's sarcoma, 57 of 171 patients received WLI for pulmonary involvement at diagnosis. WLI improved the 4-year event-free survival rate in patients with isolated pulmonary involvement (0.40 versus 0.19, $P < 0.05$) and in patients presenting with both pulmonary and bone metastasis (0.00 versus 0.27,

$P = 0.0001$). Confounding factors such as patient selection and use of high-dose myeloablative regimens are present in all the reported studies; nevertheless, current protocols do recommend WLI (12 to 15 Gy given over 8 to 10 fractions) for pulmonary metastasis.

For patients with bone metastasis, radiotherapy can be used for consolidation of the metastatic sites after systemic treatment in a definitive treatment plan. Radiotherapy can also provide excellent palliation of symptoms in patients with recurrent and diffusely metastatic disease. The radiotherapy course can be abbreviated to achieve symptom relief in an efficient manner without significant morbidity. Urgent radiotherapy should be instituted at diagnosis or at relapse for acute neurologic compromise to enhance the possibility of symptom reversal.

KEY PRACTICE POINTS

- Ewing's sarcoma should be treated in a multidisciplinary fashion.
- Surgery should be performed for local control if the procedure can be done with minimal morbidity and minimal loss of function. Radiotherapy should be used in cases in which the tumor cannot be resected or in which resection would result in incomplete tumor removal or significant morbidity.
- If surgery is considered, treatment planning must take into account the age of the patient, location of the tumor, and response to induction therapy.
- There are potential risks of loss of function and developmental damage to all organs in the irradiated field. Care must be taken to minimize these risks with appropriate modern technology.

Suggested Readings

Ahrens S, Hoffmann C, Jabar S, et al. Evaluation of prognostic factors in a tumor volume-adapted treatment strategy for localized Ewing sarcoma of bone: the CESS 86 experience. Cooperative Ewing Sarcoma Study. *Med Pediatr Oncol* 1999;32:186–195.

Bacci G, Picci P, Ruggieri P, et al. No advantages in the addition of ifosfamide and VP-16 to the standard four-drug regimen in the maintenance phase of neoadjuvant chemotherapy of Ewing's Sarcoma of bone: Results of two sequential studies. *J Chemother* 1993;5:247–257.

Burgert EO, Jr., Nesbit ME, Garnsey LA, et al. Multimodal therapy for the management of nonpelvic, localized Ewing's sarcoma of bone: intergroup study IESS-II. *J Clin Oncol* 1990;8:1514–1524.

Cotterill SJ, Ahrens S, Paulussen M, et al. Prognostic factors in Ewing's tumor of bone: analysis of 975 patients from the European Intergroup Cooperative Ewing's Sarcoma Study Group. *J Clin Oncol* 2000;18:3108–3114.

Craft AW, Cotterill SJ, Bullimore JA, et al. Long-term results from the first UKCCSG Ewing's Tumour Study (ET-1). United Kingdom Children's Cancer Study Group (UKCCSG) and the Medical Research Council Bone Sarcoma Working Party. *Eur J Cancer* 1997;33:1061–1069.

Delattre O, Zucman J, Melot T, et al. The Ewing family of tumors a subgroup of small-round-cell tumors defined by specific chimeric transcripts. *N Engl J Med* 1994; 331:294–299.

Dominikus M, Windhager R, Kotz R. Treatment of malignant bone tumors in young children-complications and revisions. *Acta Orthop Scand* 1997;276 (4 Suppl).

Donaldson SS, Torrey M, Link MP, et al. A multidisciplinary study investigating radiotherapy in Ewing's sarcoma: end results of POG #8346. Pediatric Oncology Group. *Int J Radiat Oncol Biol Phys* 1998;42:125–135.

Dunst J, Ahrens S, Paulussen M, et al. Second malignancies after treatment for Ewing's sarcoma: a report of the CESS-studies. *Int J Radiat Oncol Biol Phys* 1998;42:379–384.

Eckardt JJ, Kabo JM, Kelley CM, et al. Expandable endoprosthesis reconstruction in skeletally immature patients with tumors. *Clin Orthop* 2000;Apr:51–61.

Elomaa I, Blomqvist CP, Saeter G, et al. Five-year results in Ewing's sarcoma. The Scandinavian Sarcoma Group experience with the SSG IX protocol. *Eur J Cancer* 2000; 36:875–80.

Evans RG, Nesbit ME, Gehan EA et al. Multimodal therapy for the management of localized Ewing's sarcoma of pelvic and sacral bones: A report from the second Intergroup Study. *J Clin Oncol* 1991;9:1173–1180.

Fuchs B, Valenzuela RG, Inwards C, et al. Complications in long-term survivors of Ewing sarcoma. *Cancer* 2003;98:2687–2692.

Grier HE, Krailo MD, Tarbell NJ, et al. Addition of ifosfamide and etoposide to standard chemotherapy for Ewing's sarcoma and primitive neuroectodermal tumor of bone. *N Engl J Med* 2003;348:694–701.

Hanlon M, Krajbich JI: Rotationplasty in skeletally immature patients. Long-term followup results. *Clin Orthop* 1999;Jan:75–82.

Hoffman C, Hillmann A, Krakau H, et al. Functional results and quality of life measurements in patients with multimodal treatment of a primary bone tumor located in the distal femur. Rotationplasty versus endoprosthetic r placement. *Med Pediatr Oncol* 1998;31:202–203.

Hornicek FJ, Gebhardt MC, Tomford WW, et al. Factors affecting nonunion of the allograft-host junction. *Clin Orthop* 2001;Jan:87–98.

Kenan S, Lewis MM, Peabody TD. Special considerations for growing children. In: Simon MA, Springfield D, eds. *Surgery for Bone and Soft-Tissue Tumors*. Philadelphia: Lippincott-Raven Publishers; 1998:245–262.

Kushner BH, Meyers PA, Gerald WL, et al. Very-high-dose short-term chemotherapy for poor-risk peripheral primitive neuroectodermal tumors, including Ewing's sarcoma, in children and young adults. *J Clin Oncol* 1995;13:2796–2804.

Nesbit ME, Jr., Gehan EA, Burgert EO, Jr., et al. Multimodal therapy for the management of primary, nonmetastatic Ewing's sarcoma of bone: a long-term follow-up of the First Intergroup study. *J Clin Oncol* 1990;8:1664–1674.

Paulussen M, Ahrens S, Burdach S, et al. Primary metastatic (stage IV) Ewing tumor: survival analysis of 171 patients from the EICESS studies. European Intergroup Cooperative Ewing Sarcoma Studies. *Ann Oncol* 1998;9:275–281.

Paulussen M, Ahrens S, Dunst J, et al. Localized Ewing tumor of bone: Final results of the Cooperative Ewing's Sarcoma Study CESS 86. *J Clin Oncol* 2001;19:1818–1839.

Picci P, Bohling T, Bacci G, et al. Chemotherapy-induced tumor necrosis as a prognostic factor in localized Ewing's sarcoma of the extremities. *J Clin Oncol* 1997;15:1553–1559.

Sailer, SL, Harmon, D.C., Mankin, H.J., et al. Ewing's sarcoma: Surgical resection as a prognostic factor. *Int J Radiat Oncol Biol Phys* 1988;15:43–52.

Schiller C, Windhager R, Fellinger EJ, Salzer-Kuntschik M, Kaider A, Kotz R. Extendable tumour endoprostheses for the leg in children. *J Bone Joint Surg Br* 1995;77:608–614.

Schuck A, Ahrens S, Paulussen M, et al. Local therapy in localized Ewing tumors: Results of 1058 patients treated in the CESS 81, CESS 86, and EICESS 92 trials. *Int J Radiat Oncol Biol Phys* 2003;55:168–177.

Vosika GJ, Cornelius, D.A., Bennek, J.A., et al. Immunologic and toxicologic study of disaccharide tripeptide glycerol dipalmitoyl: A new lipophilic immunomodulator. *MolBiother* 1990;2:50–56.

Vosika, G.J., Cornelius, D.A., Gilbert, C.W., et al. Phase I Trial of ImmTher, a new liposome-incorporated lipophilic disaccharide tripeptide. *J Immunother* 1991;10:256–266.

10 RETINOBLASTOMA

Misha Faustina, Cynthia E. Herzog,
and Dan S. Gombos

CHAPTER OVERVIEW

This chapter will review the presentation, epidemiology, workup, and treatment modalities available to children with retinoblastoma. Current approaches include the use of systemic chemotherapy combined with adjuvant techniques to treat intraocular disease, reducing the need for external-beam radiotherapy. A multidisciplinary approach in which the expertise of pediatric oncologists, ophthalmologists, radiation oncologists, and geneticists is combined generally works best.

INTRODUCTION

Retinoblastoma is the most common primary intraocular malignancy of childhood, accounting for 3% of cancers in the pediatric age group. Left untreated, this malignancy is nearly universally fatal, yet survival rates and ocular salvage have greatly improved as a result of advances in its diagnosis and treatment.

EPIDEMIOLOGY AND GENETICS

Retinoblastoma occurs in approximately 1 in 15,000 live births. In the United States, approximately 350 new cases are diagnosed each year, with 5,000 cases estimated annually worldwide. Only 10% of all patients with retinoblastoma have a known family history of the disease.

Sporadic nonheritable cases constitute 60% to 70% of all retinoblastomas, in which 2 separate somatic mutations of both copies of the retinoblastoma (Rb) gene have occurred in the same retinoblast. Nonheritable retinoblastoma tends to be unilateral and unifocal, with a mean age at presentation of 24 months. In contrast, heritable disease is associated with germline mutations, bilateral and multifocal lesions, and an earlier age at onset and diagnosis (12 months). Germline mutations are inherited in an autosomal dominant manner. Varying expressivity and reduced penetrance have been noted. Germline mutations result in every cell carrying only 1 normal Rb transcript; 85% of these patients develop bilateral disease, and the others develop unilateral disease (generally but not always multifocal in nature).

Rb is located on the long arm of chromosome 13 at band 14.2 (13q14.2). It functions as a tumor suppressor gene in cell-cycle regulation between G_1 and S. Mutations can occur in any part of the gene; the cause of new mutations is not fully understood. If either allele is mutated, enough functional retinoblastoma protein may be produced by the remaining allele to maintain suppression. Knudson (1971) developed a mathematical model of retinoblastoma inheritance called the 2-hit hypothesis, which theorized that malignancy occurs when a developing progenitor cell acquires a mutation in both cellular copies of Rb.

A few general principles apply to genetic counseling for retinoblastoma. For patients with hereditary or germline retinoblastoma, the generally quoted risk of disease in each child is 45%, owing to a 50% risk of inheriting the Rb gene and a penetrance of 90%. Even if there is no known family history, siblings of a patient with retinoblastoma must be considered at risk for developing the disease. If a second affected child is born into the family, 1 of the parents must have a germline mutation, and all future children will have a 45% risk. A patient with unilateral retinoblastoma has a 15% risk of germline mutation. His or her chance of having an affected child is 7% to 15%. Formal genetic counseling is offered to all patients with retinoblastoma seen at M. D. Anderson Cancer Center.

CLINICAL FEATURES

The most common presenting sign of retinoblastoma among patients in the United States is leukocoria, or white pupillary reflex, which occurs in

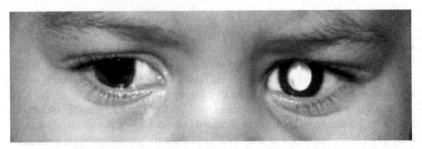

Figure 10–1. Patient with leukocoria. External photograph. Image reprinted with permission from Dr. David Abramson, New York, NY.

about 60% of the cases (Figure 10–1). Strabismus, or malalignment of the eyes, is detected in 20% to 25% of affected patients. Less common initial manifestations include inflamed eyes, orbital cellulitis, neovascular glaucoma, hyphema, and tumor hypopyon. In the developing world, extraocular and/or orbital disease with proptosis is the most common finding at presentation.

Ophthalmoscopic examination of early retinoblastoma lesions may reveal round transparent or white intraretinal lesions with white-fleck calcifications (Figure 10–2). Tumors may have an endophytic growth pattern with friable white preretinal lesions and dispersion ("seeding") into the vitreous or an exophytic growth pattern in which multilobulated white masses grow beneath the retina causing an overlying retinal detachment. Both patterns may be evident simultaneously. Extensive retinoblastoma may manifest as secondary glaucoma with rubeosis iridis, hyphema, and corneal edema or as a vitreous hemorrhage obscuring the view of posterior tumors. Tumor necrosis can cause panuveitis with severe periocular inflammation, including orbital cellulitis. Cases of orbital extension with massive exophthalmos and invasion of the surrounding bones and sinuses have been reported.

Retinocytomas, or retinomas, are benign tumors that are found in nearly 1% of parents of patients with retinoblastoma. These tumors are small translucent gray masses with central calcification that are thought to be spontaneously arrested retinoblastoma lesions in *Rb* carriers.

The germline *Rb* mutation predisposes patients to cancers throughout life. Intracranial malignancies are the most frequent cause of death in the first decade of life for patients with bilateral retinoblastoma. Trilateral retinoblastoma, which occurs in 8% to 15% of all heritable retinoblastomas, refers to bilateral retinoblastoma that is associated with a primitive neuroectodermal tumor (PNET) manifesting as a midline intracranial neoplasm. The pineal gland is the most frequent location of a PNET, but they can occur in the suprasellar and parasellar regions as well. The outcome for patients with trilateral disease is nearly universally death.

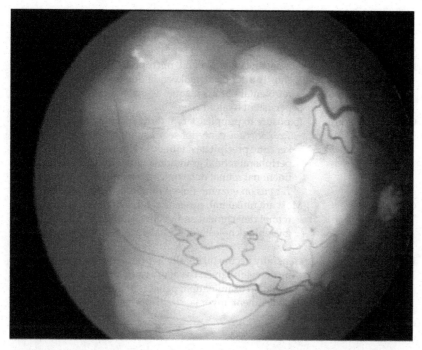

Figure 10–2. Large retinoblastoma lesion in the fundus. Photograph shows that the lesion involves the macula.

The natural history of retinoblastoma, if left undetected and untreated, is relentless progression leading to destruction of the eye, extraocular extension into the optic nerve and orbit, invasion of the brain, disseminated metastasis, and death.

WORKUP

The components of the recommended workup for retinoblastoma are as follows:

- A thorough history and physical examination by the pediatrician and the ophthalmologist
- A slit-lamp and dilated-fundus examination of the patient and his or her parents and siblings, with measurement of corneal diameter and intraocular pressures (generally under anesthesia)
- An ocular sonographic examination
- Neuroimaging of the orbit and the brain

The history and physical examination may reveal evidence of clinically silent systemic disease or the presence of constitutional signs that will aid

Table 10–1. Other Diseases to Consider When a Diagnosis of Retinoblastoma Is Suspected

Disease	Differentiating Characteristics
Persistent hyperplastic primary vitreous	Almost always unilateral; microphthalmos; detected shortly after birth; leukocoria due to opacified retrolental fibrous plaque; associated cataract and persistent hyaloid artery
Ocular toxocariasis	Exposure to puppies, larval form of canine ascarid *Toxocara canis*; anterior segment inflammation with keratitic precipitates, vitreous cells, posterior synechia, peripheral retinal granuloma with vitreous bands, and tractional retinal detachment; serum tests positive for *T. canis* on enzyme-linked immunosorbent assay
Coats' disease	Most are unilateral, congenital retinal telangiectasis with retinal detachment and yellow subretinal exudates with glistening cholesterol crystals; age 4–10 years; male sex
Retinopathy of prematurity	Generally occurs bilaterally in premature infants of low birth weight given oxygen; avascular peripheral retina noted on examination; patients at high risk for retinal detachment, myopia, strabismus, and severe loss of vision

in making a differential diagnosis (Table 10–1). Systemic evaluation for metastatic disease and for second primary cancers is also important. A thorough ophthalmic examination should document retinal findings and anterior segment involvement. An imaging study of the orbit is helpful in delineating calcific intraocular lesions and ruling out extraocular extension, and additional views of the brain are critical to rule out the presence of PNETs. Ophthalmic echography may reveal evidence of calcification, which appears as highly reflective internal echoes. The use of B-scan echography can depict the topology of the lesion, allowing for further differentiation and measurement of its dimensions. On computed tomography (CT) scans, 90% of retinoblastomas appear as calcified lesions. Magnetic resonance imaging is less likely than CT to demonstrate calcification but is superior to CT in detecting invasion of the optic nerve and midline intracranial tumors (Figure 10–3). Retinoblastoma lesions appear hyperintense on T1-weighted images (especially if the tumor is well differentiated) and hypointense on T2-weighted images.

The most commonly used staging system for retinoblastomas is the Reese-Ellsworth system, which is summarized in Table 10–2. This classification system is based on the number, size, and location of intraocular tumors. The stage (I to V) indicates the prognosis for globe conservation using external-beam radiotherapy (EBRT). With the advent of primary chemotherapy, alternative schemes, such as the International Classification

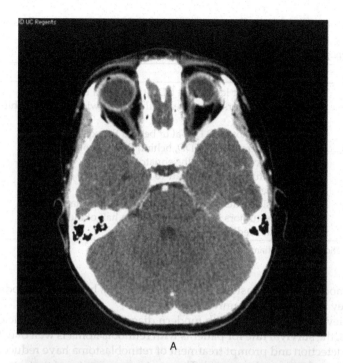

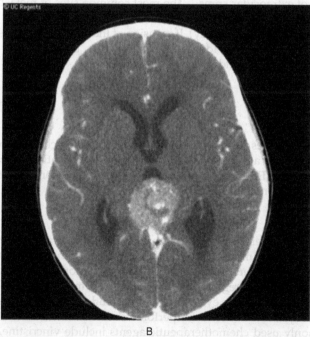

Figure 10–3. Neuroimaging of 2 patients with retinoblastoma. A, Computed tomography scan demonstrates intraocular calcified retinoblastoma. B, A magnetic resonance imaging scan depicts a midline primitive neuroectodermal tumor. Both images reprinted with permission from Dr. Joan O'Brien, San Francisco, CA.

Table 10–2. Reese-Ellsworth Grouping of Retinoblastoma

Group	Description
Ia	Solitary tumor less than 4 DD, at or behind the equator
Ib	Multiple tumors, none greater than 4 DD wide, all at or behind the equator
IIa	Solitary tumor 4–10 DD, at or behind the equator
IIb	Multiple tumors 4–10 DD, behind the equator
IIIa	Any tumor anterior to the equator
IIIb	Solitary tumor greater than 10 DD, behind the equator
IVa	Multiple tumors, some greater than 10 DD
IVb	Any lesion extending anterior to the ora serrata
Va	Massive tumors involving more than half of the retina
Vb	Vitreous seeding

Abbreviation: DD, disc diameter.

of Intraocular Retinoblastoma system (Table 10–3), have been introduced, but they are not yet used universally.

In developed countries with modern diagnostic and therapeutic capabilities, the survival rate for patients with retinoblastoma is well over 98%. Early detection and prompt treatment of retinoblastoma have reduced the incidence of extraocular spread. The most common sites of metastasis include the central nervous system (CNS), orbit, bone marrow, and viscera (especially the liver and kidney). If invasion of the optic nerve is suspected or neurologic signs are evident, lumbar puncture, bone marrow biopsy, and bone scanning are indicated.

TREATMENT

Treatment strategies for retinoblastoma have gradually changed over the past decade, with a trend away from the use of enucleation (removal of the eyeball) and EBRT and toward the use of focal, more conservative modalities combined with chemotherapy.

Chemoreduction

Chemoreduction refers to the use of systemic chemotherapy as a primary modality to shrink tumors; it is then followed by additional local treatments (e.g., laser thermotherapy, cryotherapy, plaque radiotherapy) to consolidate the response. At regular intervals during chemotherapy, the patient is anesthetized, his or her eyes are examined, and focal ablative treatment of potentially active tumor foci is performed.

Commonly used chemotherapeutic agents include vincristine, etoposide, and carboplatin. Some cancer centers use only 1 or 2 of these agents, and others also include cyclosporine to inhibit the multi-drug resistance

Table 10–3. International Classification of Intraocular Retinoblastoma (the "ABC" System)

ABC Group	Ophthalmologic Findings	Reese-Ellsworth Group
A	Tumor confined to retina	Ia
	No vitreous seeding and	Ib
	No RD	IIIa
	No tumor greater than 2 DD in any dimension	IVb
	No tumor closer than 2 DD to fovea or 1 DD to disc	
B	Tumor confined to retina	Ia
	No vitreous seeding and	Ib
	No detached retina greater than 2 DD	IIa
	from tumor base	IIb
		IIIa
	Tumor occupies no more than half of eye	IIIb
	Tumor may occupy any retinal location	IVa
		IVb
C	Minimal tumor spread from retina to adjacent spaces	IVa
	Fine vitreous seeding and/or	IVb
	RD greater than 2 DD from base of tumor to	Va
	total RD	Vb
	No viable or visible subretinal tumor implants	
	Tumor occupies no more than the two thirds of the eye	
D	Massive tumor spread from retina to adjacent spaces	IVa
	Vitreous "snowballs" or masses and/or	IVb
	RD with subretinal implants or masses	Va
	Tumor occupies no more than two thirds of eye	Vb
	Visual potential must be present	
E	Any of the following:	IVa
	More than two thirds of eye filled with tumor	IVb
	No visual potential	Va
	Neovascular glaucoma or neovascularization of iris	Vb
	Hyphema and/or vitreous hemorrhage	
	Corneal blood staining	
	Tumor in the anterior segment	
	Phthisis or pre-phthisis of eye	
	Orbital cellulitis-like presentation	
	Tumor in or on ciliary body or anterior to vitreous face	

Courtesy of Dr. Linn Murphree, Los Angeles, CA. Abbreviations: DD, disc diameter; RD, retinal detachment.

protein Pgp. Protocols vary, but generally a low-dose, 6-cycle regimen provides adequate tumor reduction. At M. D. Anderson, we use the 3-drug regimen without cyclosporine.

The most common side effect of chemotherapy is bone marrow suppression, particularly neutropenia and thrombocytopenia. The use of carboplatin is also associated with a risk of hearing loss. However, the adverse effect of most concern is the low but generally lethal risk of secondary leukemias associated with etoposide therapy. Techniques for local application of chemotherapeutic agents (i.e., subconjunctival, episcleral, or peribulbar) promise to reduce these systemic risks.

Thermotherapy

Transpupillary thermotherapy (TTT) is the newest focal treatment method for retinoblastoma, and it has largely replaced laser photocoagulation. At M. D. Anderson, TTT is delivered to the tumor via an indirect ophthalmoscope or laser-mounted microscope. The temperature delivered (i.e., 45°C to 60°C) is high enough to cause cytotoxic effects but is below the coagulation threshold (greater than 60°C).

The most common complications associated with this modality include focal iris atrophy, tractional and vaso-occlusive complications, and lens opacities. Chemotherapy and chemothermotherapy (systemic chemotherapy administered within hours of TTT) are well suited for lesions of the posterior pole.

Cryotherapy

Cryotherapy is generally reserved for treating equatorial and peripheral tumors. It is generally not effective for vitreous seeds unless they are directly adjacent to the tumor. We use a triple freeze-thaw technique in which the retinal cryoprobe is applied to the overlying sclera and opacification of the lesion is visualized using an indirect ophthalmoscope. Successful treatment leads to a flat chorioretinal scar.

Although cryotherapy is somewhat more effective than laser photocoagulation, its use is associated with uveitis, choroidal detachment, and rhegmatogenous and exudative retinal detachments.

Radiotherapy

Retinoblastomas are radiosensitive tumors. The tumoricidal effects of radiation result from destruction of the neoplasm's reproductive capabilities and the subsequent induction of programmed cell death, which is also called apoptosis. Both brachytherapy and EBRT are highly effective.

Stallard (1962) first described the use of episcleral plaque brachytherapy for retinoblastoma. The technique is most commonly indicated for solitary tumors that are smaller than 15 mm in diameter and 3 to 10 mm thick. It can be used as either a primary treatment modality or a salvage technique after other approaches have failed. An iodine-125 plaque, constructed of radioactive iodine seeds placed in a gold carrier, is commonly used. The overlying sclera is marked using indirect ophthalmoscopy, and a dummy plaque is used to aid in intraoperative localization. After the active plaque

Table 10–4. Classification of Retinoblastoma Regression Patterns

Type	Description
0	No evidence of prior retinoblastoma lesion
I	White "cottage-cheese" mass of calcification
II	Gray "fish-flesh" appearance
III	Mixed pattern (combination of types I and II)
IV	Flat chorioretinal scar

has been sutured in place, the edges are checked to ensure that there is a margin of at least 2 mm around the tumor. The active plaque delivers a total radiation dose of 40 to 45 Gy over 4 to 5 days, after which it is removed in a second procedure. These plaques provide acceptable isodose curves while minimizing collateral radiation damage.

EBRT, once considered the standard globe-conserving modality, remains an important treatment method for tumors that fail to regress after treatment with other modalities. In EBRT, radiation is typically delivered using a linear accelerator with a lateral-lens-sparing technique. A total radiation dose of 42 to 46 Gy is given in daily fractions of 1.8 to 2.0 Gy. Regression patterns following EBRT have been categorized and are described in Table 10–4. The most common characteristic is a mixed white "cottage-cheese" complex combined with a gray "fish-flesh" appearance (type III).

Long-term risks of EBRT include damage to the retina, optic nerve, lens (e.g., cataract), and midline bone hypoplasia. In germline retinoblastoma, the risk of second primary cancers increases dramatically within the field of radiation. Patients are at particularly high risk for developing tumors of the head and skull (e.g., soft-tissue sarcomas and osteosarcomas). Technologic advances using megavoltage and lower radiation doses have decreased some of these effects. However, because most radiation complications depend on the patient's age and dose, the use of EBRT is generally avoided in children younger than 12 months old.

Enucleation

Removal of the eyeball is still used in patients with tumors that fill the globe, especially when invasion into the optic nerve or choroid is suspected. Children who present with advanced unilateral disease are well suited for this approach. Enucleation is also indicated when the eye is affected by secondary neovascular glaucoma and invasion of the anterior segment and when conservative therapies have failed.

During the surgical excision, care must be taken to avoid perforating or compressing the globe. An optic nerve stump of 10 mm or more is ideal for reducing the risk of spread to the CNS. An integrated orbital implant may be placed after enucleation, providing excellent motility and cosmesis.

Complications of enucleation include perforation of the globe, breakdown of the conjunctiva, infection, and extrusion of the orbital implant.

Treatment of Metastatic Disease

Retinoblastoma can metastasize from the eye by various routes, including hematogenous dissemination, CNS involvement via the optic nerve and/or cerebrospinal fluid, and direct invasion of adjacent structures, including the orbit and sinuses. Metastatic disease, particularly with CNS involvement, should be treated aggressively with a multimodal approach that includes systemic multiagent chemotherapy, surgical excision, and whole-brain EBRT. Courses of chemotherapy lasting 6 to 18 months are generally advocated. Regimens similar to those advocated for chemoreduction have been used with favorable results.

SECOND PRIMARY TUMORS

Second primary tumors are the most common cause of mortality in patients with germline retinoblastoma. In addition to midline intracranial tumors, the *Rb* mutation predisposes these patients to osteosarcomas, soft tissue sarcomas, melanomas, brain tumors, and other neoplasms. Because patients with germline retinoblastoma carry 1 *Rb* mutation in most or all cells of the body, few additional mutations are needed for a new cancer to develop. The risk is increased in patients treated with radiotherapy and some forms of chemotherapy that damage DNA. Such patients have a lifetime predisposition (estimated at 1% per year) to develop nonocular cancers throughout the body, particularly in the bones, brain, and skin. Surveillance is essential, and annual physical examinations are suggested. Although some treatment centers advocate annual magnetic resonance imaging scans of the brain and long bones, we generally do not perform this scanning in the absence of symptoms or signs of disease.

KEY PRACTICE POINTS

- Retinoblastoma generally presents with leukocoria, strabismus, or both.
- Cure rates approach 98% to 99%.
- The primary globe-salvaging technique includes chemoreduction in which systemic chemotherapy is combined with local focal ablative modalities (e.g., laser, cryotherapy, brachytherapy).
- Patients with the *Rb* gene defects are at higher risk for second nonocular tumors. Radiotherapy before the age of 1 year increases this risk.

Suggested Readings

Abramson DH, Frank CM. Second nonocular tumors in survivors of bilateral retinoblastoma: a possible age effect on radiation-related risk. *Ophthalmology* 1998;105:573–580.

Abramson DH, Frank CM, Dunkel IJ. A phase I/II study of subconjunctival carboplatin for intraocular retinoblastoma. *Ophthalmology* 1999;106:1947–1950.

Augsburger JJ, Oehlschläger U, Manzitti JE, et al. Multinational clinical and pathologic registry of retinoblastoma: Retinoblastoma International Collaborative Study report 2. *Graefes Arch Clin Exp Ophthalmol* 1995;233:469–475.

Bagley LJ, Hurst RW, Zimmerman RA, et al. Imaging in the trilateral retinoblastoma syndrome. *Neuroradiology* 1996;38:166–170.

Balmer A, Munier F, Gailloud C. Retinoma: case studies. *Ophthalmic Paediatrics and Genetics* 1991;12:131–137.

Damato B. Retinoblastoma. In: Damato B. *Ocular Tumours: Diagnosis and Treatment.* Oxford, UK: Butterworth-Heinemann; 2000:127–149.

DiCiommo D, Gallie BL, Bremner R. Retinoblastoma: the disease, gene and protein provide critical leads to understand cancer. *Semin Cancer Biol* 2000;10:255–269.

Draper GJ, Sanders BM, Brownbill PA. Patterns of risk and hereditary retinoblastoma and applications to genetic counseling. *Br J Cancer* 1992;66:211–219.

Ellsworth RM. Retinoblastoma: an overview. In: Blodi FC, ed. *Contemporary Issues in Ophthalmology,* vol 2. New York, NY: Churchill Livingstone; 1985:1–10.

Eng C, Li FP, Abramson DH, et al. Mortality from second tumors among long-term survivors of retinoblastoma. *J Natl Cancer Inst* 1993;85:1121–1128.

Gallie BL, Budnig A, DeBoer G, et al. Chemotherapy with focal therapy can cure intraocular retinoblastoma without radiotherapy. *Arch Ophthalmol* 1996;114:1321–1328.

Gallie BL, Phillips RA, Ellsworth RM, et al. Significance of retinoma and phthisis bulbi for retinoblastoma. *Ophthalmology* 1982;89:1393–1399.

Gurney JG, Ross JA, Wall DA, et al. Infant cancer in the U.S.: histology-specific incidence and trends, 1973 to 1992. *J Pediatr Hematol Oncol* 1997;19:428–432.

Harbour JW. Overview of Rb gene mutations in patients with retinoblastoma: implications for clinical genetic screening. *Ophthalmology* 1998;105:1442–1447.

Harbour JW. Retinoblastoma: pathogenesis and diagnosis. In: Char DH. *Tumors of the Eye and Ocular Adnexa.* Hamilton, ON, Canada: BC Decker; 2001a:253–265.

Harbour JW. Retinoblastoma: treatment. In: Char DH. *Tumors of the Eye and Ocular Adnexa.* Hamilton, ON, Canada: BC Decker; 2001b:266–278.

Hayden BH, Murray TG, Scott IU, et al. Subconjunctival carboplatin in retinoblastoma: impact of tumor burden and dose schedule. *Arch Ophthalmol* 2000;118:1549–1554.

Kingston JE, Hungerford JL, Madreperla SA, et al. Results of combined chemotherapy and radiotherapy for advanced intraocular retinoblastoma. *Arch Ophthalmol* 1996;114:1339–1343.

Kingston JE, Hungerford JL, Plowman PN. Chemotherapy in metastatic retinoblastoma. *Ophthalmic Paediatrics and Genetics* 1987;8:69–72.

Knudson AG. Mutation and cancer: statistical study of retinoblastoma. *Proc Natl Acad Sci USA* 1971;68:820–823.

Marcus DM, Brooks SE, Leff G, et al. Trilateral retinoblastoma: insights into histogenesis and management. *Surv Ophthalmol* 1998;43:59–70.

Messmer EP, Heinrich T, Höpping W, et al. Risk factors for metastasis in patients with retinoblastoma. *Ophthalmology* 1991;98:136–141.

Murphree AL, Villablanca JG, Deegan WF, et al. Chemotherapy plus local treatment in the management of intraocular retinoblastoma. *Arch Ophthalmol* 1996;114:1348–1356.

Saarinen UM, Sariola H, Hovi L. Recurrent disseminated retinoblastoma treated by high-dose chemotherapy, total body irradiation, and autologous bone marrow rescue. *Am J Pediatr Hematol Oncol* 1991;13:315–319.

Shields CL, De Potter P, Himelstein BP, et al. Chemoreduction in the initial management of intraocular retinoblastoma. *Arch Ophthalmol* 1996;114:1330–1338.

Shields CL, Santos MCM, Diniz W, et al. Thermotherapy for retinoblastoma. *Arch Ophthalmol* 1999;117:885–893.

Shields CL, Shields JA. Recent developments in the management of retinoblastoma. *J Pediatr Ophthalmol Strabismus* 1999;36:8–18.

Shields CL, Shields JA, De Potter P, et al. Plaque radiotherapy in the management of retinoblastoma: use as a primary and secondary treatment. *Ophthalmology* 1993;100:216–224.

Singh AD, Shields CL, Shields JA. Prognostic factors in retinoblastoma. *J Pediatr Ophthalmol Strabismus* 2000; 37:134–141.

Stallard, HB. The conservative treatment of retinoblastoma. *Trans Ophthalmol Soc U K* 1962;82:473–534.

11 DIFFERENTIATED THYROID CANCER

Rena Vassilopoulou-Sellin

CHAPTER OVERVIEW

Thyroid nodules are relatively common in adult women but uncommon in adult men and in children and adolescents, and children are infrequently affected by differentiated thyroid cancer. When this cancer does occur in a child, the patient's prognosis is generally favorable and he or she can expect a near-normal life span; however, it can prove to be a lethal neoplasm, especially in older patients and when distant metastases are present. The survival duration for children and adolescents with differentiated thyroid cancer is substantially long despite the fact that the disease presents with extensive morbid characteristics. The varied presentations and activities of differentiated thyroid cancer in children require specific diagnostic and treatment approaches and lifelong surveillance.

INTRODUCTION

Differentiated thyroid cancer, often simply called "thyroid cancer," is an infrequent malignancy overall but the most common endocrine malignancy. At M. D. Anderson Cancer Center, less than 10% of all patients with differentiated thyroid cancer receive the diagnosis before 20 years of age. In children, differentiated thyroid cancer occurs more commonly as the papillary rather than the follicular variant, and it affects girls more often than boys. Unlike in young adults, differentiated thyroid cancer presents in children with extensive disease bulk, including multifocal primary lesions, bilateral cervical lymph node metastases, and tumor invasion into the soft tissues of the neck. Diffuse pulmonary metastases may also be present in a small subset of children with cervical lymph node metastases. Children with differentiated thyroid cancer generally have a good prognosis despite the initial extent of disease (Harness et al, 1992; Hung and Sarlis, 2002). Nevertheless, disease- and treatment-related morbidity and mortality do occur; thus, a thoughtful, comprehensive initial evaluation and treatment plan must be coupled with lifelong surveillance in all cases.

RADIATION-INDUCED DIFFERENTIATED THYROID CANCER

The risk for radiation-induced differentiated thyroid cancer is well documented. During the early decades of the twentieth century, low-dose irradiation to the head and neck was often used in the treatment of benign childhood conditions such as thymic enlargement, hemangioma, ringworm, and acne. The excess relative risk for radiation-induced differentiated thyroid cancer appears to depend on radiation dose and schedule as well as the patient's age at the time of exposure. The average time between irradiation and diagnosis of differentiated thyroid cancer is 10 years; accordingly, some cases of radiation-induced differentiated thyroid cancer will be diagnosed before the patient is 20 years old. There is no indication that radiation-induced differentiated thyroid cancer has a different clinical presentation and course than unirradiated cases of the disease. Increasing awareness of thyroid radiosensitivity, especially in children, has led to the virtual elimination of the use of irradiation for benign conditions; thus, low-dose radiation-induced differentiated thyroid cancer is expected to subside in the future.

The efficacy of external-beam radiotherapy in the management of Hodgkin and non-Hodgkin lymphoma, however, has produced high cure rates and is likely to remain an important component of therapy for these diseases. Given the near-normal life expectancy of many survivors of these childhood cancers, the potential risk for radiation-induced differentiated thyroid cancer becomes an important health concern. High-dose radiation of the thyroid gland, especially when given at a young age, has been associated with increased risk for radiologic or pathologic abnormalities and thyroid tumors, both benign and malignant. At M. D. Anderson, we have found patients to have a heightened risk for differentiated thyroid cancer after therapeutic mantle irradiation for Hodgkin lymphoma

(Vassilopoulou-Sellin, 1995). In a study of 166 patients irradiated at or before 16 years of age and for whom a minimum of 15 years of follow-up data were available, 12 patients were treated for differentiated thyroid cancer. This tumor was found 7 to 19 years after irradiation on investigation of either palpable thyroid nodules or incidental abnormalities found on diagnostic imaging scans. The presence of differentiated thyroid cancer in 7% of irradiated survivors of Hodgkin lymphoma exceeds the prevalence of the disease and suggests a possible causative relationship. Interestingly, during the same period, only 2 cases of differentiated thyroid cancer were diagnosed among 750 adults treated for Hodgkin lymphoma in our institution, emphasizing the importance of age as an independent risk factor.

Environmental radiation contamination has also been implicated in the development of differentiated thyroid cancer in children. For example, the number of childhood differentiated thyroid cancer cases increased sharply in the Ukraine after the Chernobyl nuclear accident in 1986. The tumors were overwhelmingly papillary carcinomas with a frequent incidence of cervical lymph node metastases and extrathyroidal spread. The children who were youngest at the time of the accident were more likely to develop differentiated thyroid cancer. Whereas increased vigilance may have resulted in greater appreciation of the prevalence of the disease in this population, it is generally accepted that irradiation had a causative effect.

REGIONAL LYMPH NODE INVOLVEMENT

A recent review of 117 patients younger than 20 years of age who presented at M. D. Anderson with differentiated thyroid cancer indicates that the occurrence of cervical lymph node metastases in this patient group is very common (Frankenthaler et al, 1990). Of these 117 patients, 20% had undergone neck irradiation for a variety of benign conditions, most commonly chronic adenoiditis, thymic hyperplasia, and acne. Radiotherapy preceded the diagnosis of differentiated thyroid cancer by an average of 10 years. The most common presenting sign was a painless neck mass either in the thyroid gland or in a cervical lymph node. The tumor histology was follicular variant of papillary differentiated thyroid cancer in most patients. Metastases to the cervical lymph nodes were present at the time of diagnosis in 86% of patients, and extrathyroidal or extranodal invasion of adjacent soft tissues was present in approximately 10% of patients. Although regional neck recurrence occurred in almost one third of the patients, there were no thyroid cancer–related deaths in the group.

PULMONARY METASTASES

Of 209 evaluable patients diagnosed with differentiated thyroid cancer between 1960 and 1990 and treated at M. D. Anderson, 9% had pulmonary

metastases at presentation (Vassilopoulou-Sellin et al, 1993). All these patients also had cervical lymph node metastases. The diagnosis of lung
involvement was supported by abnormal chest radiographs coupled with
diffuse, intense pulmonary radioactive iodine (RAI) uptake in half the
patients and by intense pulmonary RAI uptake despite a normal chest radiograph in the remaining patients. An abnormal chest radiograph with
negative pulmonary RAI uptake was seen in only 10% of cases with pulmonary metastases. Abnormal chest radiographs always showed a diffuse
micronodular pattern consistent with most reports of childhood differentiated thyroid cancer. Tuberculosis was initially suspected in several patients.
All patients received RAI therapy. Of 11 patients whose initial chest radiographs were abnormal, 7 had a normal chest radiograph 6 to 75 months
after diagnosis and following administration of 200 to 450 mCi RAI. With
respect to pulmonary RAI uptake, RAI-avid tissue was no longer evident
in 6 of 17 patients examined at 6 to 51 months after the therapeutic administration of 100 to 200 mCi RAI. Persistent pulmonary RAI uptake was
seen at the time of last RAI scan in the other 10 patients.

If there was no radiologic evidence of pulmonary metastases at diagnosis, none was found later. On the basis of this experience and on a broad
review of available literature, it appears that although RAI therapy can effectively clear radiologic abnormalities seen on chest radiographs, it may
not eradicate metastatic foci in many children. In these patients, asymptomatic lung metastases and prolonged life expectancy can be expected.
Therapeutic RAI should be administered with some caution to avoid RAI
toxicity, such as pulmonary fibrosis, even if pulmonary abnormalities persist. Our policy is to evaluate all children with differentiated thyroid cancer
with a total-body RAI scan after a total thyroidectomy. When pulmonary
RAI uptake is present, we recommend RAI therapy at least once. When
and how often these patients should be retreated must be determined on
an individual basis.

CLINICAL OUTCOME AND MORTALITY AFTER
PROLONGED FOLLOW-UP

Children with differentiated thyroid cancer characteristically present with
extensive regional disease. Multifocal, bilateral involvement of the thyroid, regional lymph nodes, and adjacent soft tissue is common, and lung
metastases typically develop in a substantial minority of patients. Yet, most
reviews on the subject point out that these patients' prognoses remain excellent for well beyond 10 years. The lack of documented deaths attributed to
differentiated thyroid cancer leads many investigators to propose a more-
or less-aggressive therapeutic strategy for these patients. Most investigators recognize and recommend prolonged follow-up, i.e., more than 5 or
10 years; however, it is very difficult to obtain comprehensive lifelong

follow-up information about patients. Experience with some patients, such as the one described in Case Example 1 that follows, coupled with the realization that very delayed morbidity and mortality may characterize the clinical outcome of patients with differentiated thyroid cancer, regardless of age, have prompted us to reexamine our experience for potential disease- or treatment-related mortality of patients with childhood differentiated thyroid cancer.

Of 112 patients with differentiated thyroid cancer who presented to M. D. Anderson between 1944 and 1986 who were younger than 20 years of age at the time of diagnosis and who were followed for at least 10 years, 13 died from treatment-related complications (e.g., radiation fibrosis or sarcoma) or recurrent differentiated thyroid cancer (Vassilopoulou-Sellin et al, 1998). The 99 patients who lived were a mean age of 15 years at diagnosis, had a mean follow-up duration of 25 years, and were a mean age of 41 years at the time of the most recent evaluation. There was a preponderance of girls, and 25% experienced disease recurrence some time after diagnosis. As a group, they did not differ from the patients who died with regard to age, extent of disease, or extent of follow-up data.

One patient died from complications of coexisting diabetes mellitus; another patient's cause of death was unclear. Six patients died from progressive disease at a mean age of 40 years, which is comparatively younger than adult patients in the M. D. Anderson database who died of differentiated thyroid cancer during their sixth decade of life. Four of these children had papillary (or follicular variant of papillary) differentiated thyroid cancer, and 2 had follicular differentiated thyroid cancer. Three of the children were known to have received neck irradiation during childhood for benign conditions, and none had received RAI after initial surgery. At the time of diagnosis, differentiated thyroid cancer had invaded soft tissue in 3 cases and had involved cervical lymph nodes in 2 cases, and it was considered limited to the thyroid gland in 1 case. Progressive disease included regional recurrence and distant metastases (most commonly to lungs and bones).

The deaths of the other 6 patients may be attributable to treatment-related complications. Two patients, both initially treated with surgery and external-beam radiotherapy, died from sarcomas that developed within the radiation field; one at 23 years and the other at 32 years after differentiated thyroid cancer diagnosis. One patient who was initially treated with surgery, external-beam radiotherapy, radium implants, and RAI experienced crippling tracheal stenosis and necrosis and died of airway obstruction 33 years after diagnosis. Two female patients initially treated with surgery and RAI as teenagers died of breast cancer; one at 30 years of age and the other at 32 years of age. The last patient had lung metastases and extensive RAI therapy and died from pulmonary dysfunction.

This review supports the clinical impression that children and adolescents with differentiated thyroid cancer live for many years regardless of the apparent extent of initial or recurrent disease; indeed, there were no deaths during the first 10 years of follow-up. However, prolonged surveillance of such patients reveals that 5% to 7% develop and eventually die from progressive disease, and a similar number develop and die of possible treatment-related complications or second neoplasms. The importance of lifelong surveillance cannot be overemphasized.

DIAGNOSIS, TREATMENT, AND SURVEILLANCE

Because differentiated thyroid cancer is uncommon in children and adolescents, it is not clear how to approach a child with abnormal cervical lymph nodes that can be enlarged for a variety of benign conditions. Nevertheless, persistent cervical lymphadenopathy should prompt a diagnostic investigation. History of radiation exposure or family history of nonmedullary differentiated thyroid cancer should heighten concern.

For diagnostic purposes, in addition to physical examination, a number of imaging modalities are useful. A thyroid scan with RAI can identify the few children who may have a benign condition such as Graves' disease (diffusely abnormal thyroid gland) or an autonomous benign thyroid nodule. Such patients are often thyrotoxic as well, although their thyroid hormone levels may still be in the normal range. A computed tomography or magnetic resonance imaging scan can provide a comprehensive evaluation of the neck and mediastinum and can better identify and describe lymph node metastases. An ultrasound examination of the neck, in experienced hands, provides a sensitive and detailed description of that area. In addition, fine-needle aspiration (FNA) can be done under ultrasound guidance to secure a tissue diagnosis. The FNA has emerged as a relatively simple, minimally invasive, and useful diagnostic modality in this disease. Because pulmonary metastases are relatively common in children with differentiated thyroid cancer, a chest radiograph should be part of the initial evaluation.

After the diagnosis of cancer has been obtained, surgery should follow relatively promptly. A total or near-total thyroidectomy with comprehensive lymph node dissection (as deemed appropriate on the basis of preoperative staging) is generally recommended. Because these children have a prolonged survival duration, aggressive surgery with disfiguring resection is generally avoided, even at the risk of leaving residual microscopic cancer in the neck. A preoperative serum thyroglobulin test is a useful tumor marker for postoperative surveillance of the patients.

With this age group, evaluation for RAI therapy follows surgery in almost all cases. We recommend a diagnostic RAI scan before administration of a larger therapeutic dose of RAI. This approach allows us to omit unnecessary treatment for the few children who may have limited disease and complete resection of RAI-avid tissue. The diagnostic RAI also provides information regarding the extent of RAI-avid disease and allows for better dose planning. For this initial RAI scan and treatment, we use endogenous thyroid-stimulating hormone (TSH) elevation through hypothyroidism rather than the administration of exogenous recombinant TSH to assess for the presence of RAI-avid tissue. A negative pregnancy test must be obtained in pubertal girls before RAI administration. External-beam radiotherapy is generally avoided, even in cases in which there is known or suspected residual tumor after surgery. The known prolonged life expectancy of these children and the late effects of irradiation guide this practice.

After initial surgery, we suggest lifelong surveillance. At M. D. Anderson, we generally see patients every 3 to 6 months during the first 1 to 2 years, depending on the level of clinical concern. Thereafter, if a patient is clinically stable, we usually see them once a year for the first 10 years and every other year thereafter. Each visit includes a history and physical examination, tests of thyroid function and serum thyroglobulin level, and an ultrasound of the neck, especially in patients with lymph node or other extrathyroidal involvement. A chest radiograph is done annually in most cases. The frequency and methodology of subsequent RAI scans and therapies are subjects of discussion in all cases of differentiated thyroid cancer. In children, we tend to be relatively conservative in the use of RAI, mindful of potential long-term toxicities. We obtain a whole-body RAI scan at least once after initial therapy. In this surveillance setting, we are increasingly using exogenous TSH administration rather than thyroid hormone withdrawal to prepare the patients for the scan, because it is better tolerated and apparently equally efficacious. If additional RAI therapy is needed, thyroid hormone withdrawal remains the standard of care.

Regional recurrence in the thyroid bed or cervical (and possibly mediastinal) lymph nodes may occur. A change in the physical examination, diagnostic ultrasound, or serum thyroglobulin level (i.e., elevation) should alert the physician to the need for additional evaluation and possibly treatment. Reoperation for regional recurrence and evaluation for additional postoperative RAI remains the recommended approach at this time. In general, systemic chemotherapy is seldom warranted in patients with differentiated thyroid cancer, particularly in children. Pulmonary metastases, if present, are usually detected at the time of the initial cancer diagnosis or the initial postoperative RAI evaluation. In our experience, disease progression in this area is quite uncommon. After prolonged surveillance, when patients become older adults, the pulmonary metastases may become a clinical problem. This realization, in part, guides the recommendation for lifelong surveillance of children with differentiated thyroid cancer.

After initial therapy, patients become dependent on exogenous thyroid hormone for life. Because chronic TSH elevation can theoretically stimulate the growth of thyroid cancer cells, the dose of thyroid hormone is generally adjusted to produce a relatively suppressed TSH level. However, chronic thyroid hormone excess is not without risk. It could cause irritability, which might interfere with school and social performance; menstrual irregularities, which might lead to ovarian dysfunction; and long-term bone loss. Accordingly, the goal of treatment is to provide thyroid hormone in an amount that achieves high normal thyroxine levels with relatively suppressed TSH. Overall, thyroid hormone replacement is a simple and safe undertaking. Because it is a lifelong medication, we often encounter compliance problems, especially by adolescent patients who may remain relatively asymptomatic despite taking less than the prescribed amount of thyroid hormone.

The diagnosis, treatment, and surveillance of differentiated thyroid cancer often entail rather precisely timed, protracted interventions. For example, in order to administer RAI therapeutically, the patient must remain in a hypothyroid state for at least 10 days. Even for a diagnostic RAI using recombinant TSH, several days must elapse between the first TSH injection and the body imaging scan. Such scheduling of medical care may interfere with important scholastic, social, or other developmental activities and needs. We consider it important to help children maintain a solid sense of well-being and normalcy through the duration of this chronic condition. Accordingly, if medically reasonable, we try to adjust the timing of tests and procedures to accommodate the patients' nonmedical priorities.

The following case examples illustrate some of the scenarios that may play out over time in children with differentiated thyroid cancer.

Case Example 1

A 43-year-old woman was referred to M. D. Anderson for treatment of differentiated thyroid cancer with pulmonary metastases that had been present since her childhood. When she was 9 years of age, a mass developed in her neck; the mass did not respond to antibiotics. Pertinent medical history factors included therapy with radiation for a hemangioma at 2 years of age. Pertinent findings on physical examination included 3 hard nodules on the right thyroid lobe and extensive lymphadenopathy. A chest radiograph showed diffuse micronodular opacities (Figure 11-1). The patient underwent thyroidectomy and right cervical lymph node dissection. The tumor was adherent to the trachea and encased the right recurrent laryngeal nerve, precluding complete resection. Skeletal muscle invasion was described. She received postoperative external-beam radiotherapy (30 treatments) and thyroid hormone replacement therapy. During the 10 years that followed, the patient had neither clinical nor radiologic evidence of disease recurrence or progression, but the chest radiographs remained abnormal.

At 22 years of age, the patient was reevaluated for micronodular, radiologically diffuse "miliary" appearance of the lung fields. After tuberculosis

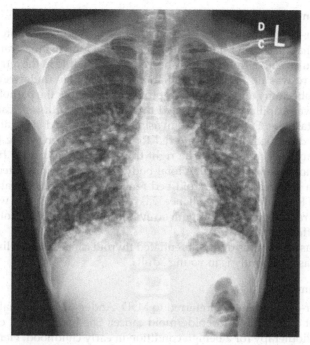

Figure 11–1. This chest radiograph of case 1 shows diffuse micronodular opacities.

was excluded and after thyroid hormone treatment was discontinued for 4 weeks, the patient underwent total-body RAI imaging, which demonstrated intense iodine uptake in the lungs. The patient was treated with 102 mCi of RAI.

During the decade that followed, the patient had 3 uncomplicated pregnancies without clinical or radiologic evidence that the differentiated thyroid cancer had deteriorated. At 40 years of age, she complained of upper-respiratory symptoms and persistent shortness of breath. In addition to stable diffuse micronodular lung lesions, she had a 1.5-cm left lung nodule that on biopsy showed papillary adenocarcinoma with positive thyroglobulin staining. A total-body RAI scan again showed intense pulmonary RAI uptake, and she received another therapeutic dose of RAI (200 mCi). Persistent xerostomia ensued. Her pulmonary function tests revealed moderate restrictive lung disease. She remained clinically and radiologically stable for the next 4 years. During this time, malignant pleural effusion developed. She chose conservative, palliative therapy and died of differentiated thyroid cancer at 46 years of age.

This case illustrates the broad spectrum of clinical presentations and outcomes associated with differentiated thyroid cancer and the potential for very delayed disease-related mortality.

Case Example 2

An 8-year-old boy who presented with upper-respiratory symptoms was found to have a left thyroid nodule. A neck ultrasound demonstrated multiple nodules, and a thyroid scan showed a cold nodule in the left thyroid lobe. There was no history of radiation exposure. He underwent a left thyroid lobectomy and cervical lymph node dissection; the pathologic diagnosis was papillary differentiated thyroid cancer with cervical lymph node metastases. Extrathyroidal invasion of the attached skeletal muscle was also described. He was referred to M. D. Anderson where the thyroidectomy was completed. The right thyroid lobe was tumor free. The chest radiograph was normal. A total-body RAI scan demonstrated iodine uptake in the area of the thyroid bed remnant, and he was treated with 50 mCi of RAI. Lifelong surveillance was recommended. The boy was clinically and radiologically stable with no evidence of disease at last follow-up, 4 years after diagnosis.

This case illustrates that differentiated thyroid cancer may be limited in children as it generally is in young adults.

Case Example 3

A 43-year-old woman was referred to M. D. Anderson for evaluation and treatment of parotid mucoepidermoid cancer. She had received external-beam radiotherapy for a benign condition in early childhood. Her history was significant for the diagnosis of differentiated thyroid cancer when she was 16 years old. The disease involved the thyroid and cervical lymph nodes as well as diffuse, micronodular lung metastases. She was treated with surgery, postoperative external-beam radiotherapy, and RAI. Stable but persistently abnormal chest radiographs were described for the next 12 years. During this time, she was treated with 150 mCi of RAI on 3 occasions because of persistent, intense pulmonary RAI uptake. Her chest radiograph was described as normal 15 years after initial diagnosis and was still normal at her last evaluation, 34 years after the diagnosis of differentiated thyroid cancer.

This case illustrates the prolonged, stable persistence of metastatic disease; the potential for delayed eradication with RAI; the risk of possible radiation-induced second malignancies; and the importance of lifelong surveillance.

CONCLUSIONS

Differentiated thyroid cancer affects a small number of children. Its presentation is characterized by extensive regional disease involvement in most cases and lung metastases in approximately 10% of cases. Total thyroidectomy and thorough cervical lymph node dissection, if lymph nodes are involved, should be the standard initial treatment. A total-body RAI scan is suggested postoperatively to diagnose and treat regional residual tissue or tumor as well as potential lung metastases, which are very RAI avid in most patients. The frequency of additional RAI scans and treatment should be individualized, taking into consideration initial disease extent and pattern, response to initial RAI administration, and the balance between long-term benefits and risks.

Whereas most patients should anticipate a normal life span, a minority of patients die from delayed disease- or treatment-related complications. All patients should be followed lifelong after a diagnosis of childhood differentiated thyroid cancer.

KEY PRACTICE POINTS

- Thyroid masses in children need thorough evaluation.
- Thyroid masses in children are more likely to be malignant than thyroid masses in adults.
- Differentiated thyroid cancer in children often presents at diagnosis as extensive disease.
- Pulmonary metastases in children are relatively common, with characteristic micronodular appearance.
- Prognosis is excellent with near-normal life expectancy.
- Lifelong surveillance is needed.

SUGGESTED READINGS

Brink JS, van Heerden JA, McIver B, et al. Papillary thyroid cancer with pulmonary metastases in children: long-term prognosis. *Surgery* 2000;128:881–886.

DeGroot LJ, Kaplan EL, McCormick M, et al. Natural history, treatment, and course of papillary thyroid carcinoma. *J Clin Endocrinol Metab* 1990;71:414–424.

Dottorini ME, Vignati A, Mazzucchelli L, et al. Differentiated thyroid carcinoma in children and adolescents: a 37-year experience in 85 patients. *J Nucl Med* 1997;38:669–675.

Frankenthaler RA, Vassilopoulou-Sellin R, Cangir A, et al. Lymph node metastasis from papillary-follicular thyroid carcinoma in young patients. *Am J Surg* 1990;160:341–343.

Harness JK, Thompson NW, McLeod MK, et al. Differentiated thyroid carcinoma in children and adolescents. *World J Surg* 1992;16:547–553.

Hung W, Sarlis NJ. Current controversies in the management of pediatric patients with well-differentiated nonmedullary thyroid cancer: a review. *Thyroid* 2002;12:683–702.

Jarzab B, Handkiewicz Junak D, Wloch J, et al. Multivariate analysis of prognostic factors for differentiated thyroid carcinoma in children. *Eur J Nucl Med* 2000;27:833–841.

Mazzaferri EL. Papillary thyroid carcinoma: factors influencing prognosis and current therapy. *Semin Oncol* 1987;14:315–332.

Mazzaferri EL, Kloos RT. Current approaches to primary therapy for papillary and follicular thyroid cancer. *J Clin Endocrinol Metab* 2001;86:1447–1463.

Robbins J, Merino MJ, Boice JD Jr, et al. Thyroid cancer: a lethal endocrine neoplasm. *Ann Intern Med* 1991;115:133–147.

Samaan NA, Schultz PN, Hickey RC, et al. The results of various modalities of treatment of well differentiated thyroid carcinoma: a retrospective review of 1599 patients. *J Clin Endocrinol Metab* 1992;75:714–720.

Schlumberger M, De Vathaire F, Travagli JP, et al. Differentiated thyroid carcinoma in childhood: long-term follow up of 72 patients. *J Clin Endocrinol Metab* 1987;65:1088–1094.

Vassilopoulou-Sellin R. Management of papillary thyroid cancer. *Oncology (Huntingt)* 1995;9:145–151.

Vassilopoulou-Sellin R, Goepfert H, Raney B, et al. Differentiated thyroid cancer in children and adolescents: clinical outcome and mortality after long-term follow-up. *Head Neck* 1998;20:549–555.

Vassilopoulou-Sellin R, Klein MJ, Smith TH, et al. Pulmonary metastases in children and young adults with differentiated thyroid cancer. *Cancer* 1993;71:1348–1352.

Vassilopoulou-Sellin R, Libshitz HI, Haynie TP. Papillary thyroid cancer with pulmonary metastases beginning in childhood: clinical course over 3 decades. *Med Pediatr Oncol Suppl* 1995;24:119–122.

Zimmerman D. Thyroid neoplasia in children. *Curr Opin Pediatr* 1997;9:413–418.

12   MEDULLARY THYROID CARCINOMA

Robert F. Gagel

CHAPTER OVERVIEW

This chapter provides an overview of the diagnosis and treatment of medullary thyroid carcinoma in young patients. Advances in the molecular diagnosis of multiple endocrine neoplasia type 2 have made it possible to diagnose this disorder with certainty in most patients during early childhood. This diagnostic capability is likely to lead to improved clinical outcomes, but it also raises a series of questions and concerns related to surgical intervention in a child. Each of these complex issues is addressed.

INTRODUCTION

Medullary thyroid carcinoma is a malignant neoplasm that is characterized primarily by its production of calcitonin and carcinoembryonic antigen (CEA). Calcitonin is a small peptide originally identified by its ability to lower the serum calcium concentration. The finding of calcitonin and CEA in a tumor with neuroendocrine features is almost always predictive of medullary thyroid carcinoma, and the finding of amyloid is confirmative. There are 2 subtypes of medullary thyroid carcinoma: sporadic and hereditary. The hereditary form is the most common subtype in the pediatric population.

HISTOLOGIC FEATURES

Medullary thyroid carcinoma in its mature form is a firm, white, sometimes chalky tumor. It is composed of parafollicular or calcitonin-producing cells. These cells originate in the neural crest during embryonic development and then migrate into the developing thyroid gland to a parafollicular location (Figure 12–1A). The greatest concentration of parafollicular cells is found in the lobes at the intersection of the upper one-third and lower two-thirds of the cephalad-caudal central axis. The anatomic location of parafollicular cells explains the typical sites of hereditary medullary thyroid carcinoma (Figure 12–1B).

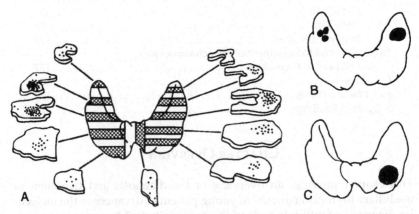

Figure 12–1. (A) Location of normal calcitonin-producing cells in the normal thyroid gland. (B) Characteristic location of medullary thyroid carcinoma in hereditary and sporadic medullary thyroid carcinoma. Reprinted from Grauer A, Raue F, Gagel RF. Changing concepts in the management of hereditary and sporadic medullary thyroid carcinoma. *Endocrinol Metab Clin North Am* 1990;19:613–635, with permission from Elsevier.

Transformed calcitonin cells are usually polyhedral or polygonal in shape and may be arranged in a variety of patterns. Amyloid is dispersed between pockets of transformed parafollicular cells, particularly in slow-growing tumors. Cellular components predominate in more rapidly growing tumors. Tumor calcification is common and may be detected by ultrasound or x-ray.

Rarely, medullary thyroid carcinomas lose their ability to produce calcitonin, which is usually predictive of a poor prognosis. The differential diagnoses of calcitonin-producing tumors include breast cancer; prostate cancer; small-cell lung carcinoma; and other neuroendocrine tumors, including pheochromocytomas, islet-cell carcinomas, and carcinoids. In addition to their differing histologic features, these tumors do not generally produce CEA, which further distinguishes them from medullary thyroid carcinoma. The one example is breast cancer, which can produce both.

Epidemiology and Tumor Subtypes

In the general population, medullary thyroid carcinoma accounts for 5% to 10% of all thyroid carcinomas, with 1,500 to 2,000 new cases diagnosed each year in the United States. Approximately 75% of these tumors are of the sporadic subtype; the remaining 25% are of the hereditary subtype. Hereditary medullary thyroid carcinoma is caused by the transmission of an autosomal dominant trait in 1 of several clinical syndromes (see Table 12–1). Although not predominant in adults, hereditary medullary thyroid carcinoma is the most common subtype of the disease in the pediatric population.

Sporadic Medullary Thyroid Carcinoma

On the initial finding of medullary thyroid carcinoma in patients younger than 20 years of age, clinicians typically consider the tumor to be of the hereditary subtype, because the sporadic subtype is rarely seen in this age group. The sporadic subtype usually presents as a thyroid nodule in adult patients, although loose stools or diarrhea may occasionally be the initial presenting complaint. The diarrhea is generally of low volume, and its frequency and severity correlate directly with tumor mass.

Distant metastasis is common in patients with sporadic medullary thyroid carcinoma. Metastasis to local lymph nodes occurs in more than 75% of patients with a palpable thyroid nodule, making lymph node dissection important even in the absence of lymph node enlargement (Moley and DeBenedetti, 1999). Metastasis is found most commonly in lymph nodes of the central neck, with eventual distribution to levels II to VI lymph nodes and the mediastinum. Hematogenous dissemination most commonly occurs later, with spread to lung, liver, and bone. The metastatic foci tend to be vascular. Hepatic metastasis may be confused with hemangiomas.

Table 12–1. Subtypes and Clinical Features of Medullary Thyroid Carcinoma

Subtype	Feature (% of cases in which this feature occurs)
Sporadic MTC	• Unilateral thyroid nodule • Lymph node metastasis common at time of presentation • Other sites of metastasis include lung, liver, and bone • Uncommon in children or young adults
Hereditary MTC (MEN2)	
MEN2A	• Medullary thyroid carcinoma (100%) • Pheochromocytoma (50%) • Parathyroid neoplasia (10% to 20%)
Variants of MEN2A	• MEN2A/Hirschsprung's disease • MEN2A/cutaneous lichen amyloidosis • Familial medullary thyroid carcinoma
MEN2B	• Medullary thyroid carcinoma (100%) • Pheochromocytoma (50%) • Absence of parathyroid disease • Marfanoid habitus (>90%) • Intestinal ganglioneuromatosis and mucosal neuromas (>90%)

Abbreviations: MEN, multiple endocrine neoplasia; MTC, medullary thyroid carcinoma.

Bone metastases are most commonly lytic. Metastasis to other tissues is less common.

Hereditary Medullary Thyroid Carcinoma

In the pediatric population, medullary thyroid carcinoma occurs most frequently in the context of a genetic syndrome. The most common syndrome is multiple endocrine neoplasia type 2 (MEN2), an autosomal dominant cancer syndrome characterized by medullary thyroid carcinoma, unilateral or bilateral pheochromocytoma, and parathyroid hyperplasia/tumors. MEN2 was first identified as a separate entity by John Sipple (1961). Medullary thyroid carcinoma occurs in all subtypes of MEN2 (MEN2A, variants of MEN2A, and MEN2B). Other manifestations of MEN2 tumors, such as pheochromocytoma, hyperparathyroidism, cutaneous lichen amyloidosis, gastrointestinal neuromas, Hirschsprung's disease, and marfanoid features, occur only with specific subtypes (Table 12-1).

MEN2A

The most common subtype of MEN2 is MEN2A, which accounts for approximately 80% of all cases of hereditary medullary thyroid carcinoma. Sipple's original kindred and the other cases he reported were all examples of MEN2A. Kindreds with this variant generally develop a palpable medullary thyroid carcinoma in the second or third decade of life, unilateral or bilateral pheochromocytoma in the second to fourth decades, and hyperparathyroidism in the third to sixth decades. At the time the syndrome was first described, the major causes of morbidity and death were cardiac arrest or stroke from a pheochromocytoma or death from widespread metastatic medullary thyroid carcinoma.

Variants of MEN2A

There are several variants of MEN2A. In one variant, MEN2A occurs with Hirschsprung's disease. Children with this disease present with obstructive symptomatology in infancy. A family history of thyroid cancer and Hirschsprung's disease in a child presenting with this symptomatology should alert the pediatrician to a possible diagnosis of MEN2A/Hirschsprung's disease.

Another variant, MEN2A/cutaneous lichen amyloidosis, is characterized by a pruritic cutaneous form of amyloid characteristically located over the upper back. Pruritus usually develops in the second or third decade, although there are examples in which localized pruritus was present in childhood before the diagnosis of MEN2A (Nunziata et al, 1989).

Familial medullary thyroid carcinoma is characterized by the presence of medullary thyroid carcinoma with no other manifestations of MEN2 (Farndon et al, 1986). Distinguishing between MEN2A and familial medullary thyroid carcinoma can be difficult; it is most important that the latter is defined by the absence of hyperparathyroidism or pheochromocytoma. Clinicians evaluating small kindreds should be aware of the possibility that a tumor that appears to be familial medullary thyroid carcinoma could actually be MEN2A disguised by 50% or less penetrance of parathyroid and adrenal manifestations. Familial medullary thyroid carcinoma generally tends to be the least aggressive form of medullary thyroid carcinoma, certainly less aggressive than the sporadic subtype.

MEN2B

The most distinctive category of medullary thyroid carcinoma, MEN2B, is considered as such because it is characterized by the presence of mucosal neuromas located over the distal tongue, in the eyelids, and throughout the gastrointestinal tract. Children with this subtype frequently have a body habitus characterized a decreased upper/lower body ratio with long, thin arms and legs, symptoms analogous to Marfan syndrome without the vascular or ophthalmologic abnormalities. These children may be identified by characteristic facial and oral neuromas, although the neuromas can be subtle, particularly early in life.

Children with MEN2B usually present with gastrointestinal discomfort. Young children may present with colic, pseudo-intestinal obstruction, diarrhea, or constipation. Mothers of these children frequently report continual visits to the pediatrician during early childhood for colic or other gastrointestinal symptomatology. Delayed puberty and slipped femoral epiphyses are common. In some children, an observant dentist or oral surgeon might identify mucosal neuromas; in others, the features of MEN2B do not raise suspicion until the child or teenager presents with a thyroid nodule.

Early identification of MEN2B is important. Metastastic medullary thyroid carcinoma in this patient group has been described during the first year of life. Local lymph node metastasis is common during this time period, and distant metastasis is seen with some regularity during the second decade. Medullary thyroid carcinoma is rarely cured by total thyroidectomy; as well, lymph node dissection is not commonly performed and is generally successful only if thyroidectomy and node dissection are performed during the first year of life. Death from metastatic medullary thyroid carcinoma in the context of MEN2B may occur in the third or fourth decade of life, although a larger experience indicates that approximately 50% of children with evidence of metastatic disease will have a long survival duration. There are reports of kindreds with 3 or more living generations of affected members.

Pheochromocytomas, unilateral or bilateral, occur in approximately 50% of patients with MEN2B, necessitating annual screening for these tumors. Hyperparathyroidism is almost never identified in MEN2B. When hypercalcemia is identified, other causes, including bone metastasis or ectopic production of parathyroid hormone-related protein by a pheochromocytoma, should be considered.

Clinical Features of MEN2-Associated Tumors

The medullary thyroid carcinoma found in MEN2A is almost always bilateral and multicentric, and it develops most commonly at the location of the greatest concentration of calcitonin-producing cells in the normal thyroid gland (Figure 12–1B). The earliest identifiable abnormality is a diffuse expansion in the number of calcitonin-producing cells followed by the development of nodules from these cells, and then microscopic foci of medullary thyroid carcinoma. These foci eventually coalesce with other foci to form the tumor. Lymph node metastasis is uncommon with both parafollicular cell (calcitonin-producing) hyperplasia and microscopic medullary thyroid carcinoma, but it is found in more than 75% of all medullary thyroid carcinomas greater than 1 cm in size (Moley and DeBenedetti, 1999).

Because the focus of therapeutic interventions for children with a hereditary subtype of this malignancy has shifted from management of metastasis to prevention of metastasis, the tumor-node-metastasis classification system is not useful for describing early thyroidal changes. Optimally, the thyroid gland will be removed at the earliest stages of tumor development.

The pheochromocytomas found in MEN2-associated tumors evolve from a background of diffuse adrenal medullary hyperplasia and are frequently multifocal. Malignant transformation is rare and is commonly associated with large tumors (Lee et al, 1996). The tumors may develop synchronously or asynchronously, with a 7- to 10-year lag between the development of the primary tumor and one in the contralateral gland (Gagel et al, 1988). There are several reports of symptomatic pheochromocytomas in the first and second decades of life (Gagel et al, 1988), although tumors are more commonly identified in the third and fourth decades.

The pheochromocytomas in MEN2-associated tumors differ from those found in sporadic or other hereditary subtypes (e.g., von Hippel-Lindau disease, hereditary paraganglioma, neurofibromatosis, or MEN1) in another important way. MEN2-related pheochromocytomas produce a disproportionately large amount of epinephrine relative to other chromaffin tumors in which norepinephrine is the predominate product (Gagel et al, 1988). This observation is relevant, because patients with MEN2-related pheochromocytomas are more likely to have adrenergic symptoms of anxiety, tremulousness, and palpitations rather than the noradrenergic finding of hypertension, particularly during their teenage years.

Hyperparathyroidism in MEN2A occurs only rarely during the childhood or teenage years and is almost never the primary manifestation of MEN2A. Hyperparathyroidism is not a component of MEN2B.

EVALUATION AND MANAGEMENT OF HEREDITARY MEDULLARY THYROID CARCINOMA

During the first decade after the initial description of MEN2, management of medullary thyroid carcinoma was focused on the identification of thyroid nodules in patients at risk for MEN2. Medullary thyroid carcinoma was rarely identified before 20 years of age. This changed, however, with the recognition that measurement of calcitonin following stimulation with intravenous calcium or pentagastrin could be used to identify medullary thyroid carcinoma before the development of a palpable mass. This finding led to the use of these agents to identify gene carriers among children at risk for development of medullary thyroid carcinoma. The knowledge that 90% of children at risk for medullary thyroid carcinoma would subsequently develop the disease led to the recommendation of prophylactic thyroidectomy. A 25-year experience with this treatment approach has demonstrated that prophylactic thyroidectomy performed between 10 and 15 years of age can positively alter the outcome of the disease in some kindreds. Whether this intervention has cured all patients is less clear. An 18-year follow-up of 1 kindred showed no evidence of recurrent disease in 28 affected children (Gagel et al, 1988), although 1 child was subsequently diagnosed with nodal metastasis in the neck, and several patients had detectable serum calcitonin values. These concerns and the recognition that metastasis can occur in the context of MEN2A as early as 6 years of age have led to several treatment recommendations. A description of these recommendations follows.

RET Proto-oncogene Mutations in MEN2

Genetic linking efforts identified a centromeric chromosome 10 locus for MEN2 in 1987 (Mathew et al, 1987), and mutations of the *RET* proto-oncogene were subsequently reported in MEN2A, familial medullary thyroid carcinoma (Mulligan et al, 1993), and MEN2B (Hofstra et al, 1994). Two groups of activating mutations have been identified. The first group affects the extracellular domain of the RET receptor. Highly conserved cysteines, important for regulation of receptor dimerization, are mutated to other amino acids (Figure 12–2). A mutation at a single codon (codon 634) accounts for 80% of all mutations found in MEN2, and mutations of codons 609, 611, 618, and 620 account for an additional 10% to 15% of mutations. These mutations cause dimerization and activation of the RET receptor complex, thereby activating downstream ERK 1/2 and JNK pathways, leading to transformation. The second group, which contains intracellular mutations, accounts for approximately 5% to 10% of all germline mutations in MEN2. A single mutation at codon 918 accounts for most of the intracellular-domain mutations. The other intracellular mutations are uncommon (Eng et al, 1996).

Genotype-Phenotype Correlations in MEN2

A codon 634 mutation is most commonly associated with classic MEN2A or Sipple's syndrome. MEN2A/cutaneous lichen amyloidosis has been found only in kindreds with codon 634 mutations. Mutations of codons 609, 611, 618, 620, or 630 may cause familial medullary thyroid carcinoma or MEN2A (Mulligan et al, 1994). The MEN2A/Hirschsprung's disease variant has been found in kindreds with mutations at codons 609, 618, and 620.

The second group of mutations associated with MEN2 affect the intracellular domain (Figure 12–2B). These include mutations at codons 768, 790, 791, 804, 883, 891, 918, and 922. The most common intracellular mutation is an M918T amino acid substitution, which is found in 95% of cases of MEN2B (accounting for approximately 5% of all mutations) (Hofstra et al, 1994). Mutations at codons 883 and 922 have also been associated with MEN2B, although rarely.

Familial medullary thyroid carcinoma without other phenotypic features of MEN2 has been found in kindreds with a mutation at codon 768, 791, or 891 or a V804M amino acid substitution. A mutation at codon 790 and a V804L amino acid substitution have been associated with familial medullary thyroid carcinoma and MEN2A.

RET Proto-oncogene Testing

RET proto-oncogene testing is widely available. A listing of certified laboratories that provide analysis can be found at www.genetests.org. Most laboratories, but not all, perform direct DNA sequencing of the 6 or 7 exons

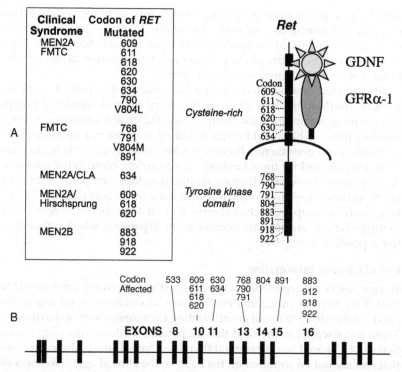

Figure 12–2. Mutations of the *RET* proto-oncogene cause hereditary medullary thyroid carcinoma. (A) The left panel shows the clinical syndrome associated with specfic *RET* codons mutated. (B) Schematic diagram of *RET* proto-oncogene showing specific codons mutated in MEN2. The germline mutations of the *RET* proto-oncogene are distributed in 7 exons that broadly encompass cysteine-rich and tyrosine kinase domains of the receptor. The most common mutations affect the extracellular cysteine-rich region (exons 8, 10, 11) with codon 634 accounting for more than 80% of all mutations in hereditary medullary thyroid carcinoma. Mutations of the intracellular tyrosine kinase domain (exons 13–16) account for approximately 7% to 10% of all mutations. Abbreviations: CLA, cutaneous lichen amyloidosis; FMTC, familial medullary thyroid carcinoma; GDNF, glial cell-derived neurotrophic factor; GFRα-1, glial cell-derived neurotrophic factor receptor alpha-1; MEN, multiple endocrine neoplasia; MTC, medullary thyroid carcinoma.

mutated in hereditary medullary thyroid carcinoma. Most laboratories initially evaluate for the presence of exon 10 and 11 mutations, because they collectively account for more than 90% of all mutations. If mutation of these exons is not identified, the analysis is extended to exons 8, 13, 14, 15, and 16. Because current recommendations for therapeutic intervention are based on *RET* analysis, the 5% or greater potential for testing error is significant.

Most of the errors are related to either sample mix-up (which occurs when one patient's sample is confused with another's) or to specific technical errors (for example, contamination of the polymerase chain reaction by mutant DNA, the failure of the polymerase chain reaction to amplify the mutant allele, or polymerase-induced errors).

An incorrect test result can be problematic for the patient. A false-positive result could lead to an unnecessary thyroidectomy. Although this would be an unfortunate circumstance, the greater concern is a false-negative result, which could result in failure to perform a necessary thyroidectomy in a gene carrier. Because routine annual calcitonin testing has been discontinued for most kindreds, gene carriers come to the attention of clinicians only when a thyroid nodule develops, the point of time in the evolution of the disease when lymph node metastasis is likely. To prevent sample mix-up and technical error, *RET* analysis should be performed twice (preferably at different laboratories) in all patients, whether the initial test is positive or negative.

Use of Genetic Information

Twenty years of experience with prospective screening for hereditary medullary thyroid carcinoma on the basis of calcitonin level has facilitated the transition to use of genetic testing for management of the disease. There is consensus in the field that all patients with an activating mutation of *RET* should be offered total thyroidectomy. There is also consensus that risk should be stratified on the basis of the clinical aggressiveness of medullary thyroid carcinoma associated with the particular *RET* mutation (Brandi et al, 2001). Although these recommendations may be limited, they are based on more than 3 decades of clinical experience with kindreds who have subsequently been shown to have specific *RET* mutations. Information gleaned from studies of in vitro transforming activity of particular *RET* mutations that roughly correlate with clinical experience have also been factored into the stratification of the 3 risk categories: highest, high, and intermediate.

Highest Risk

Children with MEN2B and a *RET* mutation at codon 883, 918, or 922 comprise the highest risk group. Metastasis may occur during the first year of life (Stjernholm et al, 1980), a finding that led to a consensus recommendation for total thyroidectomy and central lymph node dissection during the first few months of life. Levels II to VI lymph nodes should be sampled; if they are found to be positive for disease, a more extensive node dissection should be performed.

High Risk

Children with a *RET* mutation at codon 611, 618, 620, 634, or 891 are considered to be at high risk. There is consensus that these children should have a total thyroidectomy that includes the posterior capsule of the thyroid gland before 5 years of age. The basis for this recommendation is the finding by Scopsi and colleagues (1996) of microscopic medullary thyroid carcinoma in 2 children with codon 634 mutations at 2 years of age and nodal metastasis in a 6-year-old child (Graham et al, 1987). There is less consensus regarding the need for central-node dissection, although most surgeons consider it appropriate to clear the central neck during the primary surgical procedure so that it is not necessary to reenter this compartment during any subsequent operations.

Intermediate Risk

Mutations at codons 609, 768, 790, 791, and 804 are associated with less aggressive medullary thyroid carcinoma. Although lymph node metastasis and death from metastatic medullary thyroid carcinoma have been identified with each of these mutations, there is considerable evidence that a patient with 1 of these mutations is less likely to develop metastatic disease. These patients comprise the intermediate-risk group. Indeed, there are kindreds in which some of these mutations exist although there has never been a death due to medullary thyroid carcinoma, making it difficult to convince parents of the necessity for early thyroidectomy. There is no consensus regarding the appropriate management of children with this group of mutations. Two approaches are currently utilized. The first is to continue performing annual pentagastrin- or calcium-stimulated calcitonin measurements and removing the thyroid gland when the serum calcitonin rises above the normal range. An alternative approach, favored by many working in the field, is to recommend a total thyroidectomy during the teenage or young-adult years. Some clinicians combine these 2 approaches, selecting an age for performance of thyroidectomy unless calcitonin values become abnormal earlier.

Evaluation and Management of Pheochromocytoma and Hyperparathyroidism

Pheochromocytoma is uncommon in the pediatric and young-adult population, but it does occur. It is important to collect a 12- or 24-hour urine sample or measure plasma metanephrines and catecholamines before thyroidectomy and to initiate an annual screening process for pheochromocytoma. Gagel and Marx (2003) have published a detailed report on the management of pheochromocytoma.

Hyperparathyroidism is almost never seen in children, but it would be prudent to perform a serum calcium measurement at the age of 10 years and every 2 to 4 years thereafter.

Conclusions

Hereditary medullary thyroid carcinoma is one of the rare genetic malignancies in which the identification of gene carrier status leads to specific therapeutic action. Although not proven with certainty, evidence collected indicates that intervention in young children will have a positive impact on the morbidity and mortality associated with this syndrome and may lead to cure in a significant percentage of this patient population.

KEY PRACTICE POINTS

- Medullary thyroid carcinoma in children is almost always hereditary.
- Genetic testing for medullary thyroid carcinoma in the context of MEN2 provides certainty of diagnosis.
- Prophylactic thyroidectomy is indicated in children with specific *RET* proto-oncogene mutations.
- When making a treatment decision, clinicians should consider the specific *RET* codon mutated.
- Clinicians should balance the risks and benefits of prophylactic thyroidectomy in each child.
- Patients with a medullary thyroid carcinoma that is less than 1 cm in size should have a lymph node dissection.

Suggested Readings

Brandi ML, Gagel RF, Angeli A, et al. Guidelines for diagnosis and therapy of MEN type 1 and type 2. *J Clin Endocrinol Metab* 2001;86:5658–5671.

Eng CD, Clayton I, Schuffenecker G, et al. The relationship between specific RET proto-oncogene mutations and disease phenotype in multiple endocrine neoplasia type 2. International RET mutation consortium analysis. *JAMA* 1996;276:1575–1579.

Farndon JR, Leight GS, Dilley WG, et al. Familial medullary thyroid carcinoma without associated endocrinopathies: a distinct clinical entity. *Br J Surg* 1986;73:278–281.

Gagel RF, Marx S. Multiple endocrine neoplasia. In: Larsen PR, Kronenberg H, Melmed S, et al., eds. *Williams Textbook of Endocrinology.* Philadelphia, PA: WB Saunders; 2003:1717–1762.

Gagel RF, Tashjian AH Jr, Cummings T, et al. The clinical outcome of prospective screening for multiple endocrine neoplasia type 2a: an 18-year experience. *N Engl J Med* 1988;318:478–484.

Graham SM, Genel M, Touloukian RJ, et al. Provocative testing for occult medullary carcinoma of the thyroid: findings in seven children with multiple endocrine neoplasia type IIa. *J Pediatr Surg* 1987;22:501–503.

Hofstra RM, Landsvater RM, Ceccherini I, et al. A mutation in the RET proto-oncogene associated with multiple endocrine neoplasia type 2B and sporadic medullary thyroid carcinoma. *Nature* 1994;367:375–376.

Lee JE, Curley SA, Gagel RF, et al. Cortical-sparing adrenalectomy for patients with bilateral pheochromocytoma. *Surgery* 1996;120:1064–1071.

Mathew CG, Chin KS, Easton DF, et al. A linked genetic marker for multiple endocrine neoplasia type 2A on chromosome 10. *Nature* 1987;328:527–528.

Moley JF, DeBenedetti MK. Patterns of nodal metastases in palpable medullary thyroid carcinoma: recommendations for extent of node dissection. *Ann Surg* 1999;229:880–888.

Mulligan LM, Eng C, Healey CS, et al. Specific mutations of the RET proto-oncogene are related to disease phenotype in MEN 2A and FMTC. *Nature Genet* 1994;6:70–74.

Mulligan LM, Kwok JB, Healey CS, et al. Germ-line mutations of the RET proto-oncogene in multiple endocrine neoplasia type 2A. *Nature* 1993;363:458–460.

Nunziata V, Giannattasio R, di Giovanni G, et al. Hereditary localized pruritus in affected members of a kindred with multiple endocrine neoplasia type 2A (Sipple's syndrome). *Clin Endocrinol* 1989;30:57–63.

Scopsi L, Sampietro G, Boracchi P, et al. Multivariate analysis of prognostic factors in sporadic medullary carcinoma of the thyroid. A retrospective study of 109 consecutive patients. *Cancer* 1996;78:2173–2183.

Sipple, JH. The association of pheochromocytoma with carcinoma of the thyroid gland. *Am J Med* 1961;31:163–166.

Stjernholm MR, Freudenbourg JC, Mooney HS, et al. Medullary carcinoma of the thyroid before age 2 years. *J Clin Endocrinol Metab* 1980;51:252–253.

13 MELANOMA

Cynthia E. Herzog, Hafeez Diwan, Merrick I. Ross, and Victor G. Prieto

CHAPTER OVERVIEW

Melanoma rarely occurs in pediatric patients, so health care professionals must make special considerations to ensure an accurate diagnosis and to plan appropriate treatment for this age group. Because there are limited data on melanoma in pediatric patients, the guidelines presented here are based on reports of melanoma in adults. However, issues specific to the diagnosis and treatment of pediatric patients with melanoma are addressed.

INTRODUCTION

Melanoma is rare in pediatric patients, and it occurs primarily in adolescents. Surveillance, Epidemiology, and End Results data from the National Cancer Institute report annual incidence rates of 0.7 cases per 1 million children younger than 10 years of age, 2.2 cases per 1 million children 10 to 14 years of age, and 12.3 cases per 1 million adolescents 15 to 19 years of age. In the general population, the annual incidence rate is 172 cases per 1 million people. Although sun exposure is a contributing factor to melanoma development in adults, it is not clear whether sun exposure plays a role in melanoma development in pediatric patients. An exception is xeroderma pigmentosum, a genetic condition that is characterized by ultraviolet light sensitivity and the development of multiple skin cancers. A minority of pediatric patients may have a known predisposition for melanoma, such as dysplastic nevus syndrome or familial melanoma, but most have no identifiable predisposing factors.

DIAGNOSIS AND STAGING

When a child has a suspicious skin lesion, melanoma is usually not considered initially because it is rare in this age group. However, as in adults, when the lesion is irregularly colored, changes color, rapidly increases in size, or has irregular borders, removal should be considered. A conservative excision is done initially to obtain a tissue sample for pathologic evaluation. A finding of melanoma on pathologic evaluation will lead to subsequent definitive surgery. However, because melanomas can mimic nevi, the diagnosis is sometimes not established until after metastases develop.

The staging of cutaneous melanoma in pediatric patients at M. D. Anderson Cancer Center is based on the 2002 revised American Joint Commission on Cancer (AJCC) melanoma staging system (Tables 13–1 and 13–2). Although this staging system was derived primarily from data on older patients, the analyses used to establish the system included information on patients of all ages. The AJCC system combines clinical findings with pathology information about the primary tumor and possible metastases.

PATHOLOGY

Primary Skin Tumor

Because of the rarity of this disease in pediatric patients, melanoma can be a difficult pathologic diagnosis to make in this population. An

Table 13–1. American Joint Commission on Cancer Tumor-Node-Metastasis Classification System

Tumor	Thickness (mm)	Ulceration
T1	≤1.0	a: no ulceration, Clark level II/III
		b: ulceration or Clark level IV/V
T2	1.01–2.0	a: no ulceration
		b: ulceration
T3	2.01–4.0	a: no ulceration
		b: ulceration
T4	>4.0	a: no ulceration
		b: ulceration

Node	Number of Positive Lymph Nodes	Nodal Metastatic Mass
N1	1	a: micro
		b: macro
N2	2–3	a: micro
		b: macro
		c: in-transit, satellite with negative nodes
N3	≥4 matted or in-transit satellite with positive nodes	

Table 13–2. American Joint Commission on Cancer Clinical and Pathologic Staging Systems for Cutaneous Melanoma

Clinical Staging				Pathologic Staging			
Stage	Tumor	Node	Metastasis	Stage	Tumor	Node	Metastasis
0	Tis	N0	M0	0	Tis	N0	M0
1A	T1a	N0	M0	1A	T1a	N0	M0
1B	T1b	N0	M0	1B	T1b	N0	M0
	T2a				T2a		
IIA	T2b	N0	M0	IIA	T2b	N0	M0
	T3a				T3a		
IIB	T3b	N0	M0	IIB	T3b	N0	M0
	T4a				T4a		
IIC	T4b	N0	M0	IIC	T4b	N0	M0
III	Any	N+	M0	IIIA	T1–4a	N1a	M0
					T1–4a	N2a	
				IIIB	T1–4b	N1a	M0
					T1–4b	N2a	
					T1–4a	N1b	
					T1–4a	N2b	
					T1–4a	N2c	
				IIIC	T1–4b	N1b	M0
					T1–4b	N2b	
					T1–4b	N2c	
					Any	N3	
IV	Any	Any	Any	IV	Any	Any	Any

Abbreviations: M, metastasis; N, node; T, tumor; Tis, tumor in situ.

experienced dermatopathologist is needed for the pathologic evaluations of the skin lesions, because melanomas in children and adolescents present with histologic features distinct from those found in melanomas in adults.

In the revised AJCC melanoma staging criteria, the most important prognostic factors for primary disease are Breslow thickness and ulceration. Clark level of invasion is of prognostic value only in melanomas less than 1 mm in thickness. At M. D. Anderson, the pathology report for a child with melanoma contains the same prognostic criteria used for adults with melanoma: histologic subtype, Clark level, Breslow thickness, margin status, degree of inflammatory infiltrate, presence or absence of ulceration, radial growth phase, vertical growth phase, regression, satellitosis, vascular invasion, perineural invasion, and associated nevus.

Differential Diagnoses

Spitz nevus (or spindle and epithelioid cell nevi) is probably the lesion that most closely resembles melanoma in both children and adults. Spitz nevus can usually be distinguished from melanoma by a combination of histologic features (Table 13–3 and Figure 13–1). Lesions lacking these features or exhibiting necrosis, a biphasic pattern indicating a possible transformation into melanoma, or mitotic figures in the deep dermis indicate a possible Spitzoid melanoma (Figure 13–2). We recommend a conservative but complete primary excision of even routine-appearing Spitz nevi if clinically feasible, because key histologic features, including circumscription and symmetry, cannot be reliably evaluated in lesions extending to the margins.

Proliferative nodules in congenital nevi may also resemble melanoma, both clinically and histologically. Such lesions have evident growth and

Table 13–3. Histologic Features Distinguishing Spitz Nevus from Melanoma

Features	Spitz Nevus	Melanoma
Symmetry	Present	Usually absent
Circumscription	Sharp	Poor
Pagetoid spread	Absent or only in the center of the lesion	Prominent
Kamino bodies	Occasional	Rare
Cohesiveness of epidermal nests	Present	Usually absent
Melanin	Scant	Usually prominent
Vertical orientation of nests	Present	Usually absent
Maturation	Present	Rarely
"Breaking up" of nests in the dermis	Present	Rarely
Edema or telangiectasia in the dermis	Present	Usually absent

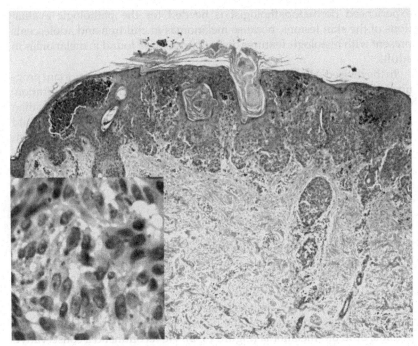

Figure 13–1. Spitz nevus. Circumscribed and symmetrical lesion. Junctional nests are evenly distributed, arranged perpendicular to the epidermal surface, and show a vertical cleft. Inset shows large epithelioid cells with prominent nucleoli.

nodularity, generally occurring in the first year of the patient's life, within large congenital nevi. Histologically, these lesions contain a discrete nodule with expansile architecture, mitotic figures, and some cytologic atypia, and they require close clinical follow-up, because there is a possibility that melanoma may arise in a congenital nevus.

The terms "typical nevus," "dysplastic nevus," and "Clark nevus" are synonymous. The National Institutes of Health Consensus Conference has recommended dropping the term "dysplastic nevus" and proposed instead "nevus with architectural disorder and cytologic atypia." Much controversy has surrounded the definition of dysplastic nevus. In essence, it is a nevus that resembles melanoma both clinically and histologically. Points of clinical similarity between dysplastic nevus and melanoma include large size (generally greater than 5 mm), poor circumscription, border irregularity, irregular or changing colors, and asymmetry. Atypical nevi occur in 2% to 9% of unselected white patients in most series. Nevi with clinical and histologic atypia are a strong, independent risk factor for development of melanoma regardless of whether the atypical nevi occur sporadically or in the context of a melanoma-prone familial predisposition (so-called

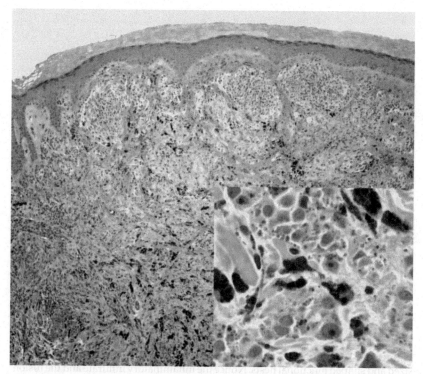

Figure 13–2. Spitzoid melanoma. Exophytic and endophytic lesion with epidermal hyperplasia. The lesion is large and has abundant melanin pigment in the deep dermis. Inset shows large cells very similar to those seen in Figure 13–1; hence the term "spitzoid."

"dysplastic nevus syndrome"). Moreover, the melanoma risk rises proportionately with the number of atypical nevi. The histopathology of atypical nevi involves abnormalities in architecture, host response, and cytology (Figure 13–3).

Sentinel Lymph Nodes

At M. D. Anderson, initial examination of the sentinel lymph nodes is done using routine hematoxylin and eosin (H&E) staining of a "breadloafed" node (a node cut into several sections). Sentinel lymph nodes that are found to be negative for melanoma on routine H&E staining are further analyzed by repeat H&E staining of a deeper tissue section and by immunohistochemical labeling with a panmelanoma antibody (human melanoma black [HMB]-45 or melanoma antigen recognized by T cells [MART]-1). The final pathology report documents the number of involved lymph nodes, the size of the tumor deposit, and whether extracapsular extension is present.

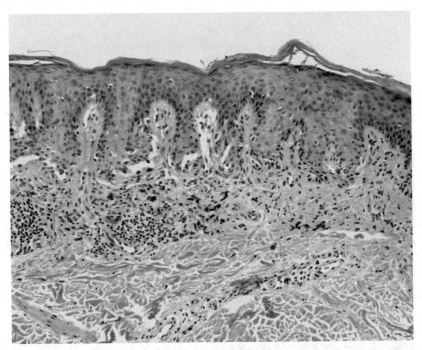

Figure 13–3. Atypical or Clark nevus. Relatively small lesion with irregularly sized and shaped junctional nests. Notice the inflammatory infiltrate and the fusion of rete ridges ("bridging").

Lymph Node Dissection

At M. D. Anderson, after a histologic diagnosis of lymph node metastasis is established, patients undergo lymph node dissection in which all lymph nodes are removed, submitted in their entirety for pathologic analysis, and evaluated histologically.

Immunohistochemisty

Antibodies against antigens typically expressed in melanocytic cells, such as S100 protein, gp100 (detected with HMB-45), or MART-1, can be used to confirm melanocytic lineage in a given neoplasm. Also, immunohisto-chemistry may help detect small clusters or even single melanoma cells within sentinel lymph node specimens (Figure 13–4).

A controversial subject is whether immunohistochemistry should be used to help differentiate between melanomas and nevus. We strongly feel that, in select cases and along with clinical and histologic criteria, immunohistochemical data are helpful in diagnosing melanocytic lesions, such as in assessing "maturation" in the dermal components. Superficial round type-A nevus cells share many immunohistochemical markers with neurons, whereas deep spindle type-C nevus cells resemble Schwann cells.

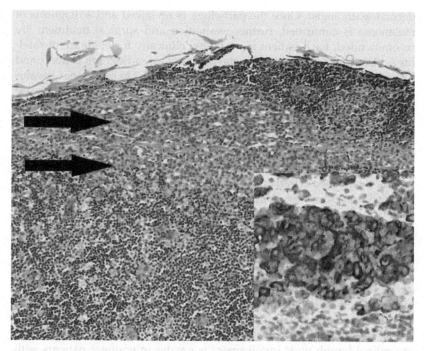

Figure 13–4. Sentinel lymph node containing a small cluster of melanoma cells (arrows), hematoxylin and eosin. Inset: These cells express melanocytic markers (gp100 [with HMB-45]). Diaminobenzidine with light hematoxylin as counterstain.

These features are seen in nevi but not in melanomas. This morphology is reflected in the decreased expression of gp100 by melanocytes located at the base of nevus and not in melanomas. Also, the almost universal lack of mitotic figures in the deep regions of nevi correlates with the very sparse expression of proliferation markers, such as Ki-67, by more deeply located melanocytes in nevi.

Using immunohistochemical expression patterns as a guide, Rudolph et al (1997) reclassified 112 lesions that on routine histologic evaluation were found to be diagnostically problematic. On subsequent clinical review, systemic progression occurred in 70.7% of the cases finally classified as melanoma and in none of those finally classified as benign lesions. These highly significant results highlight the potential usefulness of immunohistochemistry in differentiating between nevi and melanomas.

SURGICAL TREATMENT

Wide Local Excision

According to M. D. Anderson policy, the first step after an initial excisional biopsy is to have the tissue sample reviewed by an experienced dermatopathologist. Once the pathology is reviewed and a diagnosis of melanoma is confirmed, further evaluation and surgical treatment are recommended. Each patient is evaluated clinically for evidence of satellite, in-transit, or lymph node metastasis; a chest radiograph is done; and serum lactate dehydrogenase levels are measured. On preliminary evaluation, only a few pediatric patients have evidence of the spread of disease beyond the primary site. Whether the patient should be further evaluated for metastasis is determined on the basis of the risk of occult metastases associated with specific pathologic findings.

When wide local excision is performed, the surgical margins are determined on the basis of the thickness and site of the primary tumor, which are the established criteria used for adults. Generally, 1- to 2-cm margins are used for lesions less than 2 mm thick, and 2-cm margins are used for lesions thicker than 2 mm. More conservative margins are often used in anatomically restricted areas, such as the face.

Lymph Node Mapping

At M. D. Anderson, patients with melanomas more than 1 mm thick or melanomas less than 1 mm thick but with ulceration or Clark level IV or V invasion undergo lymph node mapping and sentinel lymph node biopsy (SLNB). Evidence in adult patients indicates that the incidence rate of sentinel lymph node involvement is greater in younger patients with thin melanomas than in older adults. So although lymph node mapping and SLNB are not routinely performed in adults with thin melanomas, these procedures should be considered for pediatric patients even with melanomas less than 1 mm in thickness and with no ulceration and that are Clark level II or III. An SLNB may be performed in patients with atypical Spitz nevi. Involvement of the sentinel lymph node in such a case can serve as a surrogate for a true diagnosis of melanoma.

Patients undergo preoperative lymphoscintigraphy (LS) with an intradermal injection of the radioactive tracer ^{99m}Tc-sulfur colloid. LS can identify the lymph node basin or basins at risk for involvement. It is particularly useful in regions such as the trunk or head and neck where 1 or more lymph node basins may be involved and can also detect abnormal lymph node drainage sites. At the time of surgery, isosulfan blue dye is injected intradermally in the patient to visualize the sentinel lymph node, and a hand-held gamma counter is used to detect the ^{99m}Tc-sulfur colloid. The combination of isosulfan blue dye and ^{99m}Tc-sulfur colloid results in identification of a sentinel lymph node in 99% of cases. The hand-held gamma counter is not only useful in examining the lymph node basin or basins identified by LS but also intervening areas and other lymph node basins at risk and in detecting abnormal lymph node drainage sites, which occur in about 5% of patients. Lymph nodes that localize dye or concentrate ^{99m}Tc-sulfur colloid are excised and examined histologically.

Lymph Node Dissection

When melanoma is detected clinically or pathologically in any lymph node, lymph node dissection is recommended.

EVALUATION FOR METASTASIS

Blood Tests

No blood test has been proven wholly reliable in screening for melanoma metastases. An elevated lactate dehydrogenase (LDH) level is used as a screening study, but the usefulness of this laboratory value in children and adolescents is questionable. Children normally have higher levels of LDH than adults do, so if not interpreted with caution, an elevated LDH level can lead to an unnecessary imaging study looking for metastases.

Imaging Studies

In all patients with melanoma, a routine chest radiograph is performed to look for pulmonary metastases. In patients with high-risk melanoma (greater than 4 mm thick ulceration or 1 or more positive lymph nodes), a computed tomography (CT) scan of the chest and abdomen is done to look for lung and liver metastases. Patients with high-risk melanoma of the lower extremity should also have a CT of the pelvis, and patients with high-risk head and neck melanoma should have a head and neck CT.

Positron emission tomography imaging has been approved for use in evaluating melanoma. Pediatric patients frequently have reactive lymph nodes, which raises concerns about metastatic disease. In such cases, positron emission tomography may be helpful in differentiating reactive lymph nodes from metastatic lymph nodes.

SYSTEMIC THERAPY

Adjuvant Therapy

Interferon

Patients with stage I, IIA, or IIB disease who have been treated with definitive surgical treatment but no adjuvant therapy are followed. Treatment for patients with higher-stage disease is discussed at our Melanoma Multidisciplinary Conference, with input from pathologists, melanoma surgeons, medical and pediatric oncologists, and radiation oncologists.

Adjuvant treatment with interferon is recommended for pediatric patients with stage IIC disease or for patients younger than 10 years old who have stage III disease. In our experience, treatment with interferon is generally better tolerated in pediatric patients than in adult patients.

Table 13–4.   Schedule Used to Monitor Patients Treated with Adjuvant
               Interferon

Test	Pretreatment	Week 2	Every month	Every 3–4 months	End
Complete blood count	+	+	+		+
Lytes, creatinine, serum glutamic-pyruvic transaminase, bilirubin	+	+	+		+
Thyroid function test	+			+	+
Ophthalmologic examination	+			+	+
Neuropsychologic testing	+				+

Treatment with interferon can result in significant toxicity, and patients must be monitored closely. Common toxicities in adults include fever, malaise and flu-like symptoms, fatigue, myalgia, nausea and vomiting, myelosuppression, liver toxicity, and neuropsychologic and psychiatric changes. In infants treated with interferon for hemangioma, cases of spastic diplegia have been reported. Because interferon acts as an antiangiogenic agent, concerns have been raised about the potential long-term effects it may have on a child's physical growth. Patients are also at increased risk for retinal changes. The monitoring plan used at M. D. Anderson for pediatric patients treated with interferon is shown in Table 13–4.

Biochemotherapy

Patients with stage IV melanoma may be offered biochemotherapy. Biochemotherapy is given approximately every 3 weeks and consists of dacarbazine given on day 1, cisplatin and vinblastine given on days 1 through 4, interleukin-2 given by continuous infusion on days 1 through 4, and interferon alfa-2b given on days 1 through 5.

Vaccine Therapies

Although numerous vaccine trials are ongoing in adult patients with melanoma, these therapies are generally not available to pediatric patients.

Treatment of Measurable Disease

Pediatric patients rarely have measurable disease after initial definitive surgery. For the rare patient who has metastatic or recurrent disease, treatment is individualized. Some of these patients will qualify for treatment in protocols designed for adults with melanoma.

FOLLOW-UP

Patients with melanoma are at increased risk for recurrence and need long-term follow-up. Concerns persist about the existence of predisposing

Table 13–5.   Treatment and Follow-Up Recommendations Based on Disease Stage

Disease Stage	Treatment and Evaluation	Follow-up
1A	• WLE • Consider SLNB	PE, CXR, and LDH every 6 months for 2 years and then annually.
1B, IIA, IIB	• WLE • SLNB	PE, CXR, and LDH every 3 months for 2 years, then every 6 months for 3 years, and then annually.
IIC	• WLE • SLNB • Stage with CT and PET • Consider adjuvant interferon	PE, CXR, and LDH every 3 months for 2 years, then every 6 months for 3 years, and then annually. CT and PET every 6 months for 5 years then annually.
IIIA-C	• WLE • SLNB and LND • Stage with CT and PET • Adjuvant therapy	PE, CXR, and LDH every 3 months for 2 years, then every 6 months for 3 years, and then annually. CT and PET every 6 months for 5 years and then annually.
IV	Individualized	

Abbreviations: CT, computed tomography; CXR, chest x-ray; LDH, lactate dehydrogenase; LND, lymph node dissection; PE, physical exam; PET, positron emission tomography; SLNB, sentinel lymph node biopsy; WLE, wide local excision.

genetic factors that may cause children to be at increased risk of second primary melanomas. Our recommendations for treatment and follow-up based on the stage of disease are given in Table 13–5.

KEY PRACTICE POINTS

- Practitioners should consider the possibility of melanoma in pediatric patients presenting with a suspicious skin lesion.
- Pathology must be reviewed by a dermatopathologist that is cognizant of the age of the patient.
- Definitive surgery should be performed by a surgeon familiar with the techniques of lymph node mapping and sentinel lymph node biopsy.

SUGGESTED READINGS

Bacchi CE, Bonetti F, Pea M, et al. HMB-45: a review. *Appl Immunohistochem* 1996;4:73–85.

Balch CM, Buzaid AC, Soong S-J, et al. Final version of the American Joint Committee on Cancer staging system for cutaneous melanoma. *J Clin Oncol* 2001;19:3635–3648.

Balch CM, Soong S-J, Gershenwald JE, et al. Prognostic factors analysis of 17,600 melanoma patients: validation of the American Joint Committee on Cancer melanoma staging system. *J Clin Oncol* 2001;19:3622–3634.

Binder SW, Ansong C, Paul E, et al. The histology and differential diagnosis of Spitz nevus. *Semin Diagn Pathol* 1998;10:36–46.

Ceballos PI, Ruiz-Maldonado R, Mihm MCJ. Melanoma in children. *N Engl J Med* 1995;332:656–662.

Gershenwald JE, Colome MI, Lee JE, et al. Patterns of recurrence following a negative sentinel lymph node biopsy in 243 patients with stage I or II melanoma. *J Clin Oncol* 1998;16:2253–2260.

Gershenwald JE, Thompson W, Mansfield PF, et al. Multi-institutional melanoma lymphatic mapping experience: the prognostic value of sentinel lymph node status in 612 stage I or II melanoma patients. *J Clin Oncol* 1999;17:976–983.

Handfield-Jones SE, Smith NP. Malignant melanoma in childhood. *Br J Dermatol* 1996;34:607–616.

Kirkwood JM, Ibrahim JG, Sondak VK, et al. High- and low-dose interferon alfa-2b in high-risk melanoma: first analysis of Intergroup Trial E1690/S9111/C91190. *J Clin Oncol* 2000;18:2444–2458.

Kirkwood JM, Ibrahim JG, Sosman JA, et al. High-dose interferon alfa-2b significantly prolongs relapse-free and overall survival compared with the GM2-KLH/QS-21 vaccine in patients with resected stage IIB-III melanoma: results of Intergroup Trial E1694/S9512/C509801. *J Clin Oncol* 2001;19:2370–2380.

Kirkwood JM, Strawderman MH, Ernstoff MS, et al. Interferon alfa-2b adjuvant therapy of high-risk resected cutaneous melanoma: the Eastern Cooperative Oncology Group Trial EST 1684. *J Clin Oncol* 1996;14:7–17.

Lohmann CM, Coit DG, Brady MS, et al. Sentinel lymph node biopsy in patients with diagnostically controversial Spitzoid melanocytic tumors. *Am J Surg Pathol* 2002;26:47–55.

NIH Consensus Cconference. Diagnosis and treatment of early melanoma. *JAMA* 1992;268:1314–1319.

Prieto VG, Clark SH. Processing of sentinel lymph nodes for detection of metastatic melanoma. *Ann Diagn Pathol* 2002;6:257–264.

Prieto VG, McNutt NS, Lugo J, et al. The intermediate filament peripherin is expressed in cutaneous melanocytic lesions. *J Cutan Pathol* 1997;24:145–150.

Reed JA, Finnerty B, Albino AP. Divergent cellular differentiation pathways during the invasive stage of cutaneous malignant melanoma progression. *Am J Pathol* 1999;155:549–555.

Rudolph P, Schubert C, Schubert B, et al. Proliferation marker Ki-S5 as a diagnostic tool in melanocytic lesions. *J Am Acad Dermatol* 1997;37:169–178.

Ruiz-Maldonado R, Orozco-Covarrubias M. Malignant melanoma in children. A review. *Arch Dermatol* 1997;133:363–371.

Scalzo DA, Hida CA, Toth G, et al. Childhood melanoma: a clinicopathological study of 22 cases. *Melanoma Res* 1997;7:63–68.

Su LD, Fullen DR, Sondak VK, et al. Sentinel lymph node biopsy for patients with problematic Spitzoid melanocytic lesions. *Cancer* 2003;97:499–507.

Sumner WEI, Ross MI, Mansfield PF, et al. Implications of lymphatic drainage to unusual sentinel lymph node sites in patients with primary cutaneous melanoma. *Cancer* 2002;95:354–360.

Tucker MA, Halpern A, Holly EA, et al. Clinically recognized dysplastic nevi. A central risk factor for cutaneous melanoma. *JAMA* 1997;277:1439–1444.

Walsh N, Crotty K, Palmer A, et al. Spitz nevus versus spitzoid malignant melanoma: an evaluation of the current distinguishing histopathologic criteria. *Hum Pathol* 1998;29:1105–1112.

14 NOVEL THERAPEUTIC APPROACHES

Sima S. Jeha and Laura L. Worth

CHAPTER OVERVIEW

During the latter part of the twentieth century, substantial improvements were made in the treatment of childhood cancers. Fifty years ago, most pediatric cancers were fatal. Today, however, more than 75% of pediatric patients with cancer survive the disease. Most advances have been achieved through extensive research and well-designed clinical trials. Investigators continue to explore novel therapies with the goals of providing salvage treatment to patients whose disease does not respond to current therapies and of improving the efficacy and safety of frontline regimens. Recent advances in the fields of genetics, immunology, and molecular biology have led to a better understanding of childhood cancers, which in turn has led to the rational design of drugs based on a thorough understanding of targets on or inside malignant cells. Such an approach aims to further improve cure rates and reduce toxicity. This chapter describes the novel therapies available to pediatric patients at M. D. Anderson Cancer Center. We describe the difficulties of conducting innovative research in children as well as how multidisciplinary interactions at M. D. Anderson help children quickly and safely benefit from novel therapies, including stem cell transplantation for leukemia, lymphoma, and other solid tumors.

INTRODUCTION

The sequencing of the human genome and the elucidation of many molecular pathways involved in cancer-cell proliferation, apoptosis, and metastasis have provided unprecedented opportunities for the development of anticancer agents. The challenge now is to conduct efficient evaluations of increasingly varied new agents, including small molecules, monoclonal antibodies, antisense oligonucleotides, and ribosomes.

Before a new treatment can be tested in humans, it must be shown to be effective and safe in laboratory and animal studies. Cancer clinical trials then progress in 4 phases that take about 9 years to complete. Each trial has its own eligibility criteria and often has restrictions based on the type and stage of cancer and the ages, previous treatments, and medical conditions of patients at the time the study is to be conducted.

Phase I trials are dose-finding studies that usually test a new treatment in humans for the first time. The study group is typically composed of 15 to 30 patients with cancer that is refractory to standard treatment. Researchers focus on determining the dose-limiting toxicities and maximum tolerated dose (MTD) of a new treatment in order to establish whether it is safe for use in humans. If the treatment is shown to be safe in a phase I trial, it is then evaluated in a phase II trial. In this phase, researchers assess its antineoplastic activity while continuing to monitor its safety. Phase II trials enroll fewer than 100 participants and usually focus on a particular type of cancer. A treatment that is shown to be effective in a phase II trial is then evaluated in a phase III trial where its efficacy and safety are compared with those of the standard treatment for a particular disease. Phase IV trials assess the long-term safety and effectiveness of the treatment.

In this chapter, we present the strategies followed at M. D. Anderson to resolve some of the issues that typically delay the availability of novel therapies to children and adolescents with cancer.

REALITIES OF PEDIATRIC CLINICAL RESEARCH

Several issues create challenges in the development of new drugs for pediatric patients. Here, we discuss 3: the stringent regulatory requirements, the slow accrual of children for clinical trials, and the need for more biologic correlates.

Stringent Regulatory Requirements

The first 7 decades of the twentieth century were a period of major drug discovery, new drug development, and the establishment of standards for cancer treatment and care. Limited preclinical screening procedures allowed the licensing of some very effective drugs, notably the antimicrobials, which would not have been possible with current screening procedures. The call for careful toxicology and preclinical screening in the 1970s led to stringent regulatory laws and labeling rules. As a result, the drug development process slowed considerably. This delay in research was particularly problematic for pediatric oncology because the initiation of investigational drug testing in children and adolescents usually has to await the completion of early-phase testing in adults.

The pharmaceutical industry has little impetus to study drugs in children because of the complexity of such trials and the small financial return. Instead, it is presumed that children respond to therapies the same as adults. Therefore, the anticancer therapies approved for use in adults are used to treat children, often without data to support appropriate application in the latter population.

In the past decade, an unprecedented number and diversity of novel antineoplastic therapies were introduced that must now be tested in an increasingly heavily pretreated population. The previously developed evaluation process needs to be revisited to allow the science of drug development to thrive while preserving patients' safety. Regulatory agencies are undergoing continued reorganization aimed at shortening the processes involved in bringing new drugs to the market. The Best Pharmaceuticals for Children Act provides a mechanism for the Food and Drug Administration and the National Institutes of Health to develop and fund studies in pediatric patients to gather information on off-patent drugs.

Slow Accrual

Pediatric cancer is rare, and most patients are cured with current frontline therapies. Patients who do experience first relapse are treated with salvage regimens of conventional chemotherapy. Accrual on early-phase trials is usually much slower for children than for adults, in whom cancer is more prevalent and less responsive.

Because of the high cure rate achieved in childhood cancers, most oncologists on the pediatric service are unimpressed by positive treatment responses achieved in adult patients. Hence, many of these clinicians are reluctant to refer patients who have experienced relapse for investigational therapy, especially if the therapy involves traveling to another center. Rather, they opt for the patient to remain close to home and to receive other palliative treatments from the care team with whom they are familiar. The reluctance of third-party payers to cover treatment under early-phase trials further discourages referrals to investigational protocols.

The modes of action of anticancer agents in development are increasingly varied. With the current trend of targeting aberrant genes and pathways, new drugs are expected to work in narrowly defined patient populations. This limitation presents another challenge to accrual on early-phase pediatric trials.

Patients, medical professionals, and third-party payers must recognize that higher rates of accrual to investigational trials will accelerate improvements in cancer treatment.

Need for More Biologic Correlates

Most early-phase pediatric trials lack biologic correlates. These studies typically reevaluate in children a drug that has shown efficacy and safety in adults. Biologic studies are not regularly done in children because of the desire to protect them from research testing that will not be directly beneficial. However, correlative studies are essential to better understand the drug being evaluated, which in turn leads to more rational drug development and incorporation of new drugs in combination regimens. Correlative studies are even more important with the emergence of molecularly targeted therapies, where traditional clinical end points are difficult to apply in evaluating response. There is an increasing need to define and validate surrogate markers to determine the efficacy of new agents.

NOVEL THERAPIES USED AT M. D. ANDERSON

The New Agents Working Group in the Division of Pediatrics at M. D. Anderson is composed of investigators who participate in multiple clinical trials aimed at developing novel therapeutic approaches and evaluating novel therapies, singly or in combination. Members of the New Agents Working Group have established collaborations with their colleagues in adult-care areas throughout the institution, including the Department of Leukemia, the Lymphoma and Myeloma Center, the Blood and Marrow Transplantation Program, the Sarcoma Center, and the Department of Neuro-Oncology. These close clinical collaborations in a translational-research setting facilitate ready availability of novel therapies to pediatric patients in scientifically designed trials.

In addition to being a member of the Childrens' Oncology Group, the Division of Pediatrics at M. D. Anderson collaborates with other national

Table 14–1.   New Agents Undergoing Evaluation at M. D. Anderson*

Agent	Phase	Disease Indications
Triapine + cytarabine	I	Hematologic malignancy
XL119	I	Hematologic malignancy
ABT-751	I	Hematologic malignancy
VNP 4010M + cytarabine	I	Hematologic malignancy
BMS-354825	I	Leukemia
Rosiglitazone + bexarotene	I	Hematologic malignancy
17-AAG	I	Solid tumors and leukemia
Intra-lumbar I-131	I	Leptomeningeal metastases
Deoxycytidine + valproic acid	I/II	Leukemia
PTK 787 + imatinib	I/II	Hematologic malignancy
Liposomal vincristine	I/II	Leukemia
BCX-1777	I/II	T-acute lymphoblastic leukemia or lymphoma
Aerosolized liposomal 9 nitro camptothecin	I/II	Pulmonary metastases
RAD 001	II	Leukemia
DepoCyt	II	Central nervous system prophylaxis
R115777 (Zarnestra)	II	Central nervous system tumors
DX-8951F	II	Rhabdomyosarcoma

* This list is current as of September 1, 2004.

organizations, such as the Pediatric Oncology Experimental Therapeutics' Investigators Consortium (POETIC) and the Pediatric Blood and Marrow Transplant Consortium (PBMTC). These consortia have the expertise required to expedite the development of novel therapies for pediatric malignancies through rationally designed trials.

In the discussion that follows, we present some of the novel agents whose development was made possible by the M. D. Anderson multidisciplinary environment. Table 14–1 provides a comprehensive listing of new agents available to children treated at M. D. Anderson.

Hematologic Malignancies

Although more than 75% of children with acute lymphoblastic leukemia (ALL) are cured with current chemotherapy regimens, only 50% of children with acute myelogenous leukemia have a favorable long-term outcome despite intensive therapy, including stem cell transplantation. Novel active agents are needed as salvage therapy for patients whose disease relapses and for incorporation into frontline regimens.

The adult leukemia service at M. D. Anderson is the largest unit of its kind in the world, and it is a leader in the discovery and development of novel therapies for leukemia. The Division of Pediatrics' close collaboration with colleagues in the Department of Leukemia has made it possible for children to quickly receive new active agents that would not otherwise be available to them for several years. These children benefit from the expertise of the lead investigators on site, the results obtained with a large adult sample treated with a specific agent, and informative joint meetings where the activity and toxicity of these agents are thoroughly discussed. Such high-level collaboration makes it possible to quickly provide novel agents to children that are effective and safe.

Imatinib

M. D. Anderson's collaborative environment gave our pediatricians early access to imatinib, which is used to treat chronic myelogenous leukemia (CML). This subtype of leukemia is rare in children, and both M. D. Anderson patients and consults benefited from the expertise we gained from being part of the team. At M. D. Anderson, imatinib became available for use in combination with chemotherapy to treat children with Philadelphia chromosome-positive ALL 3 years before it became widely incorporated into pediatric regimens for this disease.

Clofarabine

Clofarabine is a next-generation nucleoside analog that was developed at M. D. Anderson. When promising results with this drug were shown in adult patients with heavily pretreated relapsed and refractory acute leukemia, a parallel institutional phase I trial was activated for pediatric patients. Ordinarily, investigational drugs are started in children at a dose level equivalent to 80% of the MTD for adults. The pediatric phase I clofarabine trial was uniquely structured to promote efficacy without jeopardizing safety. In case of rapid accrual on the adult trial, skipping to higher dose levels was allowed on the pediatric trial as long as younger patients received the drug at 1 dose level below the dose that was considered safe for adult participants until an MTD was achieved in adults. Then, classic dose escalation was followed in children. With this process, the pediatric phase I study was completed shortly after the adult trial was completed. A 32% response rate was obtained in children with heavily pretreated relapsed and refractory acute leukemia. The responses were durable, which allowed the children to proceed with stem cell transplantation. The results also led to 2 multi-institutional phase II studies for pediatric acute myelogenous leukemia and ALL, which confirmed that clofarabine was active in pediatric patients with heavily pretreated refractory and relapsed leukemia.

A phase II study of clofarabine in pediatric patients with ALL is currently ongoing in Europe, and pediatric regimens containing clofarabine combinations are being developed in the United States. Other agents currently available for children with relapsed leukemia are listed in Table 14–1.

Solid Tumors

Two prominent agents used in the treatment of solid tumors at M. D. Anderson are muramyl tripeptide phosphatidylethanolamine (MTP-PE) for osteosarcoma and isotretinoin for neuroblastoma.

MTP-PE

The story of the development of MTP-PE by Eugenie Kleinerman, MD, for the treatment of osteosarcoma illustrates how novel therapies are developed at M. D. Anderson.

Pulmonary metastases are a major problem in patients with osteosarcoma. Despite treatment with multiple aggressive chemotherapeutic regimens and surgical excision, the 2-year disease-free survival rate remained stagnant at about 60%. Consequently, new approaches to the treatment of multidrug-resistant metastases were needed.

Biologic response modifiers work by activating the body's own immune system. MTP-PE is a synthetic analogue of muramyl dipeptide, the smallest component of mycobacteria capable of stimulating macrophages. By encapsulating MTP in liposomes, we provided targeted delivery of MTP-PE to the lungs, the site of metastatic disease. When macrophages (and monocytes) phagocytized the liposomes containing MTP-PE, their cytolytic activity was stimulated.

The phase I study was performed at M. D. Anderson. The MTD was determined to be 6 mg/m^2 twice weekly. Side effects included myalgia, chills, fever, malaise, and fatigue. With biologic response modifiers, the MTD is not always the biologic optimal dose. Consequently, an assay testing the activity of macrophages was incorporated into the phase I trial. An optimal biologic response dose of 2 mg/m^2 was determined on the basis of this analysis and was subsequently used for the phase II and III studies. No responses were seen with the phase I study, but this finding was not unexpected. Biologic response modifiers have optimal activity against microscopic disease, but the patients in this study had bulky disease.

The phase II study was also performed at M. D. Anderson. Later, a phase III trial was undertaken in cooperation with the Pediatric Oncology Group and the Children's Cancer Group, and more than 800 patients were enrolled. MTP-PE plus chemotherapy (ifosfamide, doxorubicin, methotrexate, and cisplatin) produced a 2-year disease-free survival rate of 80% in patients with newly diagnosed localized osteosarcoma. It was the first time in 20 years that such an impressive response had been noted for this disease.

Isotretinoin

Second to lymphoma, neuroblastoma is the most common extracranial solid tumor in children. It is a malignancy of the sympathetic nervous system that almost exclusively affects infants and young children. The current therapy for neuroblastoma is described in Chapter 6, "Neuroblastoma," of this monograph. Here, we discuss a novel agent used in treating neuroblastoma—isotretinoin.

Isotretinoin is a derivative of vitamin A that has been found to decrease the proliferation and induce the differentiation of neuroblastoma cells in vitro. Treatment with isotretinoin is initiated at the completion of chemotherapy or after recovery from bone marrow transplantation while the patient has minimal residual disease. Because its mechanism of action is different from standard chemotherapeutic agents, isotretinoin can be effective even in the presence of multidrug resistance (Matthay et al, 1999). Other than mucosal toxicity, it is uncommon to encounter complications with isotretinoin. Multiple other agents are currently under investigation at M. D. Anderson and other institutions for treatment of neuroblastoma.

Graft-Versus-Host Disease

Stem cell transplantation is increasingly being used to treat a variety of oncologic, hematologic, and immunologic diseases. As complication rates associated with allogeneic stem cell transplantation decrease, its use in the treatment of nonmalignant conditions continues to increase.

Because there is only a 1-in-4 chance of finding identical histocompatibility leukocyte antigen (HLA) typing in 2 siblings, the majority of patients requiring stem cell transplantation lack a related donor. One of the greatest challenges is finding a suitable donor for these patients. At M. D. Anderson, we consider both HLA typing and the stem cell source when selecting a donor.

Because we are a specialized cancer center, many of our patients have experienced induction failure or are at very high risk for relapse. For these patients, the 4 or more months required to prepare an unrelated donor for bone marrow or peripheral blood stem cell collection is too long. Consequently, we have turned to umbilical cord blood units from unrelated donors as an alternative source of stem cells. Lymphocytes in umbilical cord blood are immunologically naïve and require less-stringent HLA matching than bone marrow or peripheral blood stem cells. Transplants using up to 2 units of HLA mismatched umbilical cord blood produce outcomes similar to transplants using matched unrelated-donor bone marrow. This donor option expands the available donor pool to ethnic and racial minorities who are underrepresented in bone marrow registries.

Stem cell transplantation can be associated with a number of complications. Graft-versus-host disease (GVHD) continues to be a major cause of morbidity and mortality. Lack of histocompatibility is the strongest risk factor for acute GVHD. Other risk factors are the disease diagnosis, the recipient's age, the donor's age, female donor-male recipient pairing, an alloimmunized donor, a high CD34+ cell dose, and the stem cell source.

Chemotherapy and radiotherapy used to treat the primary malignancy or in the preparation for transplantation cause damage to the host tissues, resulting from the secretion of mediators such as interleukin (IL)-1 and tumor necrosis factor-α. These cytokines activate donor T cells with further recruitment of natural killer cells and cytotoxic T lymphocytes. A vicious cycle is formed that leads to further proinflammatory cytokine release and target-organ damage. The best way to treat GVHD is to prevent it. Our prophylactic regimen consists of tacrolimus and mini-methotrexate (Przepiorka et al, 2002). Methylprednisolone is the frontline treatment if GVHD occurs. Because up to 50% of cases can be refractory to steroids, M. D. Anderson is using several new agents to manage GVHD that fails to respond to steroids.

Infliximab

Infliximab is a monoclonal antibody against tumor necrosis factor-α, one of the main mediators of GVHD pathogenesis. We have studied the effect of infliximab on children with acute and chronic GVHD (Sleight et al, 2003). When infliximab was given weekly at a dose of 10 mg/kg to a group of children aged 4 months to 18 years (median age, 5 years), responses were seen in acute skin (81%), gastrointestinal (79%), and liver (33%) GVHD. In chronic GVHD, 5 of 8 children experienced an improvement. Infliximab is well tolerated. In more than 500 doses given to children for the treatment of GVHD, no infusion-related adverse event was encountered. Deaths were attributed to GVHD and infections. Currently, the Department of Blood and Marrow Transplantation at M. D. Anderson is evaluating whether infliximab will produce an additional beneficial effect when combined with methylprednisolone as frontline therapy for acute GVHD (Couriel et al, 2003a).

Rapamycin

Rapamycin is a macrolide triene antibiotic that is used to treat GVHD. It binds intracellularly to the immunophilin FK506 binding protein, inhibiting the protein kinase activity of mammalian targets of rapamycin. Rapamycin is most effective in treating chronic steroid-refractory skin GVHD. In a study of adult patients with chronic steroid-refractory GVHD (Couriel et al, 2003b), treatment with a combination of rapamycin and steroids resulted in a 68% overall response rate: 5 patients had a complete response, and 13 patients had a partial response.

The dosage of rapamycin is determined by the white blood cell count and renal function. In children, the loading dose is 3 mg/m² followed by a daily maintenance dose of 1 mg/m². Side effects include thrombocytopenia, hypertriglyceridemia, transient elevation of liver function, and a mild decrease in white blood cells. Rapamycin must be used with extreme care because it can interact with anticonvulsants (e.g., carbamazepine, phenobarbital, phenytoin), calcium channel blockers, and some antibiotics (e.g., erythromycin and rifampin).

Pentostatin

Pentostatin is currently being used to treat acute GVHD. Pentostatin is a nucleoside analog produced by *Streptomyces antibioticus*. It irreversibly inhibits adenosine deaminase in the purine salvage pathway. The accumulation of 2'deoxy-adenosine 5'-triphosphate slows cell growth and induces apoptosis. In addition, pentostatin inhibits the synthesis of IL-2 messenger RNA and the production of IL-2 and IL-2 receptors on T lymphocytes. The dose for this agent in patients with normal renal function is 1.5 mg/m^2 daily for 3 days. The patient must be premedicated with 1 L of normal saline immediately before and after pentostatin administration. In the case of a creatinine clearance of less than 50 mg/mL, the dose is decreased by 25%.

In addition to its use in treating steroid-refractory GVHD, pentostatin is also under consideration for use in preventing GVHD. In an upcoming phase I/II study, patients will receive standard tacrolimus and mini-methotrexate prophylaxis. In a randomized fashion, groups of patients will receive 1 of 3 different doses of pentostatin to determine the optimal dosage.

Photopheresis

In this procedure, a unit of whole blood is obtained to prepare a buffy coat. A photosensitizing agent (8-methoxsalen) is added to the white blood cell suspension. Ultraviolet-A light activates the photosensitizing agent that inactivates T cells. Photopheresis has efficacy in treating chronic GVHD, particularly in patients with skin and liver involvement (Apisarnthanarax et al, 2003). Until recently, this approach was available only for adults and children weighing more than 40 kg because of the large volume of blood removed extracorporeally for treatment. Physicians at M. D. Anderson have modified the procedure, performing it by continuous closed circuit. The shift in fluid status is dramatically decreased, and we are now able to offer this therapy to children weighing between 15 and 39 kg. Photopheresis is initially performed 3 times per week; the schedule is then tapered on the basis of clinical response.

IS RESEARCH IN CHILDREN ETHICAL?

One of the benefits of participation in phase I clinical trials is that the patient will be among the first to receive a new treatment that could prove effective against cancer. The risks are that the effectiveness and safety of the drug being tested in a phase I human trial is unknown. Some believe that children should not be given a drug before it is proven safe and active in adults. However, this approach delays the availability of potentially effective novel therapies to children who have run out of other options. Whereas response to investigational drugs is not guaranteed, patients do sometimes benefit from a novel treatment.

All standard agents used today were once investigational. Actually, the most effective therapy for ALL was first tested in children in the 1950s and 1960s, a time when the disease was universally fatal and amidst an uproar that the children should be left to die in dignity. Even when early-phase trials do not provide direct benefit to an enrollee, they play a crucial role in improving treatment strategies and outcome for future patients.

Because childhood cancers respond differently to treatment than do adult cancers, we might miss effective agents by relying on information generated by testing only adults. A drug that shows no activity in adult malignancies is dropped without being tested in the pediatric cancer market because, due to its small patient population, the pediatric market does not readily attract new drug development.

Quality of life in the terminally ill is a major consideration, especially in young patients. Children who are candidates for investigational agents have usually gone through multiple treatment regimens. Some feel that these children, in whom there is a slim chance that a considerable response will be achieved, should be allowed quality time rather than be enrolled in a research study. Offering palliative care is an option that should always be discussed with patients and family members, and enrolling patients in a study of investigational therapy should not negate good supportive care. Many new agents can be given in an outpatient setting if patients have no concomitant medical problems that necessitate hospital admission. Also, patients participating in investigational trials are followed very closely. Side effects and complications are documented and addressed more carefully than they are in patients who are not subjected to the close monitoring dictated by the study.

Cost can be an important consideration with investigational therapies. The patient is often responsible for travel, lodging, and medical expenses not covered by health insurance. Our social workers can help to identify resources to cover such expenses.

When a drug is initially entered into a clinical trial, it is available only in a few places. In such situations, the patient is almost always required to live away from home for long periods, which can be a considerable inconvenience, especially when the therapeutic benefits of the drug cannot be guaranteed. Patients and family members naturally wonder whether they should stay close to home and friends who can provide support during such a difficult time. We carefully advise the parents and the referring physician about the possible benefit of the investigational trial so they can make an informed decision. We also help them locate resources that may be available in other parts of the country, and we work closely with the referring physician so the patient can return home and be cared for by their primary-care team who will maintain in close contact with us.

WHEN SHOULD A CHILD BE ENROLLED IN A CLINICAL TRIAL?

Careful evaluation of pediatric patients with relapsed or refractory disease is mandatory before enrolling a child in an investigational trial. Prior regimens, responses, and toxicities should be assessed. Patients who enroll in investigational trials should not be candidates for any standard therapy and should also have adequate organ function, good performance status, and no active infections or other major medical problems at the time of enrollment. Eligibility criteria should always be strictly adhered to, and sound clinical judgment is necessary. The child's assent and his or her psychological and social status should be carefully evaluated.

With the breadth of information available on the Internet, parents commonly seek investigational agents and inquire about them even before they are indicated for clinical use in pediatric patients. On the other hand, most treating physicians tend to have a more conservative and skeptical attitude about new agents still undergoing investigation. Patients, family members, and treating physicians should be made aware of the pros and cons of all options so they can make an informed decision.

CONCLUSIONS

Close, daily interactions between investigators in basic science research and clinicians on adult and pediatric oncology services allow for the development of promising, novel therapies in a timely and rational manner. In addition, innovative statistical methods provide unprecedented means of answering questions about the efficacy and safety of new treatments. Our pediatric patients benefit from these methodologies, which only a prime cancer research center can provide. At M. D. Anderson, our patients' dignity and quality of life are never jeopardized for the sake of discovery. We take pride in offering "tomorrow's therapies today" with compassion and in collaboration with referring physicians.

KEY PRACTICE POINTS

- All current standard treatments were once investigational.
- Despite high cure rates, pediatric cancer remains the leading cause of disease-related death in children beyond the neonatal period.

- Novel approaches are needed as salvage therapy for children whose disease relapses, to improve frontline regimens, and to decrease the toxicity associated with current regimens.
- Pediatric cancer outcomes cannot be improved without clinical research, including early-phase studies of new agents.
- Investigational trials are not recommended at the cost of quality of life, and they can benefit some patients.
- M. D. Anderson offers a unique environment for the development of investigational therapeutics. Our pediatric patients benefit from the novel agents made available through our research endeavors in adults as well as through the institution's collaboration with multiple national consortia.
- Patients, family members, and referring physicians partner with us in our quest for excellence in pediatric cancer research.

SUGGESTED READINGS

Aleksa K, Koren G. Ethical issues in including pediatric cancer patients in drug development trials. *Paediatr Drugs* 2002;4:257–265.

Apisarnthanarax N, Donato M, Korbling M, et al. Extracorporeal photopheresis therapy in the management of steroid-refractory or steroid-dependent cutaneous chronic graft- versus-host disease after allogeneic stem cell transplantation: feasibility and results. *Bone Marrow Transplant* 2003;31:459–465.

Couriel DR, Hicks K, Giralt S, et al. Phase III trial with infliximab/methylprednisolone (MP) vs (MP) for the treatment of acute GVHD: preliminary findings. *Biol Blood Marrow Transplant* 2003a;9:95.

Couriel DR, Hicks K, Saliba R, et al. Sirolimus (Rapamycin) for treatment of steroid-refractory chronic graft versus host disease. *Biol Blood Marrow Transplant* 2003b;9:67.

Goldberg JD, Jacobsohn DA, Margolis J, et al. Pentostatin for the treatment of chronic graft-versus-host disease in children.*J Pediatr Hematol Oncol* 2003;25:584–588.

Jeha S, Gandhi V, Chan KW, et al. Clofarabine, a novel nucleoside analog, is active in pediatric patients with advanced leukemia. *Blood* 2004;103:784–789.

Kleinerman ES. Biological therapy for osteosarcoma using liposome-encapsulated muramyl tripeptide. *Hematol Oncol Clin North Am* 1995;9:927–938.

Matthay KK, Villablanca JG, Seeger RC, et al. Treatment of high-risk neuroblastoma with intensive chemotherapy, radiotherapy, autologous bone marrow transplantation, and 13-*cis*-retinoic acid. *N Engl J Med* 1999;341:1165–1173.

Nahata MC. Need for conducting research on medications unlabeled for use in pediatric patients. *Ann Pharmacother* 1994;9:1103–1104.

Przepiorka D, Blamble D, Hilsenbeck S, et al. Tacrolimus clearance is age-dependent within the pediatric population. *Bone Marrow Transplant* 2002;26:601–605.

Reaman GH. Pediatric oncology: current views and outcomes. *Pediatr Clin North Am* 2002;6:1305–1318.

Roberts R, Rodriguez W, Murphy D, Crescenzi T. Pediatric drug labeling. *JAMA* 2003;290:905–911.

Sleight B, Chan K, Serrano A, et al. Infliximab for GVHD therapy in children. *Biol Blood Marrow Transplant* 2003;9:96.

Somberg JC. Pediatric drug development. *Am J Ther* 2003;10:2.

15 SUPPORTIVE CARE: MYELOSUPPRESSION

Nidra I. Rodriguez Cruz, Renee M. Madden,
and Craig A. Mullen

CHAPTER OVERVIEW

The success of aggressive, curative anticancer therapies in pediatric oncology is possible only with intensive supportive-care measures. For example, antimicrobial prophylaxis can reduce infection rates in children undergoing myelosuppressive chemotherapy. Likewise, preemptive, broad-spectrum antibiotic therapy given as treatment for fever and neutropenia has been shown to reduce the mortality rate in this patient population. Furthermore, blood-product support is essential during periods of marrow suppression, and hematopoeitic growth factors, such as granulocyte colony-stimulating factor and erythropoietin, can be used to reduce the duration of pancytopenia. These interventions work together with therapeutic interventions to provide optimal outcomes for pediatric patients with cancer.

INTRODUCTION

Cancer is the second leading cause of death in children and adolescents. The prognosis for many pediatric patients with malignancies has improved significantly in the past several decades due to advancements in multimodal treatments involving surgery, radiotherapy, and chemotherapy. However, these therapies are associated with severe and prolonged bone marrow suppression and thus must be accompanied by vigorous supportive-care measures throughout the course of treatment. In this chapter, we present the policies and methods used at M. D. Anderson Cancer Center in the management of fever and neutropenia and discuss the use of antimicrobial prophylaxis in children and adolescents. Our approaches to blood-product support and hematopoietic growth factor administration are also discussed.

FEVER AND NEUTROPENIA

Fever is common in children with cancer, and is defined as a single temperature greater than 38.3°C (101.4°F) or 2 consecutive temperatures (taken at least 1 hour apart) that are greater than 38.0°C (100.4°F). Fever frequently develops in the presence of severe neutropenia, which is defined as an absolute neutrophil count (ANC) of 500/mm^3 or less or between 500 and 1,000/mm^3 but falling. ANC is calculated as the total white blood cell count × (percentage of neutrophils + bands).

Although fever in the neutropenic patient may have a noninfectious source, such as the malignancy itself or a drug- or transfusion-related reaction, sepsis should be the primary consideration in this setting. Fever is often the first and only sign of infection; other signs of inflammation may be obscure. The evaluation of patients with febrile neutropenia should proceed speedily and systematically. A complete history and a meticulous physical examination should be performed to determine whether a specified infection can be documented and to determine which investigations are required. Laboratory studies should include a complete blood cell count and blood cultures from all lumens of all indwelling central venous devices and from the peripheral vein. Cultures from urine, cerebrospinal fluid, and sputum and radiographic studies may be obtained if clinically indicated. After specimens are obtained, broad-spectrum antibiotics should be initiated, preferably within 1 hour of the patient's arrival.

About 15% to 20% of blood cultures are positive for bacterial organisms; therefore, early empiric therapy is indicated. Several antibiotic agents are available; the choice should depend on the locally prevailing organism, its antibiotic susceptibility profile, the cost of the treatment, and the patient's history of allergies. Monotherapy with a fourth-generation cephalosporin (e.g., cefepime) or a carbapenem (e.g., imipenem or meroperam) is frequently used. Empiric vancomycin administration is discouraged although it may be used for patients with a documented history of central venous catheter infection resistant to other antibiotics, patients with severe mucositis (especially after high-dose cytarabine treatment), and in hospitals with a high incidence of methicillin-resistant Stapyloccus aureus. The algorithm

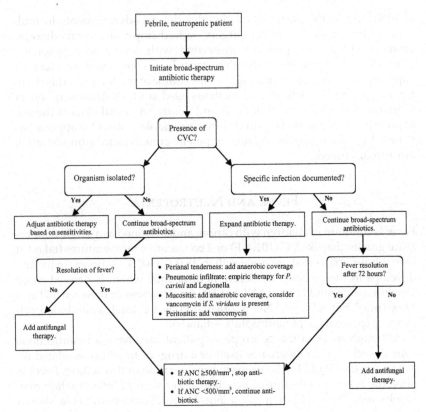

Figure 15–1. Algorithm used in the management of febrile neutropenia. Abbreviations: ANC, absolute neutrophil count; CVC, central venous catheter; IV, intravenous; *P. carinii, Pneumocystis carinii; S. viridans, Streptococcus viridans.*

used in the Division of Pediatrics at M. D. Anderson to manage febrile neutropenia is illustrated in Figure 15.1.

Other commonly used antibiotics include fluoroquinolones, extended-spectrum penicillins, and aminoglycosides; however, these agents are rarely used alone. The presence of abdominal pain, paralytic ileus, and perirectal discomfort necessitates broadening the antimicrobial coverage to include resistant gram-negative and anaerobic organisms. Antifungals may be needed if the fever persists for more than 3 to 5 days. Liposomal formulations of amphotericin, an azole (i.e., fluconazole, itraconazole, or voriconazole), or an echinocandin (e.g., capsofungin) are commonly used.

The length of antimicrobial therapy varies and is determined on the basis of the patient's clinical status, the resolution of fever, the results of

Table 15–1.   Risk Categories for Febrile Neutropenia

Low-Risk Characteristics	High-Risk Characteristics
Stable, no clinical signs of sepsis	Unstable, signs of sepsis or septic shock
No significant mucositis, pneumonia, or focal infection	Disruption of the skin or mucosal barrier, pneumonia, respiratory distress, vomiting or dehydration, hemorrhaging, or other serious condition
No serious comorbidity	Serious comorbidity
Remission status	Advanced malignant disease or undergoing leukemia induction
Adequate family support	Adverse social situation (i.e., poor compliance or reliability, language barrier, or lack of transportation or telephone), age >2 years infancy, bacteremia, bone marrow transplant, or prolonged (>5 days) or profound (ANC <0.2 × 10^9/L) neutropenia (the most important defining risk)

Abbreviation: ANC, absolute neutrophil count.

the culture studies, the focus of the identified infection, and the anticipated duration of myelosuppression.

Traditionally, pediatric cancer patients who have febrile neutropenia are admitted to the hospital and started on broad-spectrum intravenous antibiotics. They remain in the hospital until both the fever and the neutropenia are resolved. In the past decade, it has became clear that some clinical features could differentiate febrile neutropenic patients into low- and high-risk categories (Table 15.1). This categorization scheme has enabled clinicians to modify the treatment approach on the basis of risk. For example, patients at low-risk can be discharged from the hospital early, receive ongoing antibiotic administration in the outpatient setting, or be treated orally. The advantages of risk-adopted management include better quality of life, reduced antibiotic toxicity, and a cost reduction of up to 40%.

Published clinical trials have shown that both oral and intravenous antibiotics can adequately treat febrile neutropenia in low-risk pediatric patients with cancer (Orudjev et al, 2002). The choice may depend on the sensitivity profile of the local organism, the caretaker's compliance with the treatment plan, and the experience of the health care team. We currently admit the patient and administer cefepime for 24 to 48 hours at 50 mg/kg/dose (and up to 2 g/dose) every 8 hours. After observation, the stable patient may be discharged with oral ciprofloxacin with or without a gram-positive oral antibiotic (such as azithromycin or amoxicillin). Close outpatient monitoring is important because up to 15% of the children may require re-hospitalization for recurrent fever or worsening of their clinical condition (Mullen et al, 2001).

ANTIMICROBIAL PROPHYLAXIS

The efficacy of antimicrobial prophylaxis has not been universally accepted by the pediatric oncology community. Drawbacks associated with prophylaxis include induction of antimicrobial resistance and overgrowth of nonsusceptible organisms. The type of prophylaxis used should be based on the intensity of the phase of treatment and the degree of immunosuppression. It should be stressed that other precautionalry measures, such as washing hands, avoiding contact with those who are sick, eating well-cooked foods, and using boiled water, are as important as administration of antimicrobial agents.

Antibacterial Agents

The availability of oral fluoroquinolones improves the practicality and effectiveness of antibacterial prophylaxis. These agents are effective against gram-negative organisms and spare anaerobic bacteria in the bowel. Therefore, bacterial overgrowth is less problematic. Antibacterial prophylaxis may be indicated for patients who are expected to have profound neutropenia for more than 7 days and bone marrow transplant recipients undergoing myeloablative chemotherapy. Infection is most likely delayed with this approach; however, the incidence of fever is strongly associated with the duration of neutropenia.

Antiprotozoal Agents

Pneumonia caused by *Pneumocystitis carinii* is a well-recognized complication in severely lymphopenic patients. It can occur after a large volume of the bone marrow is irradiated (such as cranial irradiation) and after intensive chemotherapy. Patients with Hodgkin lymphoma and bone marrow transplant recipients are also susceptible. The chemoprophylaxis treatment of choice is trimethoprim and sulfamethoxazole (TMP/SMX) at 5 to 10 mg/kg/day divided into 2 daily doses and given on 3 consecutive days per week. For children unable to tolerate TMP/SMX or who have a history of sulfa allergy, dapsone, pentamidine, and atovaquone are acceptable alternatives. Dapsone can be given orally at 2 mg/kg/dose twice a week. Pentamidine is given at a convenient monthly dosing schedule (4 mg/kg given intravenously or 8 mg/kg given by nebulization for up to a total of 300 mg). Atovaquone is given at 45 mg/kg/day by mouth. *P. carinii* prophylaxis should be continued for up to 6 months after completion of chemotherapy or bone marrow transplantation.

Antiviral Agents

Antiviral prophylaxis can be used to prevent primary infection or the reactivation of dominant virus in patients who are seropositive. Acyclovir is used as prophylaxis against the herpes simplex virus and is recommended for the first few months in patients receiving a bone marrow transplant. Patients with a history of viral reactivation after conventional chemotherapy should also be placed on acyclovir prophylaxis during subsequent cycles of treatment. For the herpes simplex virus, the dose of acyclovir is 5 mg/kg every 8 hours. This dose is doubled if the drug is also meant to prevent herpes zoster or cytomegalovirus reactivation. Other antiviral agents include valacyclovir and famciclovir, which are prodrugs of acyclovir and appear to be as efficacious as acyclovir. These drugs can be given in once-daily doses, which is more convenient for the patient than the every-8-hour acyclovir schedule. For cytomegalovirus prophylaxis in bone marrow transplant recipients, the drug of choice is ganciclovir; however, it is now common practice to use ganciclovir for pre-emptive treatment of cytomegalovirus infection when surveillance studies (e.g., antigenemia or polymerase chain reaction assays) turn positive.

HEMATOLOGIC SUPPORT

Myelosuppression after anticancer therapy is caused by the intensity and the duration of treatment. Blood counts recover more slowly after repeated cycles of chemotherapy. Anemia and thrombocytopenia are managed by transfusion of packed red blood cells (PRBCs) and platelets. Although blood-product screening has reduced the risk for transfusion-associated infections, the problem has not been completely eliminated. Therefore, blood products should only be used when the benefits clearly outweigh the risks. The blood count level should not be used as the sole indication for a transfusion. Clinical signs and symptoms (e.g., headache, fatigue, anorexia, dyspnea, irritability, and tachycardia) are important considerations when deciding whether a blood transfusion should be ordered.

Anemia

Anemia is frequently encountered in children with cancer. Although a number of factors (e.g., tumor infiltration of the marrow, chronic inflammation, bleeding, and nutritional deficiency) may contribute to a low hemoglobin level, the anticancer treatment (e.g., chemotherapy or radiotherapy) is often the most important cause of anemia. Treatment for anemia is normally indicated when the hemoglobin level falls to the 7 to 9 g/dL range. A higher threshold may be appropriate for patients who are severely symptomatic (especially older children and adolescents), are receiving radiotherapy, have active bleeding, or have underlying cardiopulmonary comorbidities. The treatment for anemia is the transfusion of PRBCs. The volume of PRBCs transfused in pediatric patients is determined on the basis of the patient's body weight, but it ranges from 10 to 15 mL/kg (rounded to the closest number of whole units). The cells are infused over 2 to 4 hours.

The use of transfusion to raise the hemoglobin level to the normal range is not indicated for the following patients.

- Patients with white blood cell counts greater than $100,000/mm^3$ (to avoid the increase in blood viscosity and the risk for leukostasis)
- Patients with severe anemia and congestive heart failure
- Patients with chronic renal insufficiency

Anemia in some children with cancer is associated with decreased erythropoietic activity, which is caused by the direct myelotoxic effect of chemotherapy (Ruggiero and Riccardi, 2002). Recombinant erythropoietin stimulates the production of red blood cells, reducing the severity of anemia and, consequently, the need for PRBC transfusion. Although only a few clinical trials have evaluated the efficacy of erythropoietin in treating children with chemotherapy-related anemia, preliminary results are encouraging (Buyukpamukcu et al, 2002). The optimal dose, frequency, and duration of treatment with this agent in pediatric patients with cancer have not been established.

Platelet Transfusions

Platelet transfusions are used in the management of cancer- or chemotherapy-associated thrombocytopenia and are given to patients with the following clinical features.

- A platelet count of less than $10,000/mm^3$ secondary to failure of platelet production
- A platelet count of less than $50,000/mm^3$ and active bleeding or before minor surgery
- A platelet count of less than $100,000/mm^3$ and the need for major surgery

A lower threshold of platelet transfusion may used for:

- Patients with acute myeloid leukemia (the transfusion should be administered during induction chemotherapy)
- Patients with brain tumor who are receiving myelosuppressive chemotherapy
- Patients undergoing bone marrow transplantation

The average platelet dose in children is 4 units of random donor platelets/m^2, with the transfusion resulting in a rise in the platelet count of 50 to $100,000/mm^3$ (Roseff et al, 2002). However, the response to platelet transfusion can be adversely affected by fever, sepsis, ongoing bleeding, and consumptive coagulopathy. Patients with splenomegaly and prior allosensitization also respond poorly to platelet transfusion.

Granulocyte Transfusions

Granulocyte transfusions are not a routine hematologic supportive-care measure. At M. D. Anderson, granulocyte tranfusion is reserved for patients with profound neutropenia in whom a bacterial or fungal infection persists despite aggressive antimicrobial therapy. In this life-threatening situation, a granulocyte transfusion can be given to allow time for the child's own marrow function to recover. The average volume of granulocyte transfusion is 10 to 15 mL/kg, which provides approximately 1 to 2×10^9 polymorphonuclear cells/kg (Roseff et al, 2002). A much higher number of cells can be recovered if the donor receives a dose of granulocyte colony-stimulating factor (G-CSF) prior to apheresis. Because of this approach, granulocyte transfusions have been given more frequently in the past few years. For granulocyte transfusion therapy to be effective, a minimum of 4 to 5 treatments should be administered.

Other blood products may be needed in special circumstances. Either fresh-frozen plasma or cryoprecipitate is used in cases of disseminated intravascular coagulation associated with the treatment of sepsis or acute promyelocytic leukemia (Roseff et al, 2002). The dose of fresh-frozen plasma ranges from 10 to 15 mL/kg, and the dose of cryoprecipitate is 1 U for every 3 to 5 kg body weight. Antithrombin III administration is useful in patients in whom hepatic veno-occlusive disease develops after bone marrow transplant. The goal of treatment is to maintain the antithrombin III level at 100%.

Hematopoietic Growth Factors

Children receiving intensive chemotherapy are at increased risk of developing severe neutropenia. The duration of neutropenia can be reduced by the use of hematopoietic growth factors. Overall, these agents have decreased the time to marrow recovery without affecting the outcome of the associated infection and the success of cancer therapy. Filgrastim, a G-CSF, promotes the proliferation of granulocytes and decreases their rate of apoptosis. Sargramstim, a granulocyte-macrophage colony-stimulating factor (GM-CSF), increases the proliferation of granulocytes and macrophages. G-CSF may be used in conjunction with chemotherapy regimens that cause severe neutropenia for at least 7 days. It can accelerate myeloid recovery after bone marrow transplantation. The dose of G-CSF is 5 to 10 mcg/kg/day given subcutaneously or intravenously. It is often started 24 hours after the last dose of chemotherapy and continued until the ANC has adequately recovered, usually to a level of more than 2,000/mm³ for a few days.

Indications for the use of GM-CSF include the acceleration of myeloid recovery after bone marrow transplant and delayed engraftment. The GM-CSF dose is 250 mcg/m² given daily by subcutaneous injection.

A new product, pegfilgrastim, is available for use in stimulating white blood cell recovery after chemotherapy in pediatric patients with cancer. This pegylated G-CSF product is long acting, and only a single dose is needed per treatment cycle. The pegfilgrastim dose is 0.1 mg/kg. For patients weighing more than 45 kg, a fixed dose of 6 mg can be used. Pegfilgrastim should not be given less than 24 hours after completion of chemotherapy.

KEY PRACTICE POINTS

- Patients with febrile neutropenia can be classified into low- and high-risk categories. Low-risk neutopenia can be treated with less-intensive therapy than is required to treat high-risk neutropenia, e.g., oral antibiotics and early hospital discharge.
- Oral quinolones are increasingly used for patients with severe and prolonged neutropenia.
- Antifungal and antiviral prophylaxes are now possible due to the availability of oral and broad-spectrum antimicrobial agents.
- Granulocyte transfusions mobilized by G-CSF are being used more frequently and can be a beneficial adjunct in the treatment of severe sepsis.

SUGGESTED READINGS

Alexander SW, Wade KC, Hibberd PL, et al. Evaluation of risk prediction criteria for episodes of febrile neutropenia in children with cancer. *J Pediatr Hematol Oncol* 2002;24:38–42.

Alexander SW, Walsh TJ, Freifeld AG, et al. Infectious complications. In: Pizzo PA, Poplack DG, eds. *Pediatric Cancer Patients in Principles and Practice of Pediatric Oncology.* Philadelphia, PA: Lippincott, Williams and Wallace; 2002:1239–1283.

Baorto EP, Aquino VM, Mullen CA, et al. Clinical parameters associated with low bacteremia risk in 100 pediatric oncology patients with fever and neutropenia. *Cancer* 2001;92:909–913.

Buyukpamukcu M, Varan A, Kutluk T, et al. Is epoetin alfa a treatment option for chemotherapy-related anemia in children? *Med Pediatr Oncol* 2002;39:455–458.

Hughes WT, Armstrong D, Bodey GP, et al. 2002 guidelines for the use of antimicrobial agents in neutropenic patients with cancer. *Clin Infect Dis* 2002;34:730–751.

Klaassen RJ, Goodman TR, Pham B, et al. "Low-risk" prediction rule for pediatric oncology patients presenting with fever and neutropenia. *J Clin Oncol* 2000;18:1012–1019.

Kocak U, Rolston KV, Mullen CA. Fever and neutropenia in children with solid tumors is similar in severity and outcome to that in children with leukemia. *Support Care Cancer* 2002;10:58–64.

Mullen CA, Petropoulos D, Roberts WR, et al. Economic and resource utilization analysis of outpatient management of fever and neutropenia in low-risk pediatric patients with cancer. *J Pediatr Hematol Oncol* 1999;21:212–218.

Mullen CA, Petropoulos D, Roberts WR, et al. Outpatient treatment of fever and neutropenia for low risk pediatric cancer patients. *Cancer* 1999;86:126–134.

Mullen CA. Which children with fever and neutropenia can be safely treated as outpatients? *Br J Haematol* 2001;112:832–837.

Orudjev E, Lange BJ. Evolving concepts of management of febrile neutropenia in children with cancer. *Med Pediatr Oncol* 2002;39:77–85.

Roseff SD, Luban NL, Manno CS. Guidelines for assessing appropriateness of pediatric transfusion. *Transfusion* 2002;42:1398–1413.

Rossetto CL, McMahon JE. Current and future trends in transfusion therapy. *J Pediatr Oncol Nurs* 2000;17:160–173.

Ruggiero A, Riccardi R. Interventions for anemia in pediatric cancer patients. *Med Pediatr Oncol* 2002;39:451–454.

16 SUPPORTIVE CARE: SYMPTOM CONTROL

Renee M. Madden, Susannah E. Koontz-Webb,
Donna S. Zhukovsky, and Craig A. Mullen

Chapter Overview

Chemotherapy-induced emesis, poor nutrition, and pain are primary concerns with patients undergoing cancer therapy. Major advances have been made in the control of these symptoms. For example, new antiemetic agents are available that can effectively reduce nausea and vomiting after chemotherapy. Nutritional screening and early intervention, especially via the enteral route, are being used in children who experience weight loss and anorexia. A better understanding of the mechanisms of cancer pain and acceptance of the use of analgesics, by physicians and parents, also facilitate optimal symptom control in pediatric patients with cancer.

Introduction

Each year in the United States, roughly 12,000 children and adolescents are diagnosed with cancer. Despite an overall cure rate of approximately 70%, 2,200 pediatric patients die from cancer annually. Treatment successes in pediatric oncology are partly due to aggressive anticancer regimens. Equally intensive supportive-care measures have been used effectively to combat chemotherapy-, radiotherapy-, and biotherapy-related side effects, which include nausea and vomiting, poor nutrition, and pain as well as symptoms related to the tumor itself. These measures have made it possible to administer lifesaving therapies to children and adolescents in both inpatient and outpatient settings. This chapter discusses the M. D. Anderson Cancer Center approach to managing the comorbid effects of anticancer therapy in pediatric patients, including the use of antiemetic agents, nutritional support, and analgesics. Our approach to treating febrile neutropenia and to implementing hematologic supportive-care measures is discussed in Chapter 15, "Supportive Care: Myelosuppression."

Chemotherapy-Induced Nausea and Vomiting

Once considered by patients to be the most dreaded side effect of chemotherapy, chemotherapy-induced nausea and vomiting (CINV) has become a manageable consequence of cancer treatment. During the 1970s and 1980s, phenothiazines and benzamides were the mainstays of therapy for pediatric oncology patients with CINV. These agents provided only marginal relief and often produced troublesome side effects. Since the introduction of serotonin antagonists in the early 1990s, the incidence of CINV has decreased notably; however, this symptom remains a concern for patients and caregivers and continues to be an active area of research. Effective management of CINV is important because severe or persistent nausea and vomiting can prolong hospitalization, cause a variety of complications, and decrease a patient's quality of life. Because prevention of CINV has such an important impact on a patient's well-being, clinicians should have a clear understanding of the biology and effects of antiemetics.

Pathophysiology

The pathophysiology of CINV involves a complex network of neurotransmitters, neuroreceptors, and neuronal pathways in the central nervous system and in its periphery, but the exact process by which chemotherapy induces emesis remains unknown. Various neurotransmitters that play a key role in the development of CINV and their respective neuroreceptors have been identified and are targets for drug research and development. Some important neuroreceptors that have been identified to date are serotonin type 3 (5-HT_3), dopamine type 2, histamine type 1, benzodiazepine, muscarinic, and neurokinin type 1. Many antiemetics used in clinical practice block 1 or more of these receptors.

Chemotherapy appears to cause nausea and vomiting by more than 1 mechanism, as demonstrated by the varying degrees and onset of CINV among patients receiving different chemotherapeutic drugs. Although a thorough review of the mechanisms of CINV is beyond the scope of this chapter, the mediation of CINV can be summarized by 3 mechanisms: (a) stimulation of neuroreceptors in the chemoreceptor trigger zone (CTZ) by drugs, metabolites in the blood, or cerebrospinal fluid; (b) stimulation of neuroreceptors in the gastrointestinal tract that supply peripheral input to the CTZ or vomiting center through vagal afferent pathways; and (c) evocation of efferent impulses (e.g., memories, smells, sights, and sounds) from the cerebral cortex to the CTZ or vomiting center (Beckwith and Mullin, 2001).

Risk Factors

Identification of the risk factors involved in the development of CINV is the first step in managing the disorder. Not only will identifying these risk factors help determine in which patients CINV is likely to occur, but it will also assist the clinician in determining which antiemetic regimen is most appropriate for a particular patient. The risk factors can be divided into 2 groups: (a) characteristics of the patient and (b) attributes of the chemotherapeutic regimen. Notable high-risk patient characteristics include young age, female sex, fatigue, depression, anxiety or anticipation associated with chemotherapy, and a history of nausea and vomiting from previous chemotherapy.

The leading factor influencing whether a patient will experience CINV is the chemotherapeutic regimen being used. Chemotherapy agents have been classified according to the degree to which they cause CINV (Table 16–1). With this information, clinicians can determine the overall emetogenicity of a chemotherapeutic regimen and thus wisely select antiemetics that will provide the most benefit for a patient

Table 16–1. Emetogenicity Potential of Anticancer Chemotherapy Agents

High Level 5 [>90%]*	Moderate-High Level 4 [60%–90%]*	Moderate Level 3 [30%–60%]*	Moderate-Low Level 2 [10%–30%]*	Low Level 1 [<10%]*
Carmustine (>250 mg/m²)	Carboplatin	Aldesleukin	Asparaginase (all forms)	Androgens
Cisplatin (≥50 mg/m²)	Carmustine (≤250 mg/m²)	Altretamine	Cytarabine (<1000 mg/m²)	Arsenic trioxide
Cyclophosphamide (>1500 mg/m²)	Cisplatin (<50 mg/m²)	Cyclophosphamide (<750 mg/m²)	Docetaxel	Bleomycin
Dacarbazine	Cyclophosphamide (750–1500 mg/m²)	Cyclophosphamide (PO)	Doxorubicin (<20 mg/m²)	Busulfan (PO <4 mg/kg/day)
Lomustine (>60 mg/m²)	Cytarabine (≥1000 mg/m²)	Dactinomycin (<1.5 mg/m²)	Etoposide	Capecitabine
Mechlorethamine	Dactinomycin (≥1.5 mg/m²)	Daunorubicin (<50 mg/m²)	Fluorouracil (<1000 mg/m²)	Chlorambucil
Streptozocin	Daunorubicin (≥1.5 mg/m²)	Doxorubicin (20–60 mg/m²)	Gemcitabine	Cladribine
	Doxorubicin (≥60 mg/m²)	Epirubicin	Methotrexate (50–250 mg/m²)	Corticosteroids
	Irinotecan	Fluorouracil (≥1000 mg/m²)	Mitomycin	Daunorubicin (liposomal)
	Lomustine (≤60 mg/m²)	Idarubicin	Paclitaxel	Doxorubicin (liposomal)
	Melphalan (IV)	Ifosfamide	Temozolamide	Estramustine
	Methotrexate (>1000 mg/m²)	Methotrexate (250–1000 mg/m²)	Teniposide	Floxuridine
	Mitoxantrone (≥15 mg/m²)	Mitoxantrone (<15 mg/m²)	Thiotepa	Fludarabine
	Procarbazine (oral)		Topotecan	Hydroxyurea
				Interferon
				Melphalan (PO)
				Mercaptopurine
				Methotrexate (<50 mg/m²)
				Pentostatin
				Thioguanine
				Tretinoin
				Vinblastine
				Vincristine
				Vinorelbine

* Probability of emesis within 24 hours when single agent is infused over 3 hours or less without the use of prophylactic antiemetics. Abbreviation: PO, by mouth. Sources: Hesketh et al, 1997 and Beckwith and Mullin, 2001.

(see Appendix 16–1). Other chemotherapy-related risk factors to note are that: (a) bolus administration of agents is generally more emetogenic than prolonged infusions, (b) a patient's susceptibility to CINV can vary with subsequent cycles, and (c) a patient's circadian rhythm may influence whether and to what degree CINV occurs (Hesketh et al, 1997).

Phases of Symptomatology

There are 3 clearly defined components of the emetic process: nausea, vomiting, and retching. Nausea is the unpleasant feeling that may signal that vomiting is imminent. Often, nausea is accompanied by signs and symptoms of autonomic nervous system stimulation (flushing, pallor, and tachycardia) as well as peristalsis, retrograde duodenal peristalsis, and a reduction in gastric tone. Vomiting (emesis) is the forceful expulsion of gastric contents through the mouth, and it can occur without nausea. Retching, also referred to as "dry heaves," may precede, alternate with, or follow emesis.

CINV usually begins within 1 to 2 hours of the initiation of a chemotherapy infusion and can last up to 24 hours after the infusion is completed. Symptoms are at peak intensity 4 to 6 hours after initiation of an infusion, and they typically resolve within 12 to 24 hours of their onset. The primary biologic mediator of acute CINV is serotonin. This so-called serotonin (or acute) phase is more preventable and more controllable than the delayed phase of CINV. Prophylactic antiemetic regimens directed against the acute phase often include a 5-HT$_3$ antagonist combined with a corticosteroid. The serotonin phase of CINV has been the target of most antiemetic research.

Delayed CINV follows acute CINV and is frequently refractory to antiemetics. The most important determinant of whether delayed CINV will develop appears to be the presence of acute CINV. Symptoms of delayed CINV usually peak 24 to 48 hours following chemotherapy administration and resolve gradually over the course of 1 to 3 days; however, some patients experience symptoms that persist for up to 1 week. Delayed CINV occurs most frequently with certain chemotherapy agents, e.g., cisplatin, cyclophosphamide (especially if given with an anthracycline), doxorubicin, carboplatin, and mitomycin. The pathophysiologic mechanism behind the delayed CINV phase is not well defined, but it appears to differ from that of acute CINV, because 5-HT$_3$ antagonists have little impact on this problem. Mechanisms postulated to be responsible for the development of delayed CINV have included chemotherapeutic metabolites, tissue destruction, hypomagnesemia, and gastritis. Drug therapy for delayed CINV includes corticosteroid plus metoclopramide with or without the addition of a 5-HT$_3$ antagonist. For children, the use of metoclopramide often warrants the addition of an antihistamine (such as diphenhydramine) to prevent extrapyramidal side effects.

Anticipatory vomiting affects up to 40% of pediatric patients receiving chemotherapy. It is a conditioned response to stimuli such as poor control of CINV with previous treatment cycles. As such, anticipatory vomiting may become a "lifelong" condition, and patients may experience it years after the completion of treatment. Patients usually experience nausea more often than vomiting, and the nausea typically occurs in the 24 hours preceding chemotherapy. Anticipatory vomiting is not typically present at the beginning of chemotherapy but rather develops after 4 to 5 cycles of treatment. Risk factors for its development include young age, side effects from previous chemotherapy, predisposition to motion sickness, anxiety, and depression. Anticipatory vomiting can be extremely difficult to manage and often requires nonpharmacologic interventions, such as music, relaxation exercises, guided imagery, hypnosis, acupuncture, diet, avoiding noxious stimuli, and engaging in favorite activities. Drug therapy for anticipatory vomiting is targeted at cortical structures of the brain, and the cornerstones of therapy are the benzodiazepines (Gralla et al, 1999; Mullin and Beckwith, 2001).

Treatment

Upon initiation of antiemetic therapy, clinicians must continuously ascertain the effectiveness of the agents. Total control is defined as the complete absence of nausea and vomiting. Complete response is achieved when vomiting and retching cease although the patient may still experience some nausea. There are 2 types of partial response: a major response in which a patient has 1 or 2 episodes of vomiting in a 24-hour period and a minor response in which a patient has 3 to 5 episodes of vomiting in a 24-hour period. Antiemetic failure occurs when a patient experiences more than 5 episodes of vomiting in a 24-hour period. Breakthrough nausea and vomiting refers to the occurrence of CINV despite the use of prophylactic antiemetics. In these cases, additional antiemetics, or "rescue therapy," are necessary. Antiemetic regimens should be adjusted for patients with a minor response or in whom the antiemetics have failed, and considerations should be made for patients with a major response (Hesketh et al, 1998). Once the overall level of a regimen has been determined, the appropriate antiemetic therapy can be selected. Table 16–2 lists the antiemetic regimen commonly used in the treatment of pediatric patients. The doses and administration schedules and the associated side effects are also provided.

NUTRITION

Providing nutritional support to pediatric patients with cancer is a dynamic process. The aims of providing metabolic support to a child undergoing cancer therapy are to prevent nutritional deficits, support normal growth and development, and assist in the alleviation or amelioration of chemotherapy side effects. Most cancer patients experience cachexia at some point during their treatments, thus warranting nutritional

Table 16–2. Summary of Antiemetics Used for Pediatric Patients

Class	Drug	Brand	Route	Single Dose (Max)	Schedule	Side Effects	Comments
Serotonin (5-HT3) Antagonist	Ondansetron	Zofran	IV, PO	0.15 mg/kg IV (8 mg)	Q 8 hr	Headache Diarrhea	Zofran is available in an ODT form (4 mg and 8 mg) and a 4 mg/5 mL solution
				0.45 mg/kg IV (32 mg)	One time dose	Constipation	More effective if given with steroids
				$<0.4\ m^2$ 0.15 mg/kg IV/PO $0.4\text{--}1.2\ m^2$ 4 mg IV/PO $>1.2\ m^2$ 8 mg IV/PO	Q 8 hr/TID Q 8 hr/TID Q 8 hr/TID	Increases in AST/ALT Arrhythmias	
	Granisetron	Kytril	IV, PO	10 mcg/kg IV (2 mg) 10–40 mcg/kg PO (2 mg) (max dose is 2 mg/day)	QD or Q 12 hr QD or Q 12 hr		
	Dolasetron	Anzemet	IV, PO	1.8 mg/kg IV, PO (100 mg)	QD		
Corticosteroid	Dexamethasone	Decadron	IV, PO	6–10 mg/m^2 IV, PO (20 mg)	QD or Q 12 hr	Dyspepsia Euphoria Insomnia Edema	Doesn't require a steroid taper since it is given short term
				4–8 mg PO (delayed N/V)	Q 8 hr/TID	Weight gain Increased appetite Hyperglycemia	Watch chemo regimens with steroids
Substituted benzamide	Metoclopramide	Reglan	IV, PO	0.5–2 mg/kg IV/PO	Q 2–4 hr prn Q 2–4 hr prn	EPS Diarrhea Anxiety Restlessness Arrhythmias	Premed with Benadryl 15–30 minutes before dose to decrease EPS

Class	Generic	Trade	Route	Dose	Frequency	Side effects	Notes
Phenothiazine	Prochlorperazine	Compazine	PO	0.1 mg/kg PO (10 mg)	Q 6-12 hr prn	EPS Restlessness Sedation Dry mouth Constipation Blurred vision	Give Benadryl 15-30 minutes dose to before decrease EPS
	Promethazine	Phenergan	IV, PO	0.25-1 mg/kg IV, PO (25 mg)	4-6 hr prn	Orthostatic hypotension	
	Chlorpromazine	Thorazine	IV, PO	0.5-1 mg/kg IV, PO (25 mg)	Q 4-8 hr prn		
Benzodiazepine	Lorazepam	Ativan	IV, PO	0.025-0.05 mg/kg IV, PO (2 mg)	Q 6-8 hr prn	Sedation Dizziness Disorientation Hypotension	
Antihistamine	Diphenhydramine	Benadryl	IV, PO	0.5-1 mg/kg IV, PO (50 mg)	Q 4-6 hr prn	Sedation Agitation Dry mouth Constipation Blurred vision	

Abbreviations: ALT, alanine aminotransferase; AST, asparate aminotransferase; EPS, extrapyrimal side effects; hr, hours; IV, intravenously; MAX, maximum; mcg, microgram; N/V, nausea and vomiting; ODT, oral disintergating tablets; PO, by mouth; prn, as necessary; Q, every; QD, daily; TID, three times a day.

Table 16–3. National Academy of Sciences Recommended
Daily Allowances of Proteins and Calories

Group	Age (years)	Protein (gm/kg/day)	Calories (kcal/kg/day)
Infants	0.0–0.5	2.2	108
	0.5–1.0	1.6	98
Children	1–3	1.2	102
	4–6	1.2	90
	7–10	1.0	70
Men	11–14	1.0	55
	15–18	0.9	45
Women	11–14	1.0	47
	15–18	0.8	49

intervention. The reasons for cachexia are numerous and include nausea, vomiting, diarrhea, constipation, stomatitis, mucositis, alterations in taste and smell as a result of chemotherapy, pain from procedures such as radiotherapy and surgery, mechanical obstruction, production of cytokines from tumors, and stress or anxiety. A variety of nutritional interventions are available for meeting the metabolic needs of patients and supporting a child through rigorous treatments (Andrassy and Chwals, 1998; Bloch, 2000; Grant and Kravits, 2000).

Assessment

One of the first assessments that should be performed to determine whether a patient needs nutritional supplementation is a nutritional interview of the patient and the patient's caregiver. A detailed history of previous and current eating habits should be taken. Not only should the quantity of foods, eating habits, and stool patterns be noted, but the quality of the diet and the presence of any food allergies or intolerances should be evaluated (Han-Markey, 2000).

Before any nutritional intervention, the extent of malnutrition the patient is experiencing must be evaluated. The National Academy of Sciences' recommended daily allowances of proteins and calories is shown in Table 16–3. These criteria are used to assess malnutrition.

Growth and development can be ascertained easily by evaluating a child's anthropometric measurements (i.e., height, weight, body mass index, and frontal occipital circumference) and if applicable, using growth charts. Each measurement can be plotted on curves and compared with national standards. Serial measurements are the most useful because they offer a broad assessment of growth and development (i.e., growth velocity). For the most current copy of age- and sex-specific growth curves, log in at www.cdc.gov/growthcharts. A triceps skinfold measurement can also be taken to assess body-fat composition. Once measurements are taken and plotted, the Waterlow criteria can be used to characterize the child's level

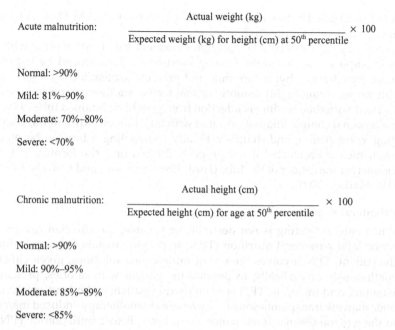

Acute malnutrition:

$$\frac{\text{Actual weight (kg)}}{\text{Expected weight (kg) for height (cm) at } 50^{\text{th}} \text{ percentile}} \times 100$$

Normal: >90%

Mild: 81%–90%

Moderate: 70%–80%

Severe: <70%

Chronic malnutrition:

$$\frac{\text{Actual height (cm)}}{\text{Expected height (cm) for age at } 50^{\text{th}} \text{ percentile}} \times 100$$

Normal: >90%

Mild: 90%–95%

Moderate: 85%–89%

Severe: <85%

Figure 16–1. The Waterlow Criteria for determining a patient's degree of malnutrition.

of malnutrition (acute or chronic). The formulas of the Waterlow criteria are illustrated in Figure 16–1.

Laboratory measurements are also used in evaluating the patient's nutritional status. Total protein, albumin, prealbumin, and cholesterol tests are useful in determining the patient's level of malnutrition. Electrolyte level and liver-function tests help clinicians monitor the efficacy of interventions and tolerance with side effects. Once the extent of malnutrition is determined, the clinician must then decide what, if any, intervention is required (Andrassy et al, 1998).

Enteral Feeding

Enteral feeding, which is the administration of nutritional products through the gastrointestinal tract, is the preferred method of feeding pediatric oncology patients, because it is a more physiologic approach, it is associated with low rates of morbidity, and it is less costly. There are a number of methods by which enteral feeds can be administered. The choice of routes depends on the patient's tolerance, the length of time nutritional support is needed, and the patient's underlying medical condition. Determinants of the appropriate enteral formula include the type of tube being used, the age and nutritional needs of the child, and the child's tolerance for the formula. The nutritional formulas currently used at M. D. Anderson are illustrated in Figure 16–2.

Although it is a desirable feeding method, enteral nutrition is not without complications. The tube-feeding syndrome, characterized by hypertonic dehydration, hypernatremia, and prerenal azotemia can be seen in patients receiving highly osmotic enteral feeds. Another complication associated with tube feeding is infection from poorly maintained tubes. Gastrointestinal complications associated with infection include nausea, vomiting, constipation, and diarrhea. Finally, the feeding tubes can become mechanically obstructed if not properly flushed or if the formula is too viscous for the caliber of the tube (Ford, 1996; Andrassy and Chwals, 1998; Han-Markey, 2000).

Parenteral Feeding

When enteral feeding is not desirable or feasible, the clinician can prescribe total parenteral nutrition (TPN) to provide metabolic support for the patient. TPN involves the use of intravenous solutions, given either continuously or cyclically, to provide the patient with calories, protein, vitamins, and minerals. TPN is often used in patients who have received bone marrow transplantation or who have a chemotherapy-induced injury to the gastrointestinal tract, pancreas, or ileus. Before initiation of TPN, venous access should be verified and established. Although TPN can be provided via a peripheral line, the most common method is through a central venous catheter. The maximum recommended dextrose concentration is 12.5% for peripheral infusion and 30% to 35% for central infusion. A step-by-step approach to providing TPN to pediatric patients is provided in Appendix 16–2.

One of the most common complications seen when initiating TPN is "refeeding syndrome" (Solomon and Kirby, 1990), a reaction characterized by several metabolic abnormalities (e.g., hypokalemia, hypophosphatemia, and hypomagnesemia) that result when glucose is reintroduced to a malnourished patient. To avoid or minimize this reaction, the TPN should be titrated slowly to the desirable goal over a few days. Other complications from TPN include the development of cholestasis, infections, and mechanical problems with the catheter. Judicious monitoring of patients during TPN administration is mandatory and includes frequent serial measurements of electrolyte level, liver function, and triglyceride levels. Weaning from TPN should begin as soon as the patient is able to take food orally or is a candidate for enteral feedings (Ford, 1996).

PAIN AND SYMPTOM MANAGEMENT

Optimal management of pain and other cancer-associated symptoms is predicated on an understanding of the multidimensional nature of

UTMDACC 2004–2005 ENTERAL FORMULARY

Product	Product Description	Kcal/ml	Pro g/L (% kcal)	CHO g/L (% kcal)	Fat g/L (% kcal)	% MCT	mOsm/kg H_2O	% Free Water	Vol for 100% RDA	Na/L mg/mEq	K/L mg/mEq	Ca/L mg	Phos/L mg	Mg/L mg
Tube Feeding Formulas														
Isosource 1.5* II	Moderate protein, volume restricted	1.5	68 (18)	170 (44)	65 (39)	30	650	78	933	1290 (56)	2250/58	1070	1070	430
Deliver 2.0* II	Calorically dense volume restricted	2	75 (15)	200 (40)	101 (45)	30	640	71	1000	800/35	1690/43	1010	1010	400
Isocal*	Isotonic, low protein	1.06	34 (13)	135 (50)	44 (37)	30	270	84	1890	530/23	1320/34	630	530	210
Isocal HN Plus*	Moderate protein	1.2	54 (18)	156 (53)	40 (29)	30	390	81	1000	1350/59	1850/47	1000	1000	400
Respalor	High nitrogen, volume restricted	1.5	75 (20)	146 (40)	68 (40)	30	400	78	1000	1270/55	1490/38	1000	1000	400
Ultracal HN Plus*	Moderate protein w/fiber, volume restricted	1.2	54 (18)	156 (53)	40 (29)	30	370	81	1000	1350/59	1850/47	1000	1000	400
Disease Specific Formulas														
Lipisorb	For malabsorption, high MCT	1.35	57 (17)	161 (48)	57 (35)	85	630	80	1180	1350/59	1690/43	850	850	340
Novasource Renal*	Renal formula	2	74 (15)	200 (40)	100 (45)	14	700 (960 diluted)	71	1000	900/39 (1500/70)	810/21 (1100/28)	1300	650	200
Impact 1.5*	High protein, critical care	1.5	84 (22)	200 (38)	69 (40)	40	550	78	1250	1280/56	1680/43	960	960	320
Nutri-Hep*	Hepatic disease failure, high BCAA	1.5	40 (11)	290 (77)	21 (12)	70	790	76	1000	1607	1320/34	956	1000	376
Elemental and Peptide Formulas														
Vivonex Plus	Elemental w/glutamine	1	45 (18)	190 (76)	6.7 (6)	–	650	85	1800	610/27	1060/27	560	560	220
Peptamen DT*	Semi-elemental	1	50 (20)	164 (65)	17 (15)	50	460	83	1500	1700/74	800/21	670	670	270
Peptamen 1.5	Calorically dense peptide-based	1.5	68 (19)	188 (49)	56 (33)	70	550	77	1000	1020/45	1860/49	1000	1000	400
Pediatric Formulas														
Enfalyte	Infant pediatric hydration solution	126/L	–	30 (100)	–	–	200	98	na	1150/50	980/25	–	–	–
Enfamil	Milk based infant formula	20oz	14.5 (9)	73 (43)	38 (48)	–	300	91	na	183/8	730/18.7	530	360	54
Kindercal	Pediatric oral/TF	1.06	30 (11)	135 (52)	44 (37)	20	345 (fl)	84	946	370/16.1	1310/34	1010	850	210
Kindercal w/Fiber	Pediatric Oral/TF with Fiber	1.06	30 (11)	135 (52)	44 (37)	20	345 (fl)	85	946	370/16.1	1310/34	1010	850	210
Lactofree	Lactose free infant formula	20oz	14.3 (8)	74 (43)	36 (49)	–	200	90	na	200/10.7	740/18.9	550	370	54
Peptamen Jr	Pediatric elemental	1	30 (12)	137.5 (55)	38.5 (33)	60	260	85	1000	460/20	1320/34	1000	800	200
Prosobee	Soy-based infant formula	20oz	17.3 (10)	73 (42)	37 (48)	–	200	91	na	240/10.4	810/21	710	560	74
Oral Supplements														
Boost Breeze	Clear liquid	0.68	34 (20)	130 (80)	–	–	900–950	89	na	210/9	970/25	633	1476	169
Boost Plus	High Kcal	1.52	59 (16)	200 (50)	58 (34)	–	720	78	946	720/31	1610/41	1390	1310	440
VHC 2.25	High Kcal, volume restricted	2.25	90 (16)	197 (35)	122 (49)	na	950	67	750	1200/52	1732/44	1232	1232	432
Choice DM Beverage	Oral diabetic	0.93	39 (17)	101 (40)	43 (43)	–	400	85	1310	850 (37)	1820 (47)	1390	1310	440
Modular Supplements (Details per 1 Tbsp (packet))														
Glutamine Powder	Free amino acid	60	10	5	0	–	N/A	N/A	N/A	15 mg	35 mg	–	–	–
Beneprotein	Modular protein	25	25	0	0	–	N/A	N/A	N/A	15 mg	15 mg	35	20	0
Benefiber	Modular fiber	16	0	4	0	–	N/A	N/A	N/A	0	0	0	0	0

Figure 16–2. *RTH, ready to hang. †Available on PRN basis only. Abbreviations: BCAA, Branch Chain Amino Acids; Ca/L, calcium per liter; CHO, carbohydrate; DM, diabetes mellitus; H_2O, water; Kcal, kilocalorie; K/L, potassium per liter; MCT, medium chained triglyceride; Mg/L, magnesium per liter; Na/L, sodium per liter; Phos/L, phosphate/liter; Pro, protein; RDA, recommended daily allowance; Tbsp, tablespoon; TF, tube feeding; Vol, volume.

symptoms. Contributing to symptom expression are medical factors (such as underlying pathophysiologic mechanisms and comorbid medical conditions) as well as psychologic, social, and spiritual factors. Consequently, optimal management is contingent on a comprehensive and systematic assessment, including a history of all domains of the symptom experience, a physical examination, and indicated diagnostic tests. Expert assessment is integral to the development of a working diagnosis and treatment plan.

Pediatric Cancer Pain

Most children with solid tumors experience pain at some point during the course of the disease. The tumor, the cancer treatment, and unrelated factors can all cause pain. The success of state-of-the-art multimodality therapies in tumor control has led to an overall shift in our focus on the management of cancer pain: from tumor-related causes to diagnostic procedure-related and treatment-related causes (Collins, 1998). Anticipation of diagnostic- and treatment-associated pain enables the clinician to use preemptive pain management strategies from the moment a diagnosis of cancer is suspected.

Pain in children is rarely an isolated occurrence; rather, it is usually accompanied by other symptoms. Systematic symptom surveys taken using validated age-appropriate tools indicate that children being treated for cancer typically experience multiple symptoms simultaneously. Using the Memorial Symptom Assessment Scale 10–18 (Collins et al, 2000) to survey pediatric patients, researchers at one comprehensive cancer center reported a mean 12.7 ($\pm$4.9) symptoms among inpatients versus 6.5 ($\pm$5.7) among outpatients. Patients who had had recent chemotherapy reported more symptoms than those no longer receiving chemotherapy (11.6 [$\pm$6.0] versus 5.2 [$\pm$5.1], respectively; $P < 0.01$). For hospitalized patients, pain was the most common symptom (reported by 84% of patients), and was highly distressing in most cases (Collins et al, 2000). In a retrospective study of dying children, researchers using similar assessment methodology identified a mean 11.1 ($\pm$5.6) symptoms experienced in the last week of life. Sixty percent of the children in the study had cancer. Pain was 1 of 6 symptoms that occurred in more than 50% of the children.

Pathophysiologic Mechanisms of Pain

The 2 primary pathophysiologic mechanisms of pain are nociceptive and neuropathic. Both mechanisms occur when chemical or mechanical stimuli activate or sensitize peripheral nociceptors or mechanoreceptors. Nociceptive pain occurs with an injury to the skin, deep tissue, or viscera and requires ongoing noxious input for its maintenance. Ablation of the nociceptive stimulus resolves the pain. Nociceptive pain can be categorized as somatic or visceral, both of which respond to therapy with opioid and nonopioid analgesics. Somatic pain occurs with injury to the skin or deep tissue. It is classically described as well localized and as an aching, throbbing, or gnawing sensation. Bone pain and pain from cutaneous metastases are examples of somatic pain. Visceral pain occurs with the stretching or distension of intrathoracic or intra-abdominal viscera. It is often poorly localized and is described as a deep ache, cramp, or pressure. Visceral pain may occur at distant cutaneous sites that can be tender to palpation. Common examples of visceral pain include abdominal pain from bowel obstruction and bladder spasms from urinary retention. Visceral pain is often associated with sympathetic nervous system hyper-reactivity such as nausea, tachycardia, and diaphoresis.

In contrast to somatic or visceral pain, neuropathic pain, which is a consequence of injury to peripheral or central nervous system tissue, may persist long after ablation of the inciting stimulus. Unlike nociceptive pain, neuropathic pain is an unfamiliar experience for most people. Qualitatively, it is characterized as burning, shooting, stabbing, paroxysmal, electric shock–like, or painful numbness. Examples include the burning pain associated with post-therapeutic neuralgia and with radiotherapy- or tumor-associated brachial plexopathy. In addition to conventional analgesics, many adjuvant analgesics benefit patients with neuropathic pain syndromes (Zhukovsky et al, 2000).

Pain and Symptom History

The components of a symptom history are a systematic symptom survey, a symptom-specific history, an oncologic history (including disease-modifying therapies), a general medical history, a psychosocial and family history (including screening for substance abuse), and a spiritual review. Individual symptoms are also assessed with validated age-appropriate measures, when available. The type and extent of symptom assessment are contingent on a child's age, developmental status, and emotional state. Parental input is important at all stages of development. The symptom-specific history assesses the following aspects of a symptom:

- Intensity
- Location
- Frequency
- Temporal features (onset, duration, pattern)
- Relieving and exacerbating features
- Associated clinical characteristics
- Prior treatment modalities and their efficacy
- Child and parent perceptions of etiology
- Importance to the child and the parents
- Impact on other symptoms, function, and quality of life
- Use of age-appropriate and developmentally appropriate measurement tools

Assessment Tools

Types of assessment tools include behavioral, numeric rating, categorical, and visual analog scales. Behavioral observation scales are the primary tools used to assess pain in neonates, infants, children younger than 4 years of age, and children with developmental disabilities. Children 3 to 8 years of age are usually able to describe their pain using "faces" scales, which are a series of photographs or drawings depicting varying degrees of facial distress. Children 8 years old and older can generally use verbal rating scales (no pain, mild, moderate, severe) and a modified version of the adult visual analog scale in which they indicate their pain using a horizontal ruler (Hester, 1993; Berde and Sethna, 2002).

Synthesis of Symptom Diagnosis and Management Plan

Once a working diagnosis is established, treatment is directed at modifying the underlying cause of the symptom or symptoms, for example, chemotherapy or radiotherapy for painful spinal cord compression or antibiotics, incision, and drainage for abscess-associated pain. Symptom-directed therapy (i.e., analgesics for pain) is often an integral component of the treatment plan when primary therapy is ineffective or while awaiting the benefit of antineoplastic therapy.

Modalities of Symptom Control

The modalities of symptom control are numerous and include disease-specific, pharmacologic, anesthetic, surgical, physiatric, cognitive-behavioral, spiritual, complementary, and alternative therapies. For cancer, disease-specific therapies include surgery, radiotherapy, chemotherapy, biologic-response modifiers, and other disease-modifying therapies. Anesthetic techniques include a variety of somatic and sympathetic nerve blocks, as well as the administration of spinal opioids and local anesthetics. One surgical modality is spinothalamic-tract cordotomy, which can be accomplished via open route or percutaneously. The optimal management plan is often multimodal. Physiatric, cognitive-behavioral, and spiritual modalities have the added benefit of providing the child with a sense of control and not contributing to the side effects of pharmacotherapy, which can limit quality of life. Involvement of child-life specialists, when available, is key to the provision of optimal care.

Treatment Assessment

Assessing the treatment of symptoms is similar to initial symptom assessment. The patient's self-report of the symptom history is key and is combined with observations of family members and involved clinicians. Use of validated measures provides a picture over time that complements patient and caregiver reports and facilitates symptom research. Changes noted on physical examination and changes in functional ability, including activities of daily living, social interactions, cognitive skills, and coping skills, provide additional data with which to assess patient outcome. The treatment plan can then be revised accordingly. Ongoing symptom assessment is mandatory for monitoring the benefits, side effects, and complications of therapy and for identifying changes in contributing pathophysiologies, as well as the development of new symptoms.

ANALGESIC PHARMACOTHERAPY

Pharmacotherapy is the mainstay of treatment for most children with cancer. The available classes of pain drugs are nonopioid analgesics, adjuvant analgesics, and opioids. Because of the paucity of analgesic studies conducted in children, pharmacotherapy use is largely based on clinical experience. From a developmental perspective, the factors that influence drug management include the ratio of body compartments, differences in plasma protein binding, development of hepatic enzyme systems for drug metabolism, extent of renal filtration and excretion of drugs and their metabolites, metabolic rate, oxygen consumption, and degree of respiratory function maturation (Berde and Sethna, 2002).

Nonopioids and Adjuvant Analgesics

Nonopioid analgesics include acetaminophen, aspirin, and nonsteroidal anti-inflammatory drugs (NSAIDs). A drug-specific dose ceiling exists for nonopioid analgesics, and doses above the ceiling increase the risk of toxicity without yielding additional analgesia. Of the nonopioid analgesics, acetaminophen is preferred over aspirin because of the increased risk of bleeding complications and Reye's syndrome associated with aspirin use. The adverse effects of nonopioid analgesics in children are similar to those seen in adults, including hepatotoxicity (acetaminophen), nephrotoxicity (acetaminophen and NSAIDs), gastric problems (NSAIDs), and platelet dysfunction (NSAIDs).

Adjuvant analgesics are a diverse group of drugs with analgesic activity but whose primary indication is for syndromes or conditions other than pain. Tricyclic antidepressants, selective serotonin reuptake inhibitors, anticonvulsants (such as phenytoin and gabapentin), oral local anesthetics, ketamine, and corticosteroids are some of the adjuvant analgesics used to manage neuropathic and other pain syndromes.

Opioids

The key factors to successful opioid use are: a) knowing the biologic phenomena of tolerance, physical dependence, and addiction and b) anticipating and preventing side effects when possible and managing them aggressively when they occur.

Tolerance, Physical Dependence, and Addiction

Tolerance to drug effects develops with regular use. Over time, larger and more frequent doses are needed to achieve the same effect. In patients with cancer, dose escalation is often the result of disease progression rather than tolerance. Clinically, patients benefit from tolerance because tolerance to side effects develops more rapidly than tolerance to analgesia. Constipation is the one exception to this rule; tolerance to constipation is rare.

Physical dependence also develops with prolonged opioid use and is defined by the development of an abstinence syndrome (withdrawal) upon abrupt drug cessation or the administration of an opioid antagonist. The manifestations of opioid withdrawal, described as "wet" syndromes, include fever, tachypnea, tachycardia, coryza, rhinorrhea, nausea, vomiting, diarrhea, and diaphoresis. When opioid analgesia is no longer required, such as after a successful nerve block, opioid withdrawal can be prevented by gradually reducing drug use over the course of a few days. To avoid drug withdrawal in patients with life-threatening respiratory depression who have developed tolerance to opioids, diluted solutions of an opioid antagonist (i.e., naloxone) can be administered to achieve the target respiratory rate.

Physical dependence is distinct from addiction, which is a psychologic and behavioral syndrome characterized by drug craving and aberrant drug use. The risk of opioid addiction is generally thought to be low in patients with no history of substance abuse. For patients with a history of addiction, there is some risk that their cancer pain will be undertreated. Experience suggests that most patients with a history of substance abuse can be safely and effectively treated with opioids. For some patients, it is critical that an addiction medicine specialist be included on the care-plan team. Addiction must be differentiated from unsanctioned drug escalation used to treat poor pain control. The latter condition is also known as pseudoaddiction.

Management of Side Effects

The side effects of opioid use, which include constipation, sedation, altered mental status, nausea, and dry mouth, are predictable. Side effects should be prevented whenever possible and managed aggressively when they occur. When opioid treatment is initiated, the patient should be encouraged to maintain adequate mobility and fluid intake if possible and should be started on a routine bowel regimen consisting of a stool softener or laxative to prevent constipation. Mild sedation, nausea, or both may occur when opioids are started, but tolerance will typically develop over the course of a few days to several days. More severe side effects that do not resolve over a few days can usually be managed with adjuvant drugs. Nausea can be treated with antiemetics, and sedation can be treated with psychostimulants, such as methylphenidate or dextroamphetamine. Psychostimulants are commonly administered in the morning and again around lunchtime. It is not advisable to administer opioids late in the day because these drugs have the potential to cause insomnia. Psychostimulants are contraindicated in children with delirium because these drugs may exacerbate confusion. Instead, antipsychotics, such as haloperidol, are the drug of choice. Dry mouth is difficult to treat but can be minimized by scrupulous oral hygiene, fluid intake, and ingestion of ice chips. If side effects remain limiting, then rotation to an alternate opioid might be beneficial. Knowledge of equianalgesic tables and dose reduction by 30% to 50% are key components of successful opioid rotation.

Principles of Analgesic Administration

Knowledge of a patient's pain syndrome and pain intensity drives the selection of analgesics. For patients with low-intensity somatic pain, acetaminophen or an NSAID is a common starting point; however, these drugs may be contraindicated if there is an increased risk for neutropenic fever or bleeding. Adjuvant analgesics are commonly used to treat neuropathic pain and certain other pain syndromes. Tricyclic antidepressants and selective serotonin reuptake inhibitors are often used to treat burning neuropathic pain, and anticonvulsants are used to treat paroxysmal electric shock-like pain; however, each of these adjuvant drugs may be effective against neuropathic pain of any quality. Opioids can be used in conjunction with nonopioid and adjuvant analgesics, as appropriate, to treat pain of any pathophysiology. For mild- to moderate-intensity pain, opioids are often administered in the form of fixed-combination tablets or elixirs with acetaminophen or NSAIDs; the dose of the nonopioid agent is limited because of its ceiling effect. The following principles should be considered when prescribing treatment for pain.

- Start 1 drug at a time, and allow an adequate trial period to assess its benefits and side effects.
- Choose the appropriate route of administration.
- Provide regularly scheduled administration for continuous pain.
- Use doses according to circumstances or "breakthrough" doses to prevent predictable incident pain and to treat pain exacerbations.
- Anticipate and manage side effects.

Routes of Administration

Administering drugs orally minimizes expense and facilitates care in the home and in other noninstitutional settings. Most patients accept and tolerate oral administration well unless they have painful mucositis, nausea or vomiting, bowel obstruction, or altered mental status precluding oral administration. Alternate routes of administration are intravenous, subcutaneous, intramuscular, spinal (intrathecal and epidural), rectal, transdermal, and oral transmucosal. The intramuscular route is rarely indicated because of associated pain and the multiplicity of other routes available.

Both the intravenous and subcutaneous routes can be used for continuous infusion of opioids and many other symptom control drugs; however, methadone has been reported to cause irritant effects when administered subcutaneously. Spinal administration of opioids may be indicated in the small percentage of patients in whom adequate analgesia cannot be achieved because of limiting side effects from systemic opioid therapy.

PALLIATIVE CARE

In 2002, the World Health Organization (WHO) revised their definition of palliative care, changing the target population from individuals with incurable illness to those with life-threatening illness. The WHO now defines palliative care as "... an approach that improves the quality of life of patients and their families facing the problems associated with life-threatening illness, through the prevention and relief of suffering by means of early identification and impeccable assessment and treatment of pain and other problems, physical, psychosocial and spiritual ... " (World Health Organization, 2002). For children, the WHO further specified the following parameters.

- Palliative care for children is the active total care of the child's body, mind, and spirit and also involves giving support to the family.
- Palliative care begins when illness is diagnosed and continues regardless of whether a child receives treatment directed at the disease.
- Health providers must evaluate and alleviate a child's physical, psychological, and social distress.
- Effective palliative care requires a broad multidisciplinary approach that includes the family and makes use of available community resources; it can be successfully implemented even if resources are limited.
- Palliative care can be provided in tertiary care facilities, in community health centers, and even in children's homes.

Palliative care has evolved considerably over the past decade and is now integrated with acute care in many medical centers. Palliative care has the potential to benefit all children with life-threatening disorders and their families, regardless of where they fall in the disease trajectory, the status of disease-modifying therapy, or where the patient is being treated. Integration of palliative care services with acute medical care services early-on facilitates expert symptom management and family support. For the unfortunate minority of patients whose disease progresses to the terminal stage, palliative care incorporates advance care planning, affording the patient and his or her family the opportunity to spend their remaining time together in a manner consistent with their values and with the goals of care.

KEY PRACTICE POINTS

- Pain and other symptoms are frequent throughout the disease course. Patients should be screened for pain and other symptoms at all clinical encounters.
- The symptom experience is multidimensional.
- The symptom assessment should include symptom-specific, oncologic, general-medicine, and psychosocial histories and a spiritual review.
- Only validated, age-appropriate symptom assessment scales should be used.
- Optimal treatment is often multidimensional and combines therapy directed at the underlying cause (e.g., disease-modifying interventions) combined with therapy directed at the symptom.
- Palliative care begins with the diagnosis of a life-threatening disease and continues throughout the disease course.

SUGGESTED READINGS

A Call for a Change: Recommendations to Improve the Care of Children Living with Life-Threatening Conditions [white paper]. Alexandria, VA: Child International Project on Palliative/Hospice Service (ChiPPS) Administrative/Policy Workgroup of the National Hospice and Palliative Care Organization; October 2001. Available at: http://www.nhpco.org.

Andrassy RJ, Chwals WJ. Nutritional support of the pediatric oncology patient. *Nutrition* 1998;14:124–129.

Beckwith MC, Mullin S. Prevention and management of chemotherapy-induced nausea and vomiting, part 1. *Hosp Pharm* 2001;36:67–80.

Berde CB, Sethna NF. Analgesics for the treatment of pain in children. *N Engl J Med* 2002;347:1094–1103.

Bloch A. Nutrition support in cancer. *Semin Oncol Nurs* 2000;16:122–127.

Borison HL, Wang SC. Physiology and pharmacology of vomiting. *Pharmacol Rev* 1953;5:193–230.

Collins JJ. Pharmacologic management of pediatric cancer pain. In: Portenoy RK, Bruera E, eds. *Topics in Palliative Care*. New York, NY: Oxford University Press; 1998:7–28.

Collins JJ, Byrnes ME, Dunkel IJ, et al. The measurement of symptoms in children with cancer. *J Pain Symptom Manage* 2000;19:363–373.

Collins JJ, Devine TD, Johnson EA, et al. The measurement of symptoms in young children with cancer: the validation of the Memorial Symptom Assessment Scale in children aged 7–12. *J Pain Symptom Manage* 2002;23:1016.

Davies B, Steele R. Families in pediatric palliative care. In: Portenoy RK, Bruera E, eds. *Topics in Palliative Care*. New York, NY: Oxford University Press; 1998:29–49.

Drake R, Frost J, Collins JJ. The symptoms of dying children. *J Pain Symptom Manage* 2003;26:594–603.

Ford EG. Nutrition support of pediatric patients. *Nutr Clin Pract* 1996;11:183–191.

Gralla RJ, Osoba D, Kris MG, et al. Recommendations for the use of antiemetics: evidence-based, clinical practice guidelines. *J Clin Oncol* 1999;17:2971–2994.

Grant M, Kravits K. Symptoms and their impact on nutrition. *Semin Oncol Nurs* 2000;16:113–121.

Han-Markey T. Nutritional considerations in pediatric oncology. *Semin Oncol Nurs* 2000;16:146–151.

Hesketh PJ, Gralla RJ, du Bois A, et al. Methodology of antiemetic trials: response assessment, evaluation of new agents and definition of chemotherapy emetogenicity. *Support Care Cancer* 1998;6:221–227.

Hesketh PJ, Kris MG, Grunberg SM, et al. Proposal for classifying the acute emetogenicity of cancer chemotherapy. *J Clin Oncol* 1997;15:103–109.

Hester NO. Assessment of pain in children with cancer. In: Chapman DR, Foley KM, eds. *Current and Emerging Issues in Cancer Pain: Research and Practice*. New York, NY: Raven Press, Ltd; 1993:219–245.

Kane JR, Himmelstein B. Palliative care in pediatrics. In: Berger AM, Portenoy RK, Weissman DE, eds. *Principles and Practice of Palliative Care and Supportive Oncology*. Philadelphia, PA: Lippincott Williams and Wilkins; 2002:1044–1061.

Levetown M. Treatment of symptoms other than pain in pediatric palliative care. In: Portenoy RK, Bruera E, eds. *Topics in Palliative Care*. New York, NY: Oxford University Press; 1998:51–69.

Mullin S, Beckwith MC. Prevention and management of chemotherapy-induced nausea and vomiting, part 2. *Hosp Pharm* 2001;36:280–302.

Physician Data Query (PDQ) Supportive Care Board. National Cancer Institute Web site. Available at: http://www.cancer.gov. Accessed.

Solomon SM, Kirby DF. The refeeding syndrome: a review. *JPEN J Parenter Enteral Nutr* 1990;14:90–97.

Waterlow JC. Classification and definition of protein-calorie malnutrition. *Br Med J* 1972;3:566–569.

World Health Organization. *National Cancer Control Programmes: Policies and Managerial Guidelines*, 2nd edition. Geneva, Switzerland: World Health Organization; 2002.

World Health Organization in collaboration with the International Association for the Study of Pain. *Cancer Pain Relief and Palliative Care in Children*. Geneva, Switzerland: World Health Organization; 1998.

Zhukovsky DS, Abdullah O, Richardson M, Walsh D. Clinical evaluation in advanced cancer. *Semin Oncol* 2000;27:14–23.

APPENDIX 16–1. PROCEDURE FOR DETERMINING THE EMETOGENICITY OF A CHEMOTHERAPY REGIMEN

Step 1	Assign emetogenic level to each agent in the regimen. See Table 16–1.		
Step 2	Identify the most emetogenic agent, and start with this number.		
Step 3	Adjust the emetogenic potential of the regimen.		
Calculate the Level of the Regimen	Make no adjustment for level 1 agents. For example: $3 + 1 = 3$ $4 + 1 + 1 = 4$ $2 + 1 + 1 + 1 = 2$ $5 + 1 = 5$	Increase by 1 level if 1 or more level 2 agents are in the regimen. For example: $3 + 2 = 4$ $3 + 2 + 2 = 4$ $2 + 2 + 2 = 3$ $4 + 2 + 2 = 5$	Increase by 1 level for each level 3 or level 4 agent in the regimen. For example: $3 + 3 = 4$ $3 + 3 + 3 = 5$ $4 + 3 = 5$ $4 + 4 = 5$

Source: Hesketh et al, 1997.

Example encountered in pediatric oncology patients:

Therapy for neuroblastoma:

Cisplatin 60 mg/m^2 intravenously on day 1 (level 5)

Etoposide 100 mg/m^2 intravenously on days 2 and 4 (level 2)

Doxorubicin 30 mg/m^2 intravenously on day 2 (level 3)

Cyclophosphamide 900 mg/m^2 intravenously on days 3 and 4 (level 4)

Emetogenicity:

Day 1 ➜ Level 5
Day 2 ➜ $3 + 2 =$ Level 4
Day 3 ➜ Level 4
Day 4 ➜ $4 + 2 =$ Level 5

Appendix 16–2. Eight-Step Process Involved in Total Parenteral Nutrition Administration

Step 1: Determine the amount of nutrients.

Age (years)	Total Calories (kcal/kg/day)*	Protein (gm/kg/day)**
0–0.5	95–110	2.2–3.2 (2.7)
0.5–1	90–100	1.6–3 (2.3)
1–3	85–95	1.2–3 (2.1)
4–6	80–90	1.1–3 (2)
7–10	70–80	1–3 (2)
11–14	60–70	1–2.5 (1.8)
15–24	45–55	0.9–2.5 (1.7)

* Amounts based on recommended daily allowance (RDA) of calories. Hospitalized
   children generally require 10% to 20% fewer calories because of their limited activity.
** Amounts based on RDA of proteins. Averages shown in parentheses.

Step 2: Determine the patient's maintenance fluid needs.

Weight	Daily Maintenance Fluids
≤10 kg	100 mL/kg
10–20 kg	1,000 mL + 50 mL/kg for patients who weigh more than 10 kg
20–30 kg	1,500 mL + 20 mL/kg for patients who weigh more than 20 kg
>30 kg	1,500–1,800 mL/m²

Step 3: Formulate macronutrient composition.

    A. Protein
        1. All protein needs are met by amino acids.
        2. Start with Travasol 10% for all patients unless they are younger than 1 year of age (in which case, use Trophamine 10%) or are fluid restricted (in which case use Aminosyn II 15%).
        3. 1 g protein = 4 kcal
    B. Lipids
        1. Generally, lipids will account for approximately 30% of total calories. Lipids should provide at least 5% of total calories (in order to avoid essential fatty acid deficiency) and no more than 60% of calories (in order to avoid ketosis).

   2. Start lipids at 0.5 to 1 g/kg/day, but do not exceed 4 g/kg/day.
   3. Lipids are generally infused over 12 hours (minimum 8 hours). If the rate of lipid infusion is less than 10 mL/hour, consider using a syringe pump to deliver the lipids or change formulations (i.e., from 20% to 10%).
   4. Most patients will tolerate 20% lipids; 10% lipids are used when patients have low fat requirements and 20% lipids cannot be infused safely.
   5. 1 mL of 20% lipids = 2 kcal; 1 mL of 10% lipids = 1.1 kcal
  C. Dextrose
   1. Ordinarily, dextrose together with lipids will provide patients with approximately 70% of total calories.
   2. Use 70% dextrose to provide calories.
   3. 1 g dextrose = 3.4 kcal.

Step 4: Compare intravenous maintenance needs to volume of total parenteral nutrition.

   1. After the macronutrients are determined, look at the volume of total parenteral nutrition (TPN) and compare to intravenous maintenance needs.
   2. The volume of amino acids + dextrose + lipids should be 60% to 80% of maintenance fluid needs. May need to add some sterile water to the TPN.
   3. When TPN is to begin, intravenous fluids should be changed to 1/2 NS or NS without electrolytes to infuse at a decreased rate.
   4. Adjust the intravenous fluid rate such that the total TPN volume + intravenous fluid does not exceed 100% of the patient's needs (you may need to allow room for intravenous medications). Exceptions to this rule are when the patient's clinical status warrants additional fluids (such as fever, nausea, vomiting, diarrhea, fistula output, etc.) or the patient is required to receive more than his/her maintenance fluid requirements as stated in the chemotherapy treatment protocol.

Step 5: Perform "safety checks."

   1. In general, approximately 30% of calories will come from lipids, and 70% will come from protein and dextrose.
   2. The final dextrose concentration should not exceed 35% for central administration. You may need to add sterile water to meet this criterion.
   3. The patient's glucose infusion rate (GIR) goal should range from 4 to 14 mg/kg/minute. A GIR above 14 mg/kg/minute can result in fatty liver, hypertriglyceridemia, hyperglycemia, and excessive CO_2 production. GIR is calculated as "mg dextrose/kg/minute."

Age (years)	GIR Range (mg/kg/minute)
0–3	11–14
4–8	8–11
9–12	6–8
13–18	4–6

4. This ratio of grams of nitrogen (N) from amino acids to total non-protein kilocalories (NPC), or the N:NPC ratio, should be 1: 150–200. For every 6.25 g of amino acid, there is 1 g of nitrogen.

Step 6: Add electrolytes.

1. To assess electrolyte needs, determine whether the current amount of intravenous fluids is sufficient.
2. Assess patient for risk of re-feeding and account for this in electrolyte additions.
3. Suggested electrolyte needs are shown in the table below. Adjustments are recommended based on clinical condition and concomitant medications.

Electrolyte	"Normal" Maintenance Requirements
Sodium	2–4 mEq/kg/day
Chloride	2–3 mEq/kg/day
Potassium	2–3 mEq/kg/day
Magnesium	0.25–0.5 mEq/kg/day
Calcium	0.5–3 mEq/kg/day
Phosphorus	0.5–2 mmol/kg/day

4. Remove electrolytes from intravenous fluid.
5. K+ infusion rate should not exceed 0.5 mEq/kg/hour for patients who are not on cardiac monitoring.
6. Perform calcium-phosphate compatibility calculations.
7. Calcium should always be considered as an additive to the TPN unless it is not feasible. Generally, 2,000 mg (9.2 mEq) is the maximum amount of calcium added to TPN.

Step 7: Add other additives.

1. Add multivitamins and trace elements per standard protocol.
2. Add famotidine to TPN at 1 to 2 mg/kg/day (usual maximum is 40 mg/day) rounded to the nearest 5 mg.

3. Most patients will not require additional zinc or other trace elements.
4. Insulin is added to TPN if patient has sustained (more than 1 measurement) glucoses levels greater than 180. As an initial guide, starting insulin doses are:

Age (years)	1 unit of insulin × gms dextrose
0–3	40–50
4–6	30–40
7–10	20–30
11–14	15–20
15–18	10–15

Step 8: Initiate/discontinue TPN.

1. Most patients will start on day 1 with 100% protein needs and 40% to 50% total calories.
2. Lipids are usually held on day 1 until a triglyceride level is ordered.
3. If patient tolerates the first day of TPN, then on day 2, the patient can receive his or her caloric goal.
4. If glucose is above 180 or electrolytes are unstable, then consider slow advance (over 2 to 3 days).
5. Weaning is usually the reverse of initiation.
6. When TPN is discontinued, change intravenous fluid accordingly, and add famotidine to regimen if necessary.

17 BEHAVIORAL MEDICINE IN CANCER CARE

Donna R. Copeland and Martha A. Askins

CHAPTER OVERVIEW

Pediatric cancer is one of the most difficult challenges a family may face. The experience will have a lasting effect on the patient and all family members. There will be some personal and shared triumphs, but there will likely be some stressful situations and encounters that could impede the child's natural developmental course and affect family dynamics. The behavioral medicine program in the Child and Adolescent Center at M. D. Anderson Cancer Center is a multidisciplinary service designed to address the many psychological, emotional, and psychosocial issues related to the experience of childhood cancer.

INTRODUCTION

Pediatric cancer is a life-altering experience for the entire family. Maintaining normalcy becomes a challenge as the child's suffering and frequent absences from home disrupt family dynamics. In addition to the physical consequences of the disease, cancer can severely affect a child's psychological, emotional, and social development and can impose significant stress on family members.

A well-designed behavioral medicine program can help pediatric patients and their family members cope with the challenges presented by cancer and its treatments. The behavioral medicine program in the Child and Adolescent Center at M. D. Anderson combines traditional interventions (e.g., counseling, psychotherapy, play therapy, and practical guidance) with contemporary interventions (e.g., creative arts, physical fitness, maternal-skills training, and cognitive remediation) to address the psychologic, emotional, and psychosocial effects of the disease. The interventions are designed to help the sick child fulfill his or her developmental course, enable the family to build or sustain strong interpersonal relationships, and provide models of effective parenting. The programs discussed in this chapter are available to all pediatric patients at M. D. Anderson. A special program, the Adolescent and Young Adult Program, has been implemented at the institution to address the issues and concerns unique to patients 15 to 21 years old. See Chapter 18 for a full description of this program.

SUPPORTIVE-CARE NEEDS OF PEDIATRIC PATIENTS AND FAMILY MEMBERS

As our awareness of the complexities of childhood cancer and its management has increased, so has our awareness of the need for appropriate behavioral medicine services. A cancer diagnosis can exacerbate a family's existing personal and shared problems and can introduce new ones. Families use a variety of resources to help them cope. Some rely on professional counselors to help them identify and work through problems, and some derive their support from relatives and from community and religious networks. Others use creative arts to promote psychological, emotional, and psychosocial healing.

The specific supportive-care needs of patients and family members vary on the basis of many variables, including the severity of the illness, the complexity of the treatments, other stresses the family may be dealing with, the family's social and economic status, whether the parents are optimistic or pessimistic about the child's condition, and the methods the family uses to manage stress. Supportive-care needs will also vary depending on the phase of treatment the patient is in: (a) the initial phase, which involves diagnosis and treatment planning; (b) the active phase, during which the patient and family settle into a treatment routine; and (c) the post-treatment or follow-up phase in which the patient is monitored for recurrent disease and late effects of treatment. At each phase of treatment, the child and the family must master specific coping skills.

In the initial treatment phase, patients and family members work with a physician to determine a treatment plan. They decide whether to participate in a clinical trial, review details of the protocol, learn about illness-related symptoms and treatment-related side effects, and become acquainted with hospital guidelines and treatment procedures. During this time, the patient and his or her family establish a rapport and working alliance with the health care team, and parents decide how parental responsibilities will be shared.

In the active treatment phase, patients and family members initiate new, normative lifestyle patterns. They must develop coping competency, achieve continuity and emotional equilibrium, assume a sense of meaning with respect to the illness, and assess career and lifestyle goals.

The post-treatment and follow-up phase is a period of watching and waiting and, in some cases, lingering anxiety. Parents worry that the disease will recur and that they might overlook the signs of recurrence. Patients struggle to come to terms with cancer-causing losses (e.g., amputation, cognitive impairment, or sterility) and to assume an identity without feeling victimized. Parents learn to let go, to allow the pediatric patient to function independently, and to encourage him or her to continue planning for the future.

At M. D. Anderson, we take an open, honest approach with patients and family members. We are attentive to their concerns at each stage of care. Our goal is to help them maintain normalcy as much as possible and to provide them with information as appropriate to help them make sound decisions.

PSYCHOLOGICAL- AND EMOTIONAL-SUPPORT
INTERVENTIONS

Through our behavioral medicine program, psychologic and emotional support are provided by a multidisciplinary team that includes child-life specialists, social workers, parent consultants, psychologists and psychiatrists, neuropsychologists, an education staff, language assistants, creative arts instructors, and clergy. These practitioners work together to provide comprehensive care designed to meet the specific needs of each family.

Child-Life Specialists

When the pediatric patient and accompanying family members enter our institution, a child-life specialist acquaints them with hospital logistics and guidelines and describes diagnostic and treatment processes. The goal of this service is to foster a sense of trust in a system that is unfamiliar and possibly daunting.

The child-life specialist explains the medical procedures the child will undergo, such as needle sticks, biopsies, diagnostic imaging, and radiotherapy, and will remain with the child during these procedures. They use hand puppets and actual medical equipment and instruments to describe treatment processes. Knowledge of the procedures and types of materials that will be used in their treatment puts the patient at ease and gives him or her a sense of being in control. Child-life specialists and volunteers also staff the playrooms, which are designed and equipped to provide patients with activities that divert their attention away from the treatment routine. The playrooms also serve as a resource for therapeutic play.

Social Workers

A social worker is assigned to each family upon their arrival at M. D. Anderson. The social worker provides emotional support for the patient and the family throughout the treatment period and supplies practical information, such as where to find lodging and how to access financial resources. Social workers are also available to accompany the patient and family to meetings with the physician to ensure that their concerns are addressed.

Parent Consultants

Parents who have endured the pediatric-cancer experience serve as consultants to new families. The parent consultants guide new families through the maze of appointments and meetings and provide them with valuable information. At a weekly session called "Coffee Time," experienced and novice parents of pediatric cancer patients meet in a support-group setting to discuss the parenting perspective of childhood cancer.

Psychologists and Psychiatrists

When patients and family members show marked signs of depression, anxiety, and other such problems, they can be counseled by a psychologist or psychiatrist. These clinicians provide therapeutic interventions to help the patient and family members cope with issues related to the disease and with preexisting circumstances, such as the separation or divorce of parents and any atypical physical and social developmental problems the child may be dealing with. Hypnotherapy is one technique clinicians use to help patients and family members relax. Psychotropic medications may be prescribed as an adjunct to counseling.

Neuropsychologists

Neuropsychologists evaluate young patients with brain tumors whose cognitive functions may have been affected by the disease or by treatments. They also evaluate young patients with other types of cancer who may have learning difficulties. Neuropsychologists monitor patients' academic progress throughout the treatment period and beyond, and they consult with teachers from community- and hospital-based schools about special provisions and accommodations that may be needed in the classroom. A full description of the neuropsychologic effects of childhood cancer, in particular the effects of radiotherapy, is provided in a subsequent section of this chapter.

Education Staff

It is important that the pediatric patient continue his or her education in order to accomplish both academic and social-development goals. Teachers from our exclusive hospital-based school and from the public school system work together to help the patient accomplish these goals. A detailed description of our education program is provided in a subsequent section of this chapter.

Language Assistants

A team of language assistants is available to interpret conversations and translate written documents for families whose native language is not English. Some of the languages for which patients commonly seek assistance are Spanish, Arabic, Vietnamese, and Chinese; however, assistance is available for numerous other languages as well.

Creative Arts Instructors

We have found that music, painting, drawing, writing, and other artistic activities are effective coping mechanisms for children with cancer. Artistic activities not only provide young patients with an avenue to express how they feel about being ill, but they are also therapeutic in that they offer the patient a sense of reassurance and joy. The following poem is an example of how young patients use the arts to communicate their feelings about the cancer experience.

Dreamer

(by Kelly Mundell, age 16)
In my dreams, I can see the world.
Take my hands and scoop the world up.
Watch all the people and see what they do.
Visit the places I want to go most.
Then take the world and make it a necklace.
Take the world with me wherever I go.
Never take the world out of my sight.

The world will become part of me.
When I get rid of the necklace,
I give it a throw.
I'll send the world to a galaxy unknown.
Just as I let it go.
I jump into the world and go for a ride.
Where we stop, I do not know.
Where I ended was in my bed.
All of a sudden, the world stops with a jolt.
I wake up, look around, and find everything the same.

Creative arts instructors help young patients discover and develop talents in many different media.

Clergy

Clergy from all religious affiliations are available to counsel and console pediatric patients and their family members. They also answer the existential questions that inevitably arise when a child becomes gravely ill.

INTENSIVE PSYCHOSOCIAL-SUPPORT INTERVENTIONS

In addition to the usual care provided through our behavioral medicine services (i.e., psychological and neuropsychological assessments; individual, child, and family therapy; hypnotherapy; and psychotropic medication), special psychosocial interventions are available for patients and parents when the child is undergoing difficult procedures (such as bone marrow transplantation) and when terminal care is initiated.

Bone marrow transplantation is a highly stressful procedure that can take several months to complete. Extended support and guidance are provided from all behavioral medicine disciplines to the patient and family members during this time. When appropriate, the patient also receives physical therapy and speech therapy.

We have found that mothers of children who are seriously ill are at greater risk for post-traumatic stress than other family members. Because the mother plays a pivotal role in helping the sick child and other family members cope, it is important to ensure that she is receiving adequate psychosocial support. One of our studies showed that when mothers are confident and skilled in problem solving, the likelihood that she will experience depression or anxiety is reduced. Through our Maternal Problem-Solving Skills Training program, we instill in mothers a positive attitude and help them identify problems and generate solutions.

When the cancer treatment is unsuccessful, the behavioral medicine staff works with physicians and nurses to ensure that the child and the family are properly informed of the options available to them. One option is hospice care; however, some families prefer to have the child cared for in their own home. Staff from M. D. Anderson's Department of Palliative Care and Symptom Control work with the primary care team to make sure that the patient is comfortable and that family members, including siblings, receive the counseling and other support services they need. After a child dies, the behavioral medicine team maintains contact with the family through cards and telephone calls. A memorial service is held quarterly in the Cancer Center Chapel for families of children and adolescents who have died in the previous 3 months. Families who attend are given a bouquet of flowers and a subscription to a periodical for bereaved families. A reception is held after the service so that families and staff can visit with each other.

Academic Interventions

Because children with cancer are likely to survive the disease, it is important for them to continue their education while they undergo treatment. Pursuing an education enables these children to continue planning their future and striving for social independence. Academic achievement is an important source of self-esteem for these young patients.

State and federal laws mandate that students who are diagnosed with cancer be provided the opportunity to complete their education. There are 4 options for educational placement: (a) community-based schooling, in which the student continues to attend the hometown school as his or her health and treatment-schedule permit; (b) homebound schooling, in which a teacher from the student's community school district teaches the child in the home; (c) home schooling, in which the student's parents take responsibility for organizing and delivering an academic curriculum that meets state guidelines; and (d) hospital-based schooling. Prior academic performance and social, emotional, and health factors should be considered when selecting the most appropriate educational environment for students with cancer.

Hospital-Based Schooling

At M. D. Anderson, a comprehensive education program has been developed to address the educational needs of students from early childhood through young adulthood. The program is designed for children who are actively receiving treatment as well as for long-term survivors who are academically challenged.

Academic Program

The academic program for the hospital-based school is based on the collaborative efforts of the M. D. Anderson education staff and staff from the student's community school district. The hospital-based school staff includes a director and certified teachers. The director, who has a background in educational psychology, is responsible for developing the program, co-ordinating educational activities, and supervising teachers. The teachers coordinate the student's referral and enrollment process, provide daily academic instruction, and evaluate the student's progress. The staff provides year-round classroom and bedside instruction, field trips, and enrichment activities that supplement the core curriculum, such as English as a second language (ESL), exercise and physical fitness, creative arts, and career counseling.

The hospital-based teachers consult with the child's community school routinely, and at an annual conference, educators from the hospital- and community-school staffs meet to coordinate the student's curriculum to ensure that he or she is on the right course of study and is receiving an optimal learning experience. As members of the behavioral medicine team, the hospital-based teachers are trained not only to help the child pursue his or her education, but to use educational endeavors as a mechanism to help them cope with cancer.

In the hospital-based school, instruction is provided in an age-appropriate setting that is located close to the inpatient area for easy accessibility. Preschool through fifth-grade students are taught in one classroom, and sixth- through twelfth-grade students are taught in a separate classroom. A learning center with a library serves as a third educational area where academic enrichment activities and cognitive remediation are taught. The classrooms and learning center are bright and inviting spaces and are located in close proximity to the inpatient area. Each classroom is equipped with a bulletin board, science exhibits, creative learning tools, and computer workstations. Videoconferencing enables students isolated in bone marrow transplantation rooms to stay connected to their respective classrooms and peers. Teachers also provide bedside instruction to students when they are in isolation or when they are too ill to participate in classroom activities.

ESL Program

The primary objective of the ESL program is to help international school-age patients learn English and acclimate to the American culture and the hospital milieu. Educators and volunteers encourage cultural exchange among the students and help the patients improve or acquire English-language skills. Workbooks, dictionaries, and computer programs are helpful ESL educational tools.

Exercise and Physical Fitness

An exercise and physical fitness program has been incorporated into the hospital-based school curriculum at M. D. Anderson. Administered by physical therapists and fitness instructors and taught in the spacious "Pediatrics Dome," the daily classes are designed to help students increase flexibility, gain strength, and maintain or develop cardiovascular fitness.

Recreational games are included in the workout to keep the program fun and interesting. Both inpatients and outpatients are encouraged to use the facility. Trainers can accommodate students with special orthopedic needs as well as those who must transport their intravenous-fluid poles with them.

Support of Homebound and Community-School Programs

The hospital-based education staff consults with homebound and community-school teachers, nurses, and counselors to familiarize them with the young cancer patient's condition and to prepare them for issues that might arise when the patient returns to the regular classroom setting. Some of the topics discussed are the patient's diagnosis, basic information about chemotherapy and other therapies, anticipated absenteeism, possible emergency situations (e.g., seizures), and how to handle inquiries from classmates.

Research has shown that children surviving brain tumors are at increased risk of experiencing social difficulties, such as isolation, even after treatment ends. These difficulties may be attributed to peer-, teacher-, and self-perceptions of cancer and its associated consequences. When the homebound and community-school educators are knowledgeable about the student's condition, they will feel more confident in supporting the students. Likewise, when the student feels supported, he or she will be more likely to succeed in academic endeavors.

Studies have also shown that the cancer patient's perception of social support from classmates is the most consistent predictor of psychological adaptation. It is important that the student's peers understand his or her condition and how they can help the student transition back to the regular school setting and adjust socially.

NEUROPSYCHOLOGICAL EFFECTS OF CANCER

Despite our efforts to promote normal psychological, emotional, and psychosocial educational development among children with cancer, some survivors may suffer neurologic consequences and learning impairment as a result of the cancer or the treatment. Children with leukemia or brain tumors are the most susceptible to learning disabilities because they receive treatment to the central nervous system (CNS). Most children with leukemia receive only intrathecal chemotherapy, which is not usually considered as damaging as radiotherapy; but many children with brain tumors must have either whole-brain or focal cranial radiotherapy (CRT).

Role of Radiotherapy

By now, it is generally agreed that CRT causes lasting damage to the developing brain, and radiotherapy is the modality most often implicated in long-term neurocognitive and academic deficits among survivors of childhood cancer. Radiotherapy creates structural changes in the brain (such as atrophy and abnormalities in the white matter and in the blood vessels), which in turn causes functional changes (slowed information processing; attention deficit; and limitations in memory, learning, and mathematics skills) that are similar to a nonverbal learning disability.

As a rule, the larger the dose of radiotherapy, the greater the adverse effect. For example, children with brain tumors who receive 50 to 60 Gy of radiotherapy may be greatly affected, whereas for children with leukemia who receive only 18 to 24 Gy, the effect may be much less profound. The effect of radiotherapy is more profound in young children, but the underlying mechanisms of this finding have not been firmly established. Most researchers support the idea that CRT is more damaging to younger children because it is administered during a period in which part of the brain is growing rapidly, which makes those structures—particularly white matter—more vulnerable to developmental interruption.

The severity of CRT side effects varies greatly among children, depending on the dose, dose schedule, size and location of the radiotherapy field, amount of time that elapses after treatment, age of the child when radiotherapy is administered, and, possibly, the child's sex. Moreover, under some conditions, the side effects of CRT seem to be potentiated or enhanced by certain chemotherapeutic agents (e.g., methotrexate), which the child may receive around the same time. Another complication associated with CRT is that adverse effects are relatively slow to appear (usually 1 to 3 years after administration) and may actually increase (or appear to increase) over time. In addition to physical and medical variables, psychosocial factors— such as the socioeconomic status of the family, the parents' marital status (children do better in 2-parent families), other family stresses that may be ongoing, and the mother's coping ability—may also cause adverse effects.

We conclude, on the basis of research of the neurocognitive effects of childhood cancer, that: a) many children who receive CNS treatment will have attention difficulties and other learning problems, b) optimal care requires a prospective neuropsychologic assessment of a wide range of abilities and skills, and c) school interventions are usually necessary. Cognitive remediation is likely to be essential while a child receives CRT.

Cognitive Remediation

The Cognitive Remediation Program involves a series of exercises designed specifically to help cancer survivors overcome learning difficulties, such as inattentiveness, that result from cancer or its treatment. Learning strategies can help patients compensate for difficulties, and psychotherapeutic interventions can help them withstand distraction and boost self-esteem and self-confidence. For example, special cognitive exercises can help patients overcome inattentiveness.

In a 2-hour session held once a week, students are engaged in 10- to 15-minute task-oriented activities. The activities are presented at a level at which the student can achieve at least 50% accuracy and are repeated until

80% accuracy is achieved; then the next level of complexity or speed is pre-sented. Students generally find these activities interesting and engaging. To avoid boredom, the therapists alter the activities with commercial games that are fun but that also incorporate attention skills. A team approach is emphasized: parents and teachers are informed of the learning strategies and are encouraged to have the student practice the task-oriented activities at home and at school. The therapist, parent, and teacher then share their observations. If the student needs extra help with schoolwork, he or she is assisted by a member of the school education team.

There is some evidence that stimulant medications, such as methylphe-nidate, may improve attention and concentration in children for whom cancer treatment is delivered to the CNS. Although the empirical evidence is still preliminary, it is possible that a number of these children could ben-efit from a stimulant, perhaps one that is provided at a lower dose than that given to healthy children with attention deficit/hyperactivity disorder. More research of stimulant medications is needed in this patient popula-tion. In a few instances at M. D. Anderson, we have found it beneficial to combine cognitive remediation and stimulant medications.

The Cognitive Remediation Program was designed to improve sur-vivors' attention skills and to improve their abilities to remember and learn. To our delight, we have found that the program contributes much more: it provides the psychological benefits of increased self-confidence and improved quality of life.

Conclusions

The various disciplines involved in the behavioral medicine program for pediatric patients and their family members collaborate closely, and the roles of the practitioners and staff often overlap. It is not uncommon for families to develop relationships with several members of the program. The members of the behavioral medicine team serve as advocates and confidantes for pediatric patients and their family members during their stay at M. D. Anderson.

KEY PRACTICE POINTS

- Psychological, emotional, psychosocial, educational, and neuropsychological support are fundamental components of the behavioral medicine program for pediatric cancer patients and their family members at M. D. Anderson.
- Through the behavioral medicine program, a full range of services are offered to help patients and family members cope with the many challenges associated with pediatric cancer, such as stress,

understanding treatment-related processes, financial concerns, family relationships, parenting skills, childhood development, educational goals, and self-expression.

· If a pediatric patient can maintain a normal developmental course, his or her psychosocial outcome will likely be optimized.

SUGGESTED READINGS

Blatt J, Copeland D, Bleyer W. Late effects of childhood cancer and its treatment. In: Pizzo P, Poplack D, eds. *Principles and Practice of Pediatric Oncology*, Revised Edition. Philadelphia, PA: J. B. Lippincott Co; 1997:1091–1114.

Butler RW, Copeland DR. Attentional processes and their remediation in children treated for cancer: a literature review and the development of a therapeutic approach. *J Int Neuropsychol Soc* 2002;8:115–124.

Fletcher JM, Copeland DR. Neurobehavioral effects of central nervous system prophylactic treatment of cancer in children. *J Clin Exp Neuropsychol* 1988;10:495–538.

Ris MD, Noll RB. Long-term neurobehavioral outcome in pediatric brain-tumor patients: review and methodological critique. *J Clin Exp Neuropsychol* 1994;16:21–42.

Searle NS, Askins M, Bleyer WA. Homebound schooling is the least favorable option for continued education of adolescent cancer patients: a preliminary report. *Med Pediatr Oncol* 2003;40:380–384.

18 THE ADOLESCENT AND YOUNG ADULT PROGRAM

Sima S. Jeha and Martha A. Askins

CHAPTER OVERVIEW

Traditionally, there has not been an oncology service dedicated specifically to the management of adolescents and young adults; rather, these patients are arbitrarily assigned to either an adult or pediatric oncology service. Thus, patients 13 to 21 years of age are usually treated by physicians who are inexperienced and perhaps uncomfortable with caring for individuals in this age range. In 1999, the Adolescent and Young Adult Program was established in the Division of Pediatrics at M. D. Anderson Cancer Center. This program has created a platform for the exchange of expertise between the pediatric and adult oncology services with the goal of providing the best medical care and psychosocial support for adolescent and young adult cancer patients. M. D. Anderson is one of only a few centers worldwide to offer this unique dimension of care. This chapter describes the Adolescent and Young Adult Program and how it is being used to improve cancer-related outcomes and quality of life for this patient group.

INTRODUCTION

Although they represent a biologically and socially distinct patient population, adolescents and young adults with cancer are arbitrarily treated on pediatric or adult oncology services because no care program has been established specifically for them. Consequently, these youth are treated on protocols designed for patients younger or older than them. Reports show, however, that emphasis on this patient group is warranted. Notably, the incidence of several cancers peaks during adolescence and young adulthood, and data from the National Cancer Institute's Surveillance, Epidemiology, and End Results database show a striking lack of improvement in survival and mortality rates from 1975 to the present among patients 15 to 44 years old. In addition, the quality-of-life issues of cancer patients between 15 and 30 years old have generally been ignored compared with those of patients younger than 15 years of age and those older than 30 years of age.

Recent reports have shown that pediatric oncologists are more likely than adult oncologists to enroll patients in clinical trials and that adolescents who are treated on protocols for pediatric patients have better outcomes than their counterparts who are treated on protocols for adult patients. Furthermore, improvements in our understanding of cancer biology and advances in cancer treatment have provided us with evidence that cancers in adolescents and young adults behave similarly and have a similar tolerance to therapy, but that the disease- and treatment-related characteristics of tumors in these youth differ from those of cancers in children and adults. Of particular concern for adolescent and young adult cancer patients and their caregivers is the fact that these patients' well being and, indeed, their survival are being threatened by disease at a critical period in their lives—the time when they are establishing a self-image and planning for the future.

In 1999, to meet the unique cancer-care needs of these youth, M. D. Anderson established the Adolescent and Young Adult (AYA) Program in the Division of Pediatrics. This innovative multidisciplinary program brings a number of departments together to address the specific medical, psychosocial, and vocational needs of cancer patients 15 to 21 years old. The program was inspired by the realization that a growing number of 15- to 30-year-old patients are surviving cancer and are being faced with 2 very challenging tasks simultaneously: learning to cope with a life-altering illness while learning to cope with normal developmental changes. The mission of the AYA Program is to improve the clinical outcome of adolescent and young adult cancer patients in an environment tailored to their physical and emotional levels of maturation.

MULTIDISCIPLINARY PROGRAM DESIGN

M. D. Anderson's high-caliber clinical and basic science research environment in which pediatric-care and adult-care oncologists coexist provided the ideal setting in which to pioneer the AYA Program. Essentially, the program aims to: (a) develop therapies to improve the outcome of adolescent and young adult cancer patients while minimizing undesirable, long-term side effects of treatment and (b) provide educational, vocational, social, and emotional support to ensure them of a desirable quality of life. The AYA Program is supported by clinicians and staff from the institution's pediatric and adult oncology services who are experts in providing therapeutic and supportive care. The program is jointly headed by a medical-pediatric physician and a pediatric psychologist. An advanced nurse practitioner assesses patients individually and coordinates their continuity of care across the spectrum of institutional departments.

IMPROVING TREATMENT OUTCOMES

Cancer is the primary cause of disease-related mortality in adolescents and young adults. In particular, 5 malignancies have the highest impact on the national mortality rate of these youth: brain tumors, lymphomas, sarcomas, germ-cell tumors, and leukemia.

Solid Tumors

Ewing's sarcoma and osteosarcoma have a peak incidence during adolescence and young adulthood. Grier et al (2003) found an interesting discrepancy in the survival rates of young patients with these tumors. In particular, they found that patients with Ewing's sarcoma who were younger than 10 years old had a 5-year event-free survival rate of 70% compared with 60% for patients 10 to 17 years old and 44% for patients 18 years old and older.

M. D. Anderson investigators recently developed uniform protocols for the treatment of Ewing's sarcoma and osteosarcoma that can be used regardless of whether the patient is being treated on the pediatric or adult oncology service. These protocols use innovative approaches, such as the administration of intra-arterial platinum by a skilled interventional radiology team in the treatment of osteosarcoma. This type of consolidated care for patients of all ages would not be possible outside a comprehensive cancer center.

Leukemia

Although the peak incidence of leukemia is bimodal (early childhood and late adulthood), it is still the most common malignant disease diagnosed during adolescence, accounting for about 20% of cancers in these patients, and it is the leading cause of disease-related deaths among adolescents and young adults.

Acute lymphoblastic leukemia (ALL) is the most common cancer in childhood. Despite the intensive treatment regimens used to treat ALL, the cure rate in adolescents is inferior to the 80% cure rate reported in children 1 to 9 years old. Patients with ALL who are older than 9 years of age are treated with more intensive regimens than are younger children. Although this approach has improved the outcome of older children with ALL, their long-term survival is still notably inferior to that of their younger counterparts.

To improve current therapeutic strategies, a better understanding is needed of the factors that influence outcome in adolescent and young adult patients with ALL. Different factors, including the disease itself, the host, and the treatment, contribute to the inferior outcomes seen in this patient group. The risk factors associated with a poor prognosis and treatment resistance are more common in adolescents than in young children. Conversely, 2 favorable prognostic indicators—hyperdiploidy and the presence of the TEL-AML1 gene fusion—are found in about 25% of pediatric patients with ALL but in less than 5% of older patients. The probability of cure is influenced by the patient's compliance with the treatment plan; the type, dose and schedule, and route of administration of the chemotherapy regimen; and the patient's ability to metabolize the chemotherapy drugs.

Because ALL is the most common pediatric cancer, most pediatric oncologists are experts in the delivery of therapeutic and supportive care for this disease. For this reason, children with ALL, who are treated on the pediatric service, have better outcomes than adolescents and young adults who are treated on the adult service and in nonuniversity settings by physicians and support staff who rarely treat leukemia. Recently, the outcomes of adolescents and young adults with ALL who are treated on either a pediatric or an adult cooperative-group protocol were compared in studies conducted in the United States and Europe. In both studies, the patients had better outcomes when treated on pediatric protocols than when treated on adult protocols.

At M. D. Anderson, patients with ALL who are younger than 30 years old at diagnosis have a 98% complete response rate and a 5-year event-free survival rate of 54% when treated on a regimen of hyperfractionated cyclophosphamide, vincristine, doxorubicin, and dexamethasone. These results are notably superior to those from the adult-cooperative protocol and might reflect the use of a more effective treatment regimen, greater expertise in a single large cancer center with a well-developed leukemia program, or both. Investigators from the pediatric and adult leukemia services at M. D. Anderson are now collaborating to design regimens of combined targeted therapies with the aim of improving outcome in adolescent and young adult patients.

IMPROVING QUALITY OF LIFE

Adolescents and young adults negotiate many important psychosocial demands as they transition toward a successful, fulfilling adulthood, including:

- Adjusting to a physically maturing body
- Achieving mature relationships with peers
- Achieving emotional independence from adults
- Establishing personal values and ethics that will serve as their guide for daily living and making important life choices
- Preparing for a career
- Preparing for marriage and family

The physical and emotional sequelae of cancer and cancer treatments can further compromise these patients' well being. Some of the disease-related consequences young patients must faced are:

- Nausea, malaise, and decreased energy
- Changes in mobility and physical functioning
- Changes in physical appearance
- Isolation from peers and usual activities
- Increased dependence on parents at a time when they would usually be gaining independence
- Absenteeism from school or work
- Feelings of loss of control
- Uncertainty about the future

The clinicians and staff who facilitate the AYA Program recognize that coping with developmental changes and a serious illness at the same time presents a unique challenge. The activities and services they offer through this program are designed to provide psychosocial support to help ensure these patients' well being.

Prior to Initiation of Therapy

Before therapy is started, the treatment options and possible treatment outcomes must be explained to the patient and family members to help them make well-informed decisions. Pertinent medical, psychosocial, and emotional issues and long-term consequences associated with therapies should be discussed.

Giving Patients Appropriate Control

Adolescence and young adulthood are typically characterized by feelings of omnipotence, idealism, and immortality. A diagnosis of cancer can be developmentally disruptive. At a time when autonomy is a key social concern, becoming a patient forces these youth to rely heavily on family members and health care providers for support. At a time when they are planning their futures, these young patients suddenly realize they may not have a future. At a time when self-esteem is of utmost importance, they find themselves facing by a potentially disfiguring and disabling disease.

Some young patients find healthy ways to cope with the challenges that cancer presents; however, some have difficulty accepting the diagnosis, which can translate into noncompliance with medical treatments or denial of the disease altogether. Therefore, it is crucial that adolescent and young adult patients receive age-appropriate support and guidance from medical, psychosocial, and other care providers as well as from family members. Positive support can help these patients maintain a sense of dignity and control during their battle with cancer.

Family members and the medical team are advised to maintain open communication with the patient to make sure that he or she is fully informed about the disease and the potential benefits and consequences of different treatment options and to encourage the patient to participate in treatment decisions. Care providers spend time alone with the patient during each visit so they can address certain issues privately.

Some families tend to be overprotective and request that the patient be shielded from unpleasant information. In such cases, the medical care provider, acting as a patient advocate, must make sure that the patient is treated with respect and is allowed to give input into care decisions. Such assurance gives the patient a sense of self-control, promotes a receptive working alliance between the patient and the caregiver, and encourages the patient to comply with the treatment plan.

Looking Beyond Therapy

When the diagnosis and treatment options are discussed with adolescent and young adult patients, members of the AYA Program team help them look beyond the treatment phase and visualize their future after surviving cancer. They address their concerns about maintaining friendships, completing their education, obtaining a job, getting married, having children, and achieving other important goals. Team members help them continue their education and career development. Infertility is discussed as a possible consequence of certain treatments. Whereas the fertility-preserving options currently available to young women are tedious and experimental, modern techniques, such as sperm banking, can preserve fertility for most young men treated with chemotherapy, pelvic surgery, or considerable radiotherapy doses to the testicles. The Department of Behavioral

Medicine at M. D. Anderson is involved in a National Cancer Institute-funded project to develop a CD-ROM to educate physicians, patients, and family members about sperm banking. The CD-ROM has a section for on-cologists that explains the value of sperm banking and how to counsel patients and family members about this option. Other sections provide information specifically for patients, their parents, and their spouses or significant others. There are also sections that provide information about advance directives and on how to determine whether to include parents in certain discussions.

During Therapy

During therapy, peer support becomes an important factor in patients' continued well-being. Cancer is a unique challenge at this young age, and sharing experiences and coping skills can be invaluable. Through the AYA Program, socialization is encouraged, and special accommodations are provided to facilitate peer interaction.

Age-Appropriate Interaction and Support

To provide adolescent and young adult patients with a facility where they can share their experiences and support each other during the treatment phase, we created an age-appropriate recreation room called Kim's Place. The center is designed exclusively for patients 15 to 25 years old and their family members and friends who are in the same age group. At Kim's Place, visitors enjoy the use of a pool table, a large-screen plasma TV, a kitchenette, a library/media room, and other recreational amenities. Patients are provided pagers that allow them to wait for appointments in this relaxed setting with others whose lives have been affected by cancer. Construction of the facility was made possible by a donation from the Women's National Basketball Association's Houston Comets in honor of Kim Perrot, a Comets guard who died of lung cancer at M. D. Anderson in 1999.

Body Image and Relationships

At the critical age when physical appearance is of utmost importance, some adolescents and young adults with cancer lose their hair, are fitted with in-dwelling catheters, gain or lose weight, and undergo radical and sometimes disfiguring surgeries. At a time when their sexual identity is evolving, these patients struggle with impaired body image and worry about reproductive capabilities. Helping these youth maintain their self-esteem is paramount. Through the AYA Program, patients are counseled about body image, rela-tionships, sexuality, and fertility. Separate weekly support group meetings are held for adolescents (ages 13 to 18) and young adults (ages 19 to 25) to help patients develop social-support networks, address issues about cos-metic and functional changes, and express their personal feelings about having cancer. A more structured group—the AYA Forum—meets weekly. At these sessions, adolescent and young adult patients are counseled about practical matters, such as how to handle relationships and how to manage personal finances. Support groups are facilitated by licensed psychologists or therapists.

In conjunction with the Department of Rehabilitation Medicine, the Division of Pediatrics provides a physical-exercise program for adolescent and young adult patients. The program is staffed by physical therapists and athletic trainers. Fitness training and physical rehabilitation are important in maintaining patients' physical strength, flexibility, and mobility. In addition to promoting overall well being among patients, the program assists those who acquire difficulties with gross- or fine-motor skills as a result of cancer or its treatment.

Planning for the Future

One of the most important challenges young people with cancer face is staying academically competitive. These youth worry about missing school and falling behind in their coursework. With the help of counselors and teachers in the AYA Program, patients can continue attending their community schools, receive a homebound education, or enroll in the hospital school, which collaborates with the Houston Independent School District to ensure that students stay on task and at grade level. Students receive individual assessments, instruction, tutoring, career planning, and vocational guidance. Counselors help students prepare for college entrance exams and guide them through the admission and scholarship application processes. The program also helps patients with cognitive and physical disabilities find appropriate educational and career opportunities. Patients have access to computers, educational programs, and creative arts classes. To accommodate our many foreign students, English-as-a-second-language courses are available. See Chapter 17, "Behavioral Medicine in Cancer Care," for a full description of the academic interventions available to young cancer patients at M. D. Anderson.

Year-Round Social Activities

The AYA Program sponsors year-round social activities that give adolescent and young adult patients the opportunity to socialize and enjoy a respite from the treatment routine. In the Teen Hangout, patients can meet with peers, relax, wait for appointments, and enjoy activities such as listening to music, watching movies, surfing the Internet, and playing foosball. Under the direction of child-life specialists, patients participate in activities such as Teen Grill and enjoy outings to theaters, festivals, professional sports events, and recreational theme parks. Two popular outings are the Lombardi Awards college football banquet and the Houston Livestock Show and Rodeo. At multicultural celebrations at which the costumes, artwork, language, history, and traditional meals of ethnic groups are featured, patients learn about the diverse lifestyles of different populations. Camp AOK ("Anderson's Older Kids") is a weeklong summer camp for

M. D. Anderson patients and siblings 13 to 18 years old. It is held at a beautiful, full-service camp site 40 miles north of Houston. At a yearly ski trip, patients who have lost limbs to cancer learn to brave the slopes. All of these activities are provided to help adolescent and young adult patients channel their energy into preserving self-esteem, gaining stamina, and learning to overcome perceived limitations. These diverse activities are funded by proceeds from M. D. Anderson's Children's Art Project and various philanthropic donations.

After Therapy

On completion of treatment, the supportive-care services provided through the AYA Program focus on monitoring for disease recurrence and second malignancies and providing long-term follow-up evaluations and care.

Monitoring for Recurrence and Secondary Malignancies

Various combinations of chemotherapy, radiotherapy, and surgery are used to bring about disease remission, which could lead to a cure. However, the cost of remission, whether it continues indefinitely or ends in relapse, is often high. At our long-term follow-up clinic, we monitor patients for recurrences, secondary malignancies, and other long-term sequela of cancer. The young patients are informed of the importance of regular follow-up visits, which facilitates early detection of complications.

Addressing Long-Term Sequela

Cancer survivors may have permanent physical or mental deficits resulting from the malignancy or the treatment. Whereas the effect of amputation is an immediate loss, the adverse effects of other therapies, such as sterility, organ damage, bone-growth abnormalities, and neurologic or endocrine problems, may be delayed.

Radiotherapy-induced hypothyrodism occurs more often in children than in adults, suggesting that the thyroid gland is more sensitive in rapidly growing preadolescents and adolescents than in adults. Thyroid nodules, Graves' disease, and thyroid cancer are rare sequelae resulting from radiotherapy. Spontaneous reversal or substantial improvement of thyroid injury occurs in about 36% of adolescent and young adult patients, but the rest require lifelong hormone-replacement therapy. Radiotherapy-induced physical deformities and mental impairment after brain irradiation are also usually more severe in patients treated at a young age than in older patients.

Cardiac failure is a major complication following chest irradiation and anthracycline treatment. Young patients who have received radiotherapy to the chest wall during childhood are at increased risk for breast cancer at an early age. With our current treatment regimens, we avoid irradiation whenever possible. When radiotherapy is necessary, we use newer techniques and megavoltage equipment to attenuate or eliminate adverse effects.

Infertility is another concern associated with cancer treatment. Both radiotherapy and chemotherapy can affect fertility. Chemotherapy-induced sterility and amenorrhea are more common in adolescents than in children and are reversible with less intensive treatments. Informing young long-term survivors about risks for infertility, complicated pregnancies, and unhealthy babies is important. In the AYA Program, we counsel young women about ovarian-tissue transposition and ovarian cryopreservation, which can provide young girls with some assurance of fertility preservation. We also inform them about the probability of early menopause and advise them not to delay starting a family. We inform young men about the ability to cryopreserve semen that can be implanted via in vitro fertilization to achieve impregnation. Sperm banking likely remains underused because many oncologists either do not mention it or do not present it in a positive and competent manner. Indeed, in a busy oncology clinic, it may be difficult to prioritize any issue other than those concerned with diagnosis and treatment of cancer. The counselors in our AYA Program are experienced at providing information about sperm banking and other fertility issues and supporting patients through the difficult decision process.

Psychosocial issues are also very important for long-term survivors. Long after completing therapy, some patients experience loss of energy, a diminished interest in sex, and impaired body image. The dearth of information about sexual self-image and functioning in survivors of pediatric and adolescent malignancies is surprising, particularly given the growing number of long-term survivors of childhood and adolescent cancers in the general population. Some boys and girls may need to take replacement hormones to stimulate puberty. Some will experience permanent changes in appearance, including limb amputation, facial deformities, or short stature. Damage to cognitive function could affect occupational success and could cause a delay in the initiation of dating and sexual relationships. Others may react to their disease by engaging in risky sexual behaviors. Our AYA Program counselors, who have become familiar with the patients, help long-term survivors cope with these and other psychosocial issues.

Ensuring Reintegration

Long-term survivors have to learn how to develop the life skills and judgment needed to cope with sequelae such as disfigurement, neurologic problems, intimacy issues, altered sexual function, sterility, organ damage, and the specter of relapse. They may also suffer a personal financial loss; for example, their parents may use their college savings to pay for costly treatments. Survivors also often face social and workplace discrimination and have problems obtaining and retaining health and life insurance. M. D. Anderson's social services staff assists in the AYA Program by serving as advocates for these young people, providing valuable assistance in the form of information and social support.

Promoting Awareness of Issues Specific to Adolescents and Young Adults

Because of the lack of published information from investigators and specialists about cancer in adolescents and young adults, a gathering of the experts was needed to develop effective treatment strategies associated with treating this patient population. M. D. Anderson hosted the first international symposium addressing the complex medical, emotional, psychosocial, and legal issues of adolescent and young adult cancer patients and their caregivers. The symposium led to the creation of a network of care providers eager to improve current standards of care for adolescents and young adults by exchanging ideas and frequently updating resources. The second such symposium held at M. D. Anderson in 2002 focused on leukemia and was co-chaired by the institution's Division of Pediatrics and Department of Leukemia. National and international experts in pediatric and adult leukemia presented study outcomes, and a panel of experts debated treatment options and plans to improve outcomes in this age group.

Conclusions

Adolescent and young adult oncology is emerging as a distinct field of study. The AYA Program pioneered at M. D. Anderson is the first of its kind and is aimed at providing more consistent medical treatment and supportive care addressing the unique educational, social, and emotional needs of this patient population. We are committed to continuing our multidisciplinary approach in which the expertise and resources of pediatric and adult oncology services are combined to improve outcome and quality of life for these young patients.

KEY PRACTICE POINTS

- Programs such as M. D. Anderson's AYA Program enable clinicians to provide specialized medical care and support services to adolescent and young adult cancer patients who represent a distinct oncologic entity with unique medical, psychosocial, and emotional needs.
- Sperm banking and other fertility-preserving approaches should be explained and encouraged.
- Peer socialization is an important therapeutic resource.
- Adolescents and young adults should be encouraged to participate in determining their care plan, and they should be provided with information about the disease, treatment options, and disease- and treatment-related consequences so they can make informed decisions.

Suggested Readings

Albritton K, Bleyer WA. The management of cancer in the older adolescent. *Eur J Cancer* 2003;39:2584–2599.

Bhatia S, Yasui Y, Robison LL, et al. High risk of subsequent neoplasms continues with extended follow-up of childhood Hodgkin's disease: report from the Late Effects Study Group. *J Clin Oncol* 2003;21:4386–4394.

Bleyer A. Older adolescents with cancer in North America: deficits in outcome and research. *Pediatr Clin North Am* 2002;49:1027–1042.

Bleyer WA. Cancer in older adolescents and young adults: epidemiology, diagnosis, treatment, survival, and importance of clinical trials. *Med Pediatr Oncol* 2002;38:1–10.

Bleyer WA, Tejeda H, Murphy SB, et al. National cancer clinical trials: children have equal access; adolescents do not. *J Adolesc Health* 1997;21:366–373.

Ganz PA. Why and how to study the fate of cancer survivors: observations from the clinic and the research laboratory. *Eur J Cancer* 2003;39:2136–2141.

Gatta G, Capocaccia R, De Angelis R, et al. Cancer survival in European adolescents and young adults. *Eur J Cancer* 2003;39:2600–2610.

Grier HE, Krailo MD, Tarbell NJ, et al. Addition of ifosfamide and etoposide to standard chemotherapy for Ewing's sarcoma and primitive neuroectodermal tumor of bone. *N Engl J Med* 2003;348:694–701.

Gurney JG, Ness KK, Stovall M, et al. Final height and body mass index among adult survivors of childhood brain cancer: childhood cancer survivor study. *J Clin Endocrinol Metab* 2003;88:4731–4739.

Jeha S. Who should be treating adolescents with acute lymphoblastic leukemia? *Eur J Cancer* 2003;39:2579–2583.

Jeha S, Kantarjian H. Treatment of acute lymphoblastic leukemia in adolescents and young adults. In: Pui CH, ed. *Treatment of Acute Leukemias: New Directions for Clinical Research*. Totow, NJ: Humana Press Inc; 2002:113–120.

Schover LR, Brey K, Lichtin A, et al. Knowledge and experiences regarding cancer, infertility, and sperm banking in younger male survivors. *J Clin Oncol* 2002;20:1880–1889.

Schover LR, Brey K, Lichtin A, et al. Oncologists' attitudes and practices regarding banking sperm before cancer treatment. *J Clin Oncol* 2002;20:1890–1897.

Searle NS, Askins M, Bleyer WA. Homebound schooling is the least favorable option for continued education of adolescent cancer patients: a preliminary report. *Med Pediatr Oncol* 2003;40:380–384.

INDEX